# THINKING IT THROUGH

## CLINICAL REASONING, CLINICAL JUDGEMENT, AND DECISION MAKING IN CANADIAN NURSING

# THINKING IT THROUGH

## CLINICAL REASONING, CLINICAL JUDGEMENT, AND DECISION MAKING IN CANADIAN NURSING

**Karin L. Page-Cutrara,** RN, PhD, CCNE, CCSNE, FCNEI

Associate Professor, Teaching Stream, School of Nursing;
Associate Dean, Learning, Teaching and Academic Programs
Faculty of Health
York University
Toronto, Ontario
Canada

ELSEVIER

Thinking It Through: Clinical Reasoning, Clinical Judgement, and Decision Making in Canadian Nursing

ISBN: 978-0-443-12526-3

---

### Notice

---

*Senior Editor (Acquisitions, Canada):* Roberta A. Spinosa-Millman
*Content Development Specialist:* Lenore Gray-Spence
*Publishing Services Manager:* Julie Eddy
*Senior Project Manager:* Cindy Thoms
*Design Direction:* Patrick Ferguson

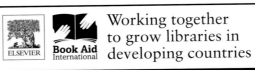

Working together to grow libraries in developing countries

www.elsevier.com • www.bookaid.org

Printed in India
Last digit is the print number: 9 8 7 6 5 4 3 2 1

To all Canadian nursing students and professional nurses.

# CONTENTS

# ABOUT THE AUTHOR

Karin Page-Cutrara, RN, PhD, CCNE, CCSNE, FCNEI is an Associate Professor, Teaching Stream, School of Nursing and Associate Dean of Learning, Teaching and Academic Programs in the Faculty of Health at York University in Toronto, Ontario, Canada. Karin obtained a Bachelor of Nursing Science at Queen's University in Kingston, Ontario, and a Master of Nursing at Athabasca University, Alberta. Her doctoral work, at Duquesne University, Pittsburgh, Pennsylvania, USA, focused on the use of simulation prebriefing in undergraduate nursing education. She has taught as a perioperative clinical nurse educator in the hospital setting and in perioperative nursing programs in various colleges. Karin currently uses simulation in teaching thinking skills and for developing nursing competencies among baccalaureate nursing students. Karin also has an interest in course and curriculum development and revision. She has co-developed and teaches in the Canadian Association of Schools of Nursing nurse educator certificate program and is co-editor of a textbook for nurse educators in Canada. Karin is committed to addressing the challenges of teaching and learning in the academic setting in her current role as Associate Dean, and to facilitating undergraduate nursing student learning and competency development. Karin is co-author of *Elsevier's Canadian Comprehensive Review for the NCLEX-RN® Examination.*

# REVIEWERS

**Olga Ahmad, RN, BSN, MN**
Simulation Educator
Faculty of Nursing
Langara College
Vancouver, British Columbia

**Patricia Bradley, RN, MEd, PhD, CCNE**
Professor Emeritus
School of Nursing
York University
Toronto, Ontario

**Tanya Spencer Cameron, RN(EC), BScN, NP-PHC, MSc(QIPS), CCNE**
Professor
BScN Collaborative Program Co-ordinator and Professor
School of Health Sciences and Emergency Services
Northern College
Timmins, Ontario

**Huasheng (Jimmy) Chen, RN, BScN, MSc**
Professor
School of Community and Health Studies
Centennial College
Toronto, Ontario

**Shelley Cobbett, RN, BN, GnT, MN, EdD**
Assistant Professor
Nursing and BScN Site Administrator
School of Nursing—Yarmouth Campus
Dalhousie University
Yarmouth, Nova Scotia

**Amy Horton, BScN, MN, NP-PHC**
Associate Director
Undergraduate BScN Programs;
Lecturer Collaborative, CTF, and PHCNP Program
Arthur Labatt Family School of Nursing
Western University
London, Ontario

**Mohamed Toufic El Hussein, RN, BSN, MSN, PhD, NP**
Professor
School of Nursing and Midwifery
Faculty of Health
Community and Education
Mount Royal University
Calgary, Alberta;
Adjunct Associate Professor
Faculty of Nursing
University of Calgary
Calgary, Alberta;
Acute Care Nurse Practitioner Medical Cardiology
Coronary Care Unit—Rockyview General Hospital
Calgary, Alberta;
Director of Education
Nurse Practitioner Association of Alberta
Calgary, Alberta

**Hellen Jarman, RN(EC), BScN, MN, GNC(C), PhD(c), NP-PHC**
Professor
School of Health and Life Sciences
Conestoga College Institute of Technology and
    Advanced Learning
Kitchener, Ontario;
Lecturer (Adjunct)
School of Nursing
Faculty of Health Sciences
McMaster University
Hamilton, Ontario

**Treva Job, RN(EC), BScN, NP-PHC, MA Ed, PhD, CCSNE, CHSE**
Simulation Lead
Health, Wellness, and Sciences
Georgian College
Barrie, Ontario

**Marnie Kramer, RN, BScN, MEd, PhD**
Assistant Professor
College of Nursing
University of Manitoba
Winnipeg, Manitoba

**Michelle LeGall-Vandepoele, RN, MN**
Instructor, Faculty of Health
University College of the North
Manitoba, Canada

**Wendy Lynch, RN, MSc (AH)**
Instructional Associate IV
Department of Psychiatric Nursing
Faculty of Health Studies
Brandon University
Brandon, Manitoba

**Laurel MacIsaac, RN, BScN, MN**
Manager
School of Health and Human Services;
Mi'kmaw and Indigenous Practical Nursing Cohort Lead
Nova Scotia Community College
Dartmouth, Nova Scotia

**Genevieve Erin MacNeil, RN, BA, BScN, MA**
Nurse Educator
Faculty of Long-Term Care
Nova Scotia Health Learning Institute for Health Care
    Providers
Nova Scotia Health Authority
Halifax, Nova Scotia

**Farhana Madhani, RN, PhD**
Assistant Professor
Faculty of Applied Health Sciences
Department of Nursing
Brock University
St. Catharines, Ontario

**Kim Tekakwitha Martin, RN, BSN**
Instructor
Faculty of Nursing
John Abbott College
Montreal, Quebec

**Michelle Morley, RN, BScN, MScN**
Professor
School of Health and Community Studies
Algonquin College
Ottawa, Ontario

**Beth Perry, RN, PhD**
Professor
Faculty of Health Disciplines
Athabasca University
Athabasca, Alberta

**Kara Sealock, RN, EdD, MEd, CNCC(C), CCNE**
Associate Professor
Faculty of Nursing
University of Calgary
Calgary, Alberta

**Debbie Sheppard-LeMoine, RN, BN, MN, PhD**
Dean
Faculty of Nursing
University of Windsor
Windsor, Ontario

**Elizabeth Ubaldi, RN, BA, MN, CCNE, DNP**
Professor
Nursing Department
Sault College of Applied Arts and Technology
Sault Ste. Marie, Ontario

**Nicole van Doornik, RN, MSN**
Lecturer
Daphne Cockwell School of Nursing
Toronto Metropolitan University
Toronto, Ontario

## STUDENT REVIEWERS

The author would like to extend a special thank you to these nursing students and recent graduates who took time from their studies to provide valuable feedback on the manuscript:

**Charlotte Allan**
Practical Nursing Program
School of Nursing
Fanshawe College
London, Ontario

**Leanne Arellano**
RN Program, 4-Year Bachelor of Science in Nursing (BScN)
York University
Toronto, Ontario

**Dilpreet Birdi**
RN Program, 4-Year Bachelor of Science in Nursing (BScN)
York University
Toronto, Ontario

**Crystal Chang**
RN Program Graduate, 4-Year Bachelor of Science in Nursing (BScN)
York University
Toronto, Ontario

**Anna Chau**
RN Program, 2nd Entry BScN
York University
Toronto, Ontario

**Tony Curcio**
Practical Nursing Program
School of Nursing
Fanshawe College
London, Ontario

**Ryan Gladwin**
RN Program, 4-Year Bachelor of Science in Nursing (BScN)
York University
Toronto, Ontario

**Catalina Gracia Bolivar**
Practical Nursing Program
School of Nursing
Fanshawe College
London, Ontario

**Maral Hangopian**
RN Program, 4-Year Bachelor of Science in Nursing (BScN)
York University
Toronto, Ontario

**Mariam Iordachescu**
RN Program, 4-Year Bachelor of Science in Nursing (BScN)
York University
Toronto, Ontario

**Andrea Laturski**
RN program
Collaborative BScN
York University
Toronto, Ontario

**Mary Oppong**
RN Program, 4-Year Bachelor of Science in Nursing (BScN)
York University
Toronto, Ontario

**Nidhi Patel**
RN Program
Collaborative BScN
York University
Toronto, Ontario

**Navpreet Sahi**
RN Program, 4-Year Bachelor of Science in Nursing (BScN)
York University
Toronto, Ontario

**Venus Versoza**
RN Program, 4-Year Bachelor of Science in Nursing (BScN)
York University
Toronto, Ontario

**Jessica Yefremov**
RN Program, 4-Year Bachelor of Science in Nursing (BScN)
York University
Toronto, Ontario

## Why a Textbook on Thinking in Nursing?

Let's be clear from the start—learning to become a nurse is challenging work. As students in undergraduate nursing and practical nursing programs, you are faced with an enormous amount of complex information that you must integrate into practice in a relatively short period of time. Nurses must demonstrate a safe understanding of that knowledge once they graduate. Topics such as nursing theory; the physical, social, and psychological sciences; research and data; and specific nursing practice knowledge that is applied using simulation and real client experiences are basic to most nursing curricula. Putting all this information together and thinking it through can be difficult.

Exposure to multiple ways of thinking and decision making can prepare you for complex and varied practice situations. The process of finding information and gathering or collecting data; interpreting and prioritizing that information to make decisions; determining client-centred plans and collaborating with health care professionals to implement and deliver competent and ethical care; and reflecting on what has been done are essential to nursing practice. If students are taught various processes for thinking and decision making early on in their nursing education, they will be better able to apply critical thinking skills, develop mental models, and begin to identify what works for them—and the clients they care for.

Nursing skills and nursing-related topics are introduced and developed in programs so that students will know the what, why, and how of taking care of clients. A strong grasp of foundational knowledge is essential to the safe performance of nursing care and is an expectation of the public for the nursing professional. Without an understanding of important concepts, students will not be able to identify what is expected or unexpected in a client's condition, for instance. This necessary knowledge is also needed to think critically and clearly, and to provide reasoning and rationale for justification of any actions.

It is crucial to provide a rationale for any and all actions selected in the role of a nurse. A sound rationale is needed to explain interventions to clients, in client teaching, and when communicating with nursing colleagues and other health care professionals. It is also a requirement to meet the standard of care set by provincial and territorial regulatory bodies. A sound rationale is a necessary precursor to any good decision or outcome.

The way nursing students have been taught about thinking has not changed for decades. They are often presented with client case studies, simulation experiences, and other reality-based activities and asked to think them through or problem-solve to find a solution. The challenge for students is to learn what process to use when working out solutions.

When learning about nursing practice, students often ask, *How will I know what to do next as I care for a client?* and *How do I make clinical decisions?* Solid decision-making skills that create a safe, ethical, and evidence-informed outcome can be learned. They are particularly important in more complex environments and in relation to clients, families, or community groups with multiple health concerns.

The overarching message in this textbook is that learning and practising how to think well—in a collaborative, comprehensive, contextually based, culturally safe manner—can help students participate in shared, safe, ethical, and competent decisions. This approach in itself can be viewed as an act of advocacy for all clients.

## Who Is This Textbook for?

This textbook is for all nursing students preparing to enter nursing practice in Canada. It is centred on Canadian nursing entry-level practice for undergraduate baccalaureate students and practical nursing students.

The use of this textbook should be situated within a full nursing curriculum. It can be used at any point during a nursing student's course of study. It will benefit those beginning to learn about nursing and how professional nurses think and those later in their program who have more experience with nursing concepts and clinical practice. Newly graduated nurses may also refer to this textbook as a refresher when entering practice and adapting to new health care environments.

## Organization of the Textbook

This textbook takes a slightly different approach to thinking like a nurse and introduces a unified process for thinking. It identifies decision making as a key thinking activity. To address a client's main concern, a decision to direct the overall course of care needs to be made by the nurse in collaboration with others, including the client. Making smaller decisions, however, occur *at every point* of a nurse's care process. For example, nurses decide what to assess first, what the client's needs are, what is most important, what to do next, and what to change in the future care of the client.

The goal of this textbook is to bridge the current gap that exists in nursing education, learning to think. It provides an overview of useful tools and nursing and non-nursing frameworks and models in a process-oriented approach. A general introduction to thinking concepts and theories, examples of thinking frameworks and models, a process for thinking that summarizes and unifies various nursing models, and topics that relate to this process are captured in this textbook.

This textbook is intended to be used alongside other nursing and practice-related courses in a nursing program. It is not meant to provide a review of medical–surgical nursing, community and public health practice, or nursing theory content covered in other courses in an accredited nursing program. It does not cover details on aspects of culture, ethical principles, or diversity in the Canadian population. The focus is on thinking and processes for thinking and making decisions.

This textbook is divided into three parts. Part A covers concepts, frameworks, and models for thinking in nursing practice. Part B describes the processes for thinking that involve clinical reasoning, decision making, and clinical judgement. Finally, Part C presents contexts for thinking it through in nursing, taking a closer look at complex decision making and areas that must be integrated into contemporary Canadian nurses' reflective practice, such as Sustainable Development Goals (SDGs); equity, diversity, and inclusion (EDI); and the Truth and Reconciliation Commission's Calls to Action.

Each chapter follows a similar structure and includes an introduction, chapter-specific learning outcomes, and a glossary of important terms. A summary, key points to remember, and a conclusion wrap up each chapter and prepare you for what comes next. Learning resources that include suggested class activities and discussion questions, case study reviews, evidence-informed thinking activities, and multiple-choice questions to check understanding are valuable additions. A final reflection and online resources and references round out each chapter's content.

Part A provides a foundation for learning about thinking. In Chapter 1, fundamental information on thinking about thinking is presented and introduces the concepts of critical thinking, metacognition, decision making, clinical reasoning, and clinical judgement. How one learns (learning style) and acquires graduate attributes, and how these attributes can be developed and nurtured are emphasized. Understanding these ideas is essential to big-picture thinking. As well, the importance of self-efficacy and self-regulation in nursing practice is also explained.

Chapter 2 presents common models used for thinking in nursing practice. These models include the scientific and the research process, and the reflective cycle. Nursing-specific models such as the nursing process and those related to clinical reasoning, clinical judgement, and ethical decision making are described and compared to highlight similarities in the skills they use when thinking it through. This chapter introduces a broad framework for presenting information at each step of the thinking and decision-making process and organizing thinking in nursing practice. It covers *n*ursing knowledge, professional *r*oles, *c*lient context, and the health care *e*nvironment (NRCE). This NRCE framework, which is applied in Chapters 3 to 6, identifies the primary components that nurses consider at every step when making decisions about client care and professional nursing issues. As a way of summarizing and representing all models and frameworks for thinking, a unified process for thinking and decision making is introduced. The application of this flexible, unified process is illustrated in Chapters 3 to 6. The chapter also discusses the NCLEX Clinical Judgement Measurement Model (NCJMM).

Part B comprises Chapters 3 to 6. Each chapter demonstrates how to apply a step in the thinking and decision-making process. In these four chapters, clinical reasoning skills, barriers to thinking, strategies to overcome barriers, and the NRCE framework are used to demonstrate thinking activities used in the particular step of the thinking and decision-making process. To summarize the step that is highlighted in each chapter, a case study on a nursing situation in which a nursing model is applied is included to show how you can use it in practice. Chapter 3 looks at the first step in the unified process for thinking and decision making: finding information. As such, it focuses on assessing, noticing, recognizing, and collecting data and information. In this chapter, the clinical reasoning cycle is used to think through this step.

Chapter 4 looks at the second step in the unified process for thinking and decision making: deciding what to do. This step focuses on analyzing, interpreting, synthesizing, and prioritizing information. In this chapter, an ethical decision-making model is applied to a case study to demonstrate how decisions can be made in practice.

Chapter 5 looks at the third step in the unified process for thinking and decision making: acting on decisions. Action flows from decisions that were made in the previous phase and includes planning, implementing, and responding. In this chapter, the nursing process is applied to a case study to illustrate the thinking involved while acting on decisions.

Chapter 6 looks at the final step in the unified process for thinking and decision making: reviewing actions. It focuses on evaluating, reflecting, judging, and concluding. In this chapter, a clinical judgement model is applied to a case study to illustrate how actions can be reflected on in practice.

Part C takes a closer look at thinking through complex decisions and developing reflective practitioner skills. Chapter 7 identifies factors that increase the complexity of decision making in practice and ways to organize your thinking to address complex situations and make competent decisions. Chapter 8 explores thinking like a reflective practitioner. It underscores the importance of the role of reflection for developing clinical reasoning skills and clinical judgement in nursing. Also, it emphasizes that meeting client needs requires big-picture thinking and an awareness of contemporary practice requirements. These requirements are SDGs that support a healthy planet and equitable and inclusive care for all groups, including Indigenous peoples and racialized populations. Addressing both complexity and reflective practice rely on integration of the foundational thinking concepts and the thinking and decision-making process presented in preceding chapters. Finally, examples of the application of models, frameworks, concepts and skills are provided in the appendix. Three different nursing activities are used to put it all together. Each illustrates how thinking *BIG* and *small* can unfold over various timelines. A helpful glossary is included that summarizes concept descriptions.

Students: refer to other courses you are taking (or have taken) and think about how all the nursing knowledge you are acquiring (or acquired) is needed when thinking and making decisions as a nurse. What you have learned about medical–surgical nursing, ethics, Indigenous peoples, anti-racist practice, community and public health nursing, and other topics will support you as you "think it through."

## Features of This Textbook

This textbook is centred on Canadian nursing entry-level practice for undergraduate baccalaureate students and practical nursing students. Many Canadian citations and references—authored or co-authored by nurses and faculty in health care agencies and postsecondary educational institutions in Canada—provide evidence for how thinking can be learned. Use of currently published literature grounds the textbook's descriptions of evidence-informed nursing care and thinking. Cited literature on Indigenous topics is authored or co-authored by Indigenous scholars.

Students as learners are at different stages and must self-assess their own knowledge and readiness to adapt their thinking. To support the application of knowledge, case studies are included and designed for discussion based on the needs of the class and learner, and the focus of the course. They are meant to encourage thinking it through and offer a basis for discussion. Often, there is no single answer.

Language was selected intentionally. Gender-neutral language (i.e., *they/them*) was used in this textbook and in the case study descriptions. The use of *nurse* may refer to registered nurse, practical nurse, and/or psychiatric nurse, and *student* may refer to one studying to enter these areas of nursing practice, or one who is a lifelong learner. *Client* is used to mean a person or individual, a family, group, community, or population, depending on the focus of the nurse's practice. The word *client* is currently used in all provincial and territorial entry-to-practice documents in Canada, and so was selected for use in this textbook. Specific names were not assigned to clients in the textbook's case studies; readers can insert a name as desired if that will focus their achievement of specific learning outcomes with regards to cultural backgrounds, challenging assumptions, or other learning needs.

*Reflective Practice Moments*, opportunities to *Focus on Technology, Toolboxes for Thinking*, and *Knowledge Check-ins* are also included, as well as other activities that provide opportunities for thinking it through. Each chapter includes suggested class activities and review questions, as well as online resources that offer students background information on the content covered in the chapter.

## Meeting the Needs of Instructors and Students

This textbook includes feedback from extensive review and input from nursing instructors, students, and new graduates. The current context of Canadian nursing practice was acknowledged by including relevant references to SDGs, EDI, and the Truth and Reconciliation Commission's Calls to Action from 2015. While the aim of this textbook does not include coverage of detailed information on these topics, discussions in classrooms and with your peers about thinking in nursing—the process of how and why decisions are made—can expand on any of these topics. Instructors and students should draw on other helpful resources when studying different ways of knowing, or when thinking about collaborating on care with racialized populations, for instance. As an instructor or as a student, think about where you are teaching and learning and how the health care context and client demographics can influence discussions on decision making as a nurse.

The work of becoming a nurse and "thinking it through" does not end with graduation from your program. It continues throughout your nursing career as new situations with clients arise and with changes in health care and population needs.

## An Important Note

The author of this text recognizes and acknowledges the diverse histories of the first peoples of the lands now referred to as Canada. It is recognized that individual communities identify themselves in various ways; within this text, the term *Indigenous* is used to refer to all First Nations, Aboriginal, Inuit, Métis, and non-status people within Canada. It is also recognized that knowledge and language concerning sex, gender, and identity are fluid and continually evolving. The language and terminology presented in this text endeavour to be inclusive of all people and reflect what is, to the best of our knowledge, current at the time of publication.

## Elsevier eBooks

More than just words on a screen, Elsevier eBooks on Vital-Source come preloaded with interactive learning features that empower students to engage with course content in entirely new ways.

Ideal for use both inside and outside the classroom, Elsevier eBooks on VitalSource gives students the ability to access textbook content any time, any place via desktop computer, laptop, tablet, or smartphone.

It includes study aids such as highlighting, e-note-taking, and the ability to share notes with other students or with instructors. Even more importantly, it allows students and instructors to do a comprehensive search within the specific text or across several titles. Please check with your Elsevier sales representative for more information.

# ACKNOWLEDGEMENTS

I would like to gratefully recognize those amazing individuals who have helped me realize this passion project. The idea of this textbook, and for presenting alternative and detailed ways to learn about thinking and making decisions, has been germinating for a decade.

Thank you to my work colleagues at York University's School of Nursing, whose conversations have motivated my thinking about nursing education and how students learn.

A special thanks needs to go to all the nursing students, past, present, and future, who I have had the sincere pleasure of teaching and learning with and from. Your successes and desires to be the best nurses you can be are inspirational.

Thanks especially to the Elsevier support team of Roberta Spinosa-Millman, Senior Editor (Acquisitions, Canada), Lenore Spence, Content Development Specialist, and Cindy Thoms, Senior Production Manager, for believing in the value of this work and for their patience and expert guidance.

To all my family, thank you for your support, encouragement, and understanding as I worked on this textbook.

Finally, to all Canadian nurses who are dedicated to thinking it through and to providing the safest, most evidence-informed and collaborative nursing care that they can—to any and all who need it—thank you for your collective wisdom.

I would like to acknowledge that I engage in work as an uninvited guest on the traditional, unceded lands of the area known as Tkaronto. It has been caretaken by the Anishinabek Nation, the Haudenosaunee Confederacy, and the Huron-Wendat and is now home to many First Nations, Inuit, and Métis communities. I acknowledge the current treaty holders, the Mississaugas of the Credit First Nation. I identify as a Canadian by birth who has benefited from Canada's colonial structures.

# Frameworks and Models for Thinking in Nursing

This first section of the textbook aims to provide you with foundational information for understanding thinking and its associated concepts. The concepts are interrelated and are applied when using frameworks and models in nursing practice.

Chapter 1 introduces thinking and what it is. Everyday thinking and thinking in the professional context of nursing practice are presented and compared. Critical thinking traits from many sources are described; you will be encouraged to consider how the traits that you have help you think and learn best. General challenges and influences on how nurses think are described.

In Chapter 2, thinking in nursing is described in more depth. Ways to think in nursing that use frameworks and models are outlined. In this textbook, a special NRCE framework is used to explain how you can think through every step of the thinking process. It will remind you to holistically consider your nursing knowledge (N), your professional role (R), the entire client context (C), and the health care environment (E) in which you practice – wherever that may be. A sampling of several general and nursing-specific models is described. The nursing models are compared, and you are encouraged to start thinking about what makes sense for you to use in your nursing practice. A unified process for thinking and decision making summarizes the steps, concepts, and skills from all the nursing models. This unified process will be used to present information in Part B.

**Part A will help you answer the questions,** *what is thinking* **and** *what is thinking in nursing practice?*

# Introduction to Thinking Critically in Nursing Practice

## LEARNING OUTCOMES

*After reading this chapter, you will be able to:*

- Define *critical thinking*.
- Identify critical thinking traits.
- Describe critical thinking skills that are needed in problem solving and decision making.
- Compare the concepts of critical thinking, clinical reasoning, and clinical judgement.
- Relate the importance of critical thinking to nursing entry-to-practice competencies.

## GLOSSARY

**Clinical judgement:** the outcome of thinking and decision-making activities that are focused on and respond to the client's health care needs; also, "an interpretation or conclusion about a client's needs, concerns, or health problems, and/or the decision to take action (or not), use or modify standard approaches, or improvise new ones as deemed appropriate by the patient's response" (Tanner, 2006, p. 204)

**Clinical reasoning:** a goal-oriented and purposeful process for thinking about a client's care

**Critical thinking:** the purposeful, informed, and self-regulated thinking about connected ideas to increase the likelihood of a desired outcome; a particular attitude, thinking skills, and knowledge are needed to think critically

**Cultural safety:** a critical awareness, where health care professionals and organizations engage in ongoing self-reflection and hold themselves accountable for providing culturally safe care, as defined by the client themself and as measured through progress toward achieving health equity

**Decision making:** selecting the best option from the alternatives that are available; in nursing, a process that requires the use of both critical thinking and clinical reasoning

**Metacognition:** the ability to reflect on and become aware of what we know and what we do not know and to use this understanding when continuing to learn (Halpern, 2014)

**Problem solving:** a process for generating reasonable options to overcome identified barriers that are preventing the attainment of a goal or outcome

**Self-efficacy:** the overall belief in one's ability or competence to manage challenges or changes in life

**Self-regulation:** the ability to reflect on thinking and identify one's learning needs, set goals, select useful resources, and self-evaluate accomplishments and subsequent development that is required to improve

**Thinking:** a cognitive activity that can include many elements, including feelings and emotions

---

This introductory chapter provides a foundation for thinking and making decisions in nursing practice. Knowing what thinking can look like and the specific skills it involves will help you begin to understand critical thinking as it applies to client-focused situations. Critical thinking is essential to addressing many professional nursing and health care issues.

## WHAT IS THINKING?

Every person has the capacity to think. No matter the mental capability, cognitive skill level, range of experiences, or professional education, everyone thinks. However, when learning to think in nursing practice, it is important to understand more about what thinking is.

Thinking is a cognitive activity that can include many elements, including feelings and emotions. It is a *process* of mentally sorting, or sifting through, ideas and information. There are different ways to think, and each way of thinking happens in certain situations and requires certain skills.

One way of thinking can be directionless or free form (like daydreaming). This kind of thinking is uncontrolled, unplanned, and not monitored. It can be creative, but has no goal, and may be based on past experiences, anticipated events, emotions, and desires, or other wants or needs. Because there is no goal, the outcome of this way of thinking is variable.

On the other hand, thinking that is automatic (such as when brushing your teeth), occurs during routine activities. This kind of thinking happens frequently and is easier (and is perhaps "mindless") because of the associated activity's familiarity. Automatic thinking, even though there is a purpose to organizing the needed information, does not require significant planning or monitoring. The outcome of an activity that is supported by automatic thinking is usually reliable or always the same.

Thinking can also be goal oriented, controlled, and purposeful. This kind of thinking is very different from daydreaming or brushing one's teeth. It occurs when a big or small problem needs to be solved, a dilemma with many options needs to be considered, or a new situation arises where it is unclear what to do. Thinking through problems, dilemmas, and new situations requires different skills and strategies. Learning to think like a nurse means learning to think in an intentional and meaningful way.

Many students want to be fast thinkers—to make decisions quickly and to know what to do right away, in every circumstance. In health care, where a client may be in crisis, this seems like a desirable skill. The truth is that in complex situations, this sort of thinking—for example, more intuitive thinking, which does not rely on an obvious process of weighing options or considering alternatives—usually occurs after acquiring a great deal of experience. Nursing students likely will not be able to develop fully intuitive thinking about nursing care during their nursing program. Although quick and clear thinking is necessary when providing care to clients, intuition is not always required to accomplish care goals.

Consider, instead, that thinking can be fast or slow. Fast thinking, or *System 1 thinking,* is intuitive, reflexive, and seemingly effortless; and when it is associated with good outcomes, it is often attributed to expertise (Halpern, 2014; Kahneman, 2011). Slow thinking, or *System 2 thinking,* is deliberate, effortful, and provides the foundation for the ability to think fast (Halpern, 2014; Kahneman, 2011). To develop the less obvious cognitive patterns and pathways for thinking intuitively in a professional context, a person would have to become very good at thinking slowly. Generally, if fast thinking is associated with intuition, then slow thinking is associated with critical thinking. See Figure 1.1 for a comparison.

Critical thinking is the purposeful, informed, and self-regulated thought process about connecting ideas to increase the likelihood of a desired outcome. It is effortful—it takes mental work and time. Critical thinking is needed to solve real-world problems, formulate inferences, calculate the probability of something occurring, and make complex decisions (Halpern, 2014). The skills and strategies used to think critically are relevant to and effective in

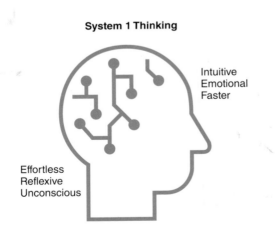

**System 1 Thinking**

Intuitive
Emotional
Faster

Effortless
Reflexive
Unconscious

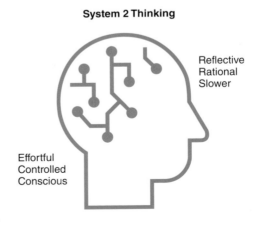

**System 2 Thinking**

Reflective
Rational
Slower

Effortful
Controlled
Conscious

Fig. 1.1 System 1 Versus System 2 Thinking Characteristics. (Adapted from Kahneman, 2011.)

a specific context, which means that they are applied in a particular way depending on the situation.

Elder (2007) describes critical thinking as a "self-guided, self-disciplined thinking which attempts to reason at the highest level of quality in a fair-minded way. People who think critically consistently attempt to live rationally, reasonably, empathically" (p. 1). Everyone is capable of critical thinking in this way, and you perform these mental processes daily. To think critically, several components are needed:

- an *attitude* or way of thinking about a certain situation (e.g., a frame of mind or disposition) that includes flexibility, curiosity, persistence, collaboration, self-correction, self-regulation, and self-awareness of biases and assumptions;
- the *knowledge* needed to understand the information that is available; and
- the *thinking skills* or abilities to make inferences, projections, calculations, comparisons, or evaluations about that information.

> Attitude + Knowledge + Thinking Skills = Critical Thinking

For example, in everyday life, you may have to think about what groceries to purchase based on your budget for food and your nutritional needs, or you may have to think about which college or university program to apply to where you may be most satisfied and successful. Other situations, such as thinking about whether to consent to a nonurgent medical treatment or to buy a house, could have significant consequences and are more complex. Solutions to these situations would require information to be sorted through in a more thoughtful and logical manner.

What are some everyday examples of critical thinking?
- A coach of a sports team works with the players during a huddle to devise a new tactic for winning the next point.
  - A coach who tells the team to continue on with tactics that are not yielding good results is not thinking critically.
- A writer arranges ideas for characters, plots, and subplots to create an engaging and believable storyline.
  - A writer who puts ideas on paper just to fill pages, without a plan for how the story will unfold, is not thinking critically.
- A business owner proposes a new plan to overcome multiple issues with supply chain disruptions and hiring vacancies.
  - A business owner who relies solely on hope and the good intentions of trusted customers during an economic downturn is not thinking critically.
- A health care worker collaborates with a client and their family to identify needs, priorities, and standards of care to choose the best solution for care from available options.

- A health care worker who insists that a client follow a standardized regimen, without incorporating the client's capacity to learn and cultural preferences, is not thinking critically.

An effective critical thinker is able to do the following:
- Ask vital questions about relevant issues or problems, framing them clearly, accurately, and concisely
- Gather relevant information and assess it proficiently using abstract and concrete thinking
- Communicate effectively and appropriately with others when analyzing options to problems
- Arrive at conclusions or solutions using logic and evidence-informed reasoning, and validate these against appropriate standards
- Think open-mindedly using systems or models of thought, while recognizing strengths and limitations in themselves and the system or model (The Foundation for Critical Thinking, 2021).

---

**KNOWLEDGE CHECK-IN**
- Describe the different types of thinking: directionless, automatic, and intentional and controlled.
- How is intuitive thinking based on experience?
- Explain how a critique of available information and the situation results in slower, thoughtful thinking.

---

## WHAT ARE CRITICAL THINKING TRAITS AND SKILLS?

What qualities does a person need to become a good or *effective* critical thinker? Educators, psychologists, and researchers have identified a number of traits and skills that support thinking in a purposeful and controlled manner.

### Critical Thinking Traits

Consider the traits of people who have well-developed critical thinking skills. They have a certain disposition and particular characteristics that make critical thinking skill acquisition and development easier. An individual's disposition and characteristics are affected by factors including family relationships, birth order, cultural experiences and exposure, their generation, a perceived personality type, and emotional intelligence (EI). For example, an individual can be significantly influenced by strong identification with a cultural group, their Indigenous culture and history, or their experience with immigration to Canada. Everyone's influences are different, and their effects on a person's world view and, therefore, critical thinking, are important to pay attention to.

Table 1.1 presents traditional views on the traits required to think critically. They help answer the question, "What are the characteristics or qualities of a critical thinker?" The

### TABLE 1.1   Examples of Critical Thinking Traits

| Critical Thinking Disposition[a] | Habits of the Mind[b] | Intellectual Traits[c] | Disposition for Effortful Thinking and Learning[d] | Seven Traits of Highly Effective Critical Thinkers[e] |
|---|---|---|---|---|
| Truth seeking | Confidence | Intellectual humility | Willingness to plan | Curiosity |
| Open-mindedness | Contextual perspective | Intellectual courage | Flexibility | Compassion |
| Analyticity | Creativity | Intellectual empathy | Persistence | Awareness |
| Systematicity | Flexibility | Intellectual perseverance | Willingness to self-correct, admit errors, and change your mind when the evidence changes | Decisiveness |
| Critical thinking | Inquisitiveness | | | Honesty |
| Self-confidence | Intellectual integrity | Intellectual autonomy | | Willingness |
| Inquisitiveness | Intuition | Intellectual integrity | | Creativity |
| Maturity | Open-mindedness | Confidence in reason | Being mindful | |
| | Perseverance | Fair-mindedness | Consensus-seeking | |
| | Reflection | | | |

[a]Facione, N. C., Facione, P. A., & Sanchez, C. A. (1994). Critical thinking disposition as a measure of competent clinical judgment: The development of the California critical thinking disposition inventory. *Journal of Nursing Education, 33*(8), 345–350.

[b]Scheffer, B. K., & Rubenfeld, M. G. (2000). A consensus statement on critical thinking in nursing. *Journal of Nursing Education, 39*(8), 352–359.

[c]Paul, R., & Elder. L. (2019). *The miniature guide to critical thinking concepts and tools* (8th ed.). The Foundation for Critical Thinking Press.

[d]Halpern, D. (2014). *Thought and knowledge: An introduction to critical thinking* (5th ed.). Psychology Press.

[e]Crockett, L. (2018). The 7 most common traits of highly effective critical thinkers. *Focused Learning Network.* http://blog.futurefocusedlearning.net/7-characteristics-effective-critical-thinkers.

traits listed here are examples from the literature on critical thinking; undoubtedly, additional traits also exist.

Although the lists in this table are distinct, when read carefully, there are common themes. Traits of open-mindedness, curiosity, confidence, creativity, and a willingness to change or be flexible are evident in several of the lists. These views also share the idea that critical thinking traits can be cultivated, modelled, encouraged, and, therefore, developed.

### Critical Thinking Skills

Critical thinking skills are slightly different from but are related to these traits. Critical thinking skills can be taught, facilitated, practised, and measured in the classroom, the laboratory, and clinical settings. If a person possesses strong critical thinking traits, they are likely able to perform or demonstrate critical thinking skills.

Many skills can assist with better critical thinking. For instance, Scheffer and Rubenfeld (2000), who described the "habits of the mind" traits of critical thinking in nursing, also identified seven skills of critical thinking in nursing:

1. *Information seeking*: searching for evidence, facts and knowledge using relevant sources, and collecting appropriate data (subjective, objective, historical, current)
2. *Discriminating*: identifying differences and similarities in situations and carefully distinguishing according to category/rank

3. *Analyzing*: breaking down a whole into parts to understand relationships and functioning of a concept or situation
4. *Transforming knowledge*: adapting or converting the nature, form or function of a concept, depending on the context; synthesizing
5. *Predicting*: visioning and anticipating a plan and its consequences
6. *Applying standards*: judging according to approved professional or social rules/criteria, or identified personal values
7. *Logical reasoning*: drawing inferences or conclusions that are based on confirmed evidence

These authors indicated that their study of critical thinking was a "beginning step" (Scheffer & Rubenfeld, 2000, p. 358). Research on critical thinking in nursing is ongoing. Later chapters in this textbook will provide examples of critical thinking skills that nurses apply in the practice setting specifically.

Why do we need to worry about critical thinking skills? As you likely know, critical thinking skills are useful in everyday life for solving problems. Problem-solving skills are often associated with critical thinking. A problem occurs when there is a barrier between where you are and where you want to be (Halpern, 2014); so, **problem solving** is necessary to generate options to overcome that identified barrier. Problem solving is specific and focused on identifying reasonable options. Good knowledge, sound logic, and a certain degree of creativity (which are associated with critical thinking skills) are essential to coming up with options that are potentially useful.

## DEVELOPMENT OF CRITICAL THINKING SKILLS

Critical thinking skills are developed through an understanding of how you think and learn, participate in educational programs, engage in practice, and receive feedback on demonstrated thinking. When it comes to developing these skills, practice, practice, and more practice are essential. An increased awareness of yourself and your own performance, and how you "think about your thinking" are vital. Everyone is unique.

### Understanding How You Learn

Everyone has different abilities and capacities for development. To develop your critical thinking skills, it helps to understand your approach to thinking, your learning preferences, your strengths, and the areas you need to improve on when thinking and learning. In a professional role, you will be thinking about your thinking continuously.

*Learning* can be described as a relatively permanent change in behaviour or knowledge as a result of an experience. While not all learning requires critical thinking and effort (it is easy to learn that if you place your hand on a hot surface, you should pull your hand back), the intentional and purposeful learning inherent in formal education (like nursing) is required to make changes to your existing knowledge and usual actions.

Confirm your learning style. What is your favourite way to learn something new? One easy way to do this is to consider whether you learn best by observing, reading, or writing (a visual learner), by listening (an auditory learner), or by actively participating in or experiencing hands-on practice (a kinesthetic learner). As a critical thinker, you should also ask yourself why you prefer to learn in a particular way.

You may have discovered that you prefer to learn using a variety of methods—that you have no true, single preference. As such, you may be a more holistic learner and learn better when combining different approaches. For many people, this is the case (VARK Learn Limited, 2022). For those who have multiple perspectives of learning and for Indigenous students, a more integrated view may be preferred (Antoine et al., 2018). Neurodivergent thinkers may have other ways of approaching thinking and learn with the same critical and analytical results as neurotypical thinkers.

All learning styles can lead to learning. It is important to understand this point so that you can take advantage of all learning opportunities that are available to you. Take time to carefully consider your own learning preferences by referring to Box 1.1.

When thinking critically about learning preferences, it is important to understand that the way one prefers to learn and the way that leads to the most effective, efficient learning may be different. For example, if a person prefers to learn through reading but must learn to sing a song, reading about the song instead of listening to it may not result in optimal learning.

Consider the following when engaging in learning:

- Use the general critical thinking skills that have been identified so far.
- Find meaning in what you read by trying to understand ideas more deeply. Why did the author write these ideas, and where did they come from?
- Ask questions after listening to others talk about their practice. How can a better understanding of others' experiences help you in your future practice?

Often, a learner will become so involved in learning a relatively small concept that they forget how it applies to other concepts and how it "fits" into the larger idea of client health and health care. Remind yourself that tasks or objectives accomplished while learning often support the achievement of a larger goal (thinking *BIG* and *small* at the same time). To analyze something, for example, you need to pull all available information together and synthesize it to create a new, bigger understanding. Thinking *BIG* and *small* when learning is an important way to develop new knowledge.

### Participating in Educational Programs

Educational programs help students learn and think critically. They also offer different ways to engage in learning that can meet learners' preferred styles and knowledge requirements. You may recognize the following examples of learning activities from courses that you have taken:

- Rephrase a problem in several ways.
- Create a concept or mind map to describe relationships between a concept and its subconcepts.
- Categorize a large amount of information.
- List multiple options for solving a specific problem, and associated pros and cons.
- Rationalize the best option for solving a problem.
- Engage in or listen to a debate during class.
- Explain why the right answer is correct and why the wrong answers are incorrect in a multiple-choice question.

These types of learning activities help students understand course content and successfully complete a course. All of the learning activities in a nursing program help graduates meet entry-to-practice competencies and program outcomes.

In addition to specific nursing program outcomes, other generic learning occurs in all educational programs—no matter the discipline. Called "graduate attributes" (characteristics that are acquired by graduates by the end of their program), they look a lot like traits developed through

## BOX 1.1    Learning Preferences Activity

Review each style and the indicators of that style. Note that critical thinking skills can be associated with indicators of each learning style—it is possible to think critically no matter which style you prefer. Consider your preferred style (there may be more than one) and note how you like to learn. Does the way you like to learn change depending on what you need to learn?

| Learning Style | Style Indicators | Examples of Associated Critical Thinking Skills |
|---|---|---|
| **Visual** Observing an activity, reading, note-taking or highlighting text, interpreting graphs or diagrams | **When learning, I prefer to:** <br>• Imagine myself completing an activity <br>• Watch my peers attempt a new skill before I try it <br>• Group ideas together in order to recall them more easily when note-taking or reading <br>• Write out flashcards when studying <br>• Draw or look at a flow chart | • *Discriminating:* categorizing <br>• *Predicting:* visioning and anticipating consequences <br>• *Analyzing:* breaking down the whole |
| **Auditory** Listening to a live or recorded lecture, reading out loud, discussing concepts with others | **When learning, I prefer to:** <br>• Make up rhymes to remember facts <br>• Listen to a lecture without taking any notes, so I can fully understand concepts <br>• Talk about and justify ideas with a study group or peer <br>• Explain concepts aloud to myself when studying | • *Logical reasoning:* drawing conclusions based on evidence <br>• *Applying standards:* judging concepts in terms of criteria and values |
| **Kinesthetic** Doing an activity oneself, moving while learning, practising directly with supplies in the lab | **When learning, I prefer to:** <br>• Go to the lab for hands-on practice instead of only reading about a skill <br>• Draw images or charts of new concepts to better understand them <br>• Move, or walk around the room and gesture with my hands when studying for a test <br>• Exercise when listening to a recorded lecture | • *Information seeking:* actively searching for evidence <br>• *Transforming knowledge:* adapting concepts to the physical world and understanding context |
| **Holistic, Multiperspective** Integrating multiple ways of knowing at the same time | **When learning, I prefer to:** <br>• Hear a full story that illustrates the ideas <br>• Make connections to my own experiences and background <br>• Situate the learning beyond the classroom when possible | • *Information seeking:* actively searching for evidence <br>• *Transforming knowledge:* adapting concepts to the physical world and understanding context <br>• *Two-eyed seeing:** seeing from one eye with the strengths of Indigenous knowledge and ways of knowing, and from the other eye with the strengths of Western (and/or scientific) knowledge and ways of knowing while learning to use both eyes together for the benefit of all |

*https://www.migmawei.ca.
Bartlett, C., Marshall, M., & Marshall, A. (2012). Two-eyed seeing and other lessons learned within a co-learning journey of bringing together indigenous and mainstream knowledges and ways of knowing. *Journal of Environmental Studies and Sciences, 2,* 331–340. https://doi.org/10.1007/s13412-012-0086-8.

### TABLE 1.2 Graduate Attributes

| Attributes | Related Attributes |
| --- | --- |
| Collaboration | Openness to diversity; interpersonal skills; adaptability and compromise; individual contribution |
| Communication | Writing skills; oral skills; visual communication; multilingualism or use of professional terminology; technology skills |
| Confidence | Leadership and empowerment; independence; initiative; resilience |
| Creativity | Imagination; innovation; divergent thinking; artistic sensibility |
| Critical thinking | Analytic and synthetic reasoning; interpretive proficiency; intellectual curiosity; information literacy |
| Ethical responsibility | Global citizenship; community engagement; social and environmental awareness; professionalism |
| Scholarship | Knowledge breadth and depth; intra- and interprofessional knowledge; lifelong learning; investigation |

Adapted from ElAtia, S., Ipperciel, D., Zaiane, O., et al. (2020). Graduate attributes assessment program. *International Journal of Information and Learning Technology, 38*(1), 117–134 (p. 122). doi:10.1108/IJILT-03-2020-0025. https://www.yorku.ca/wp-content/uploads/sites/300/2020/10/Graduate-Attributes-Assessment-Program-2020.pdf.

critical thinking (Table 1.2). These attributes are interrelated, which means that each attribute supports another.

By fully participating in formal, well-designed nursing educational programs, you will be able to develop the critical thinking skills needed in nursing, as well as postsecondary graduate attributes. Educational program instructors provide an evaluation of the critical thinking skills and attributes you demonstrate so that you can improve your performance.

### Engaging in Practice and Receiving Feedback

Practice and performance feedback support the development of critical thinking skills. The activity practised and the type of feedback provided relate to specific learning expectations. For instance, if you are learning to administer a medication via intramuscular injection, you will practise this action and will likely be given feedback on your psychomotor skills *and* the decisions that you made while performing the administration of the medication. Learning through practice in an educational program is course specific and, ultimately, aimed at meeting the broader program's goals. All practice and feedback in an educational program should be provided based on the program's goals in some way, so that your performance and your progress toward those goals (or graduate attributes) can be determined. Because organized learning activities and program outcomes are intentionally associated with critical thinking skills, you can track your development of these skills through the feedback you receive over time. Always keep feedback in a special file to refer to later. This feedback will enable you to self-assess your performance, identify barriers to your thinking and to develop a reflective stance.

### Self-Assessment of Critical Thinking

Self-assessment is an important aspect of feedback. Take the initiative (a sign of a critical thinker) to conduct periodic self-assessments to understand how you are developing your critical thinking skills and identify any obstacles encountered. To start, consider a challenge you faced in the past in relation to a particular problem, whether in your personal life or in a course. How would you assess the critical thinking skills you applied to that problem at the time? What feedback did you receive? Were you *unable* to:

- Discern the real issue?
- Gather enough (or relevant) information about the problem?
- Identify reasonable options or solutions?
- Decide between available options?
- Prioritize what to do first?
- Think within the available timeline?

If you answered "yes" to any of the above questions, you may have been influenced by obstacles, or barriers, to critical thinking, which resulted in the problem you experienced. Refer to Table 1.3. Do you identify with any of these obstacles? Have you experienced any of these effects on the thinking process?

### Self-Efficacy, Self-Regulation and Metacognition

Strong critical thinking skills used when engaging in practice and receiving feedback also require the broader reflective skills of self-efficacy, self-regulation, and metacognition. These skills provide students with insight into their weaknesses and strengths in learning and obstacles to critical thinking.

Once you understand how learning preferences, your educational program, practice, and feedback affect critical thinking skills, you will be equipped to further develop entry-to-practice competencies more independently. Self-efficacy and self-regulation are vital to success in a professional discipline such as nursing and will help with this development.

Self-efficacy is about believing in yourself and your ability to grow and develop as a thinker—which involves recognizing when you are progressing and when you are not, and that you can change as needed. General self-efficacy can be

## TABLE 1.3    Obstacles to Critical Thinking and Their Effects on the Thinking Process

| Obstacles | Effects |
| --- | --- |
| Lack of foundational knowledge, and not knowing enough science or theory; unable to break down a complex situation into parts: "I just don't know." | Poor grasp of significance of problems with difficulty in initiating any further thinking |
| Overconfidence in ability to address a problem, or a desire to be "first" or "best": "I can do it without anyone's help." | Little collaborative input (including databases or other people) and incomplete information to address a problem |
| Biased viewpoint; set in assumptions; a lack of self-awareness: "My way of thinking is best." | Omission of an important component that could negatively affect the outcome |
| Thinking in one way only; unaware of, and not using evidence: "I see that there is only one answer." | Inability to identify more than one relevant option, resulting in a lack of creative solution or a less optimal outcome |
| Unable to admit errors in thinking; desire to maintain status: "I will lose others' respect if I ask for help." | Inability to select the required action to address the problem and achieve the desired outcome |
| Desire to conform; pressured by time limitations, distractions, or others' needs: "I must follow the norms, no matter what." | Missing important steps in thinking about solutions to the problem and risking a less optimal outcome |
| Fear of repercussions or lack of confidence based on past negative experiences from generational trauma or system inequities: "If I ask for help, I will be judged or punished." | Weakened self-efficacy and confidence, and a significantly reduced capacity for growth in thinking (i.e., analysis paralysis) |

described as the overall belief in one's ability or competence to manage challenges or changes in life. When learning a new skill, this characteristic (see Table 1.1 for traits similar to self-efficacy) helps students sustain their efforts to succeed. Mentors, instructors, peers, and coaches can help you build self-efficacy. Pay attention to the feedback they offer and your perceived self-efficacy during learning and practice.

**Self-regulation** is the ability to adapt your thinking and to change behaviour when faced with a challenge or with new, relevant information. Self-regulated learning refers to a student's ability to diagnose their own learning needs, set goals, select useful resources, and self-evaluate their accomplishments and subsequent development. Continually reassessing learning needs requires reflection on any obstacles that arise and how they affect learning (see Table 1.3). This ongoing process also involves a sense of self-efficacy, self-motivation, and behavioural engagement (Zimmerman, 1995). Notice that self-efficacy is needed for self-regulation, or being responsible for monitoring one's own development.

It is possible to become a self-regulated learner—but how? One process that can be used consists of three cyclical phases that relate to one's own actions (Zimmerman, 2002):

- *Forethought phase:* This phase, which occurs *before* learning takes place, is about building your learning supports. It considers what is needed when approaching a potential problem, learning opportunity, or change, including assessing your own motivation and beliefs, analyzing the tasks to be completed, and setting goals to increase performance and success.
- *Performance phase:* This phase, which occurs *during* learning, is about keeping track of your progress while it is happening. It considers what occurs when addressing a problem, engaging in learning, or initiating a change. It includes self-observation and self-monitoring (taking notes).
- *Self-reflection phase:* This phase, which occurs *after* learning, is about reviewing the actions taken. It considers how successful you were and what could be done differently next time. It also includes self-judgement and self-evaluation (based on one's past performances and in relation to others' performances) and self-reaction (based on personal satisfaction—positive or negative feelings that can affect future motivation).

**Metacognition** is the ability to reflect on and become aware of what we know and what we don't know, and to use this understanding as we continue to learn (Halpern, 2014). Metacognition is known as an *executive function,* a set of skills that underlies the capacity for self-regulation, critical thinking, skill performance, and clinical practice. It is predictive of academic potential.

Metacognition is a broad concept, but it is extremely important. As a student, it is likely that you have been asked to provide a rationale and evidence for your actions or clinical performance in a certain situation. In your explanation, you must be attuned to the quality of your thinking (or your *metacognition*), which uses all of the traits and skills presented in this chapter. Metacognition enhances your capacity for self-awareness in relation to your learning and development, and can be improved through self-regulated learning strategies (Kuiper & Pesut, 2004).

Table 1.1 started you thinking reflectively—a sign of a System 2 critical thinker. Continuous exploration of how you think, what skills you need to develop, how you need to hone your thinking skills, how you learn, and what you know about your own thinking (or not) contributes to the development of professional behaviours and competencies. Metacognition means that when thinking and acting, you are always thinking about your thinking and asking yourself questions such as:

- What do I want to achieve here?
- Should I seek more information?
- Who could I ask for help?
- Is this similar to what I have experienced in the past?
- What should I do first?
- Am I on the right track?
- What can I do differently?

Now that you have a good grasp of what sort of skills are needed to think critically, you may be wondering if this looks any different in the practice of nursing and caring for clients.

---

**KNOWLEDGE CHECK-IN**
- Consider how understanding learning preferences can help you access ways to learn that work best for you. Note that your preferred way may not be the optimal way to learn in some circumstances.
- How does active involvement in an educational program provide you with options to learn specific skills and practise knowledge?
- Explain the connection between active engagement in programs and feedback aimed to help you continually improve.
- How is being accountable to feedback helpful to professional development and self-regulation skills?
- Describe how metacognition is related to self-regulation and critical thinking.

---

## WHAT IS THINKING IN NURSING?

Many professions require their members to be intentional and deliberate, skillful, accountable, and reflective about how they think. These requirements demonstrate part of what is needed to be a competent practitioner. Students enter nursing educational programs with varied personal knowledge, experience, and critical thinking skills, which must be developed so that these skills can be professionally applied. Solid thinking skills are required when caring for all clients in complex and dynamic health care environments.

In nursing textbooks, a variety of terms are associated with thinking in nursing practice, and they are often used interchangeably. For example, nurses and nurse educators use *critical thinking, clinical reasoning, decision making,* and *clinical judgement* to describe the essential cognitive work that nurses perform during client care. Students may be left wondering, *What sort of thinking am I supposed to use in practice?* These terms are defined in this chapter, but they can also be explored further by referring to the prominent literature available in nursing education and other sciences.

Thinking in nursing practice involves critical thinking. To align with *professional* requirements, critical thinking in nursing must have a focus on health and the client. This thinking must be skillful and incorporate a reasonable breadth and depth of knowledge to achieve safe and competent client care.

When a nurse who is caring for a client in a professional capacity engages in critical thinking about that client's care, the term **clinical reasoning** is often used. This term is an applied definition in nursing practice and in other health care professions. Like critical thinking, it is goal oriented, controlled, and purposeful. It occurs in the specific context of client care. It refers to processes for thinking about a client's health issues and challenges and has been described as:

> the process by which nurses and other clinicians make their judgements, and includes both the deliberate process of generating alternatives, weighing them against the evidence, and choosing the most appropriate, and those patterns that might be characterized as engaged, practical reasoning (e.g., recognition of a pattern, an intuitive clinical grasp, a response without evident forethought).
>
> **(Tanner, 2006, pp. 204–205)**

What does this definition of *clinical reasoning* really mean? It describes a goal-oriented and purposeful process for thinking about a client's care, as well as the more expert and intuitive processes. It can be considered as "critical thinking at the bedside."

Here is an alternate definition of *clinical reasoning:*

*a complex cognitive process that uses formal and informal thinking strategies to gather and analyze patient information, evaluate the significance of this information and weigh alternative actions. Core essences of this concept include cognition, metacognition and discipline-specific knowledge.*

*(Simmons, 2010, p. 1155)*

This definition indicates that knowledge, thinking ability, and a certain frame of mind or awareness are required in clinical reasoning. Clinical reasoning entails identifying and prioritizing options, and applying research and best practices. All of this supports decisions and final judgements about client care. As an example, reflect on a scenario where clients experiencing homelessness often miss or are late for their health appointments at a community clinic. The clinic nurse demonstrates clinical reasoning by considering this health issue and the clients' ability to attend, as well as the challenges of public transit, weather, and possible distrust of the health care system. After reviewing available options, a flexible drop-in schedule is created to efficiently accommodate these clients' needs.

Remember that clinical reasoning and client-focused thinking, depending on a nurse's clinical experience and years in practice, can be slower (methodical, discovering patterns) or faster (intuitive).

## Professional Requirements

In nursing, the skills required to think critically are adapted to the health care setting, so that client-focused professionalism is achieved when thinking. Such clinical reasoning skills, or competencies, must be applied to a nurse's practice, as required by nursing regulatory bodies across Canada. Regulatory bodies may use different terms to describe thinking competencies in nursing care delivery. You have likely encountered many of these terms already. Table 1.4 presents references to critical thinking skill requirements in a number of regulatory body standards documents.

| TABLE 1.4 Examples of Regulatory Body Requirements for Critical Thinking Skills | |
|---|---|
| **Regulatory Body and Standards Document** | **References to Critical Thinking Skill Requirements** |
| **British Columbia College of Nurses and Midwives**<br>*Nurse Practitioners and Registered Nurses Professional Standards* (2020) | "Uses critical thinking when collecting and interpreting data, planning, implementing and evaluating nursing care"; and "Uses decision support tools appropriately to assess and make decisions about client status and plan care" (p. 12) |
| **College of Nurses of Ontario**<br>*Entry-to-Practice Competencies for Registered Nurses* (2019) | "Entry-level RNs apply the critical thinking process throughout all aspects of practice." (p. 4); and "critical inquiry to support professional judgment and reasoned decision-making" (p. 5) |
| **College of Registered Nurses of Newfoundland and Labrador**<br>*Standards of Practice for Registered Nurses and Nurse Practitioners* (2019) | "uses critical inquiry to assess, plan, intervene and evaluate client care"; and "exercises reasonable judgement in the application of evidence-informed practice" (p. 6) |
| **Nova Scotia College of Nursing**<br>*Standards of Practice for Registered Nurses* (2017) | "Attaining, maintaining and demonstrating the appropriate competencies (knowledge, skills and judgment) to practise safely and provide client-centred care"; and "Exercising reasonable judgment" (p. 9) |
| **Registered Nurses Association of the Northwest Territories and Nunavut**<br>*Standards of Practice for Registered Nurses and Nurse Practitioners* (2019) | "uses critical inquiry to assess, plan, intervene and evaluate client care and related services"; and "exercises reasonable judgment" (p. 7) |
| **Saskatchewan Registered Nurses Association**<br>*Registered Nurse Practice Standards* (2019) | "Demonstrating . . . problem-solving strategies, decision-making..." (p. 4); and "Using an ethical and reasoned decision-making process" (p. 5) |

As Table 1.4 indicates, nurses are required by regulatory bodies to use critical thinking in practice. Nurses do so when they correctly apply professional standards and provide safe, competent, and ethical care to clients, families, groups, communities, and populations. Thinking that facilitates a culturally safe environment is one example of how nurses are expected to demonstrate professional standards. Cultural safety requires nurses to acknowledge and address factors that may affect the quality of care provided, such as their own biases, attitudes, assumptions, stereotypes, prejudices, and characteristics, as well as health care and other structures (Curtis et al., 2019; Hart-Wasekeesikaw, 2009). It calls on nurses to think about and define cultural safety from the client's viewpoint. Cultural safety involves metacognitive skills and an ability to acknowledge and address power imbalances in the nurse–client relationship and inequity in health care delivery.

Nurses must engage in critical thinking continually. This thinking is not reserved just for big problems, complex client health issues, and challenging practice environments—it applies *all the time* to a nurse's practice. It is purposeful and is part of the clinical reasoning and decision-making process. Nurses must think critically to make competent, safe, and ethical choices, both individually and collaboratively. Doing so is essential to client advocacy and optimal client health.

## THINKING AND DECISION MAKING IN NURSING: HOW DO THEY RELATE?

In nursing, decision making is a process that requires critical thinking and clinical reasoning. Decision making entails *selecting the best option from the available alternatives.* The goal of decision making is to choose a way forward based on options generated through problem solving. Decision making is always context based, which means that a decision must incorporate the specific circumstances of a situation. In other words, the best option must "fit" the particular situation. Context-based thinking enables nurses' decisions to be client-centred, ethical, socially just, flexible, and accountable.

Critical thinking, problem solving, clinical reasoning, and decision making happen together. Because they are interdependent, these concepts are difficult to separate. Thinking and decision making in nursing practice that is focused on and responds to clients' health care needs results in clinical judgement.

Clinical judgement in nursing practice is "an interpretation or conclusion about a patient's needs, concerns, or health problems, and/or the decision to take action (or not), use or modify standard approaches, or improvise new ones as deemed appropriate by the patient's response" (Tanner, 2006, p. 204). It is also described as "the ways in which nurses come to understand the problems, issues, or concerns of clients/patients, to attend to salient information and respond in concerned and involved ways" (Benner et al., 2009, p. 200). It is a holistic concept, which means that it incorporates many types of thinking, nursing knowledge, health care concepts, and the context. It involves an assessment of the entire situation and thinking process.

The full process of thinking involves critical thinking, clinical reasoning, clinical decision making, and clinical judgement. The initial stages build on and support the final outcome of clinical judgement (Figure 1.2). Client outcomes, and other clinically related or health care related outcomes, are supported by this thinking.

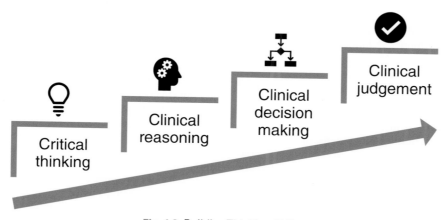

Fig. 1.2 Building Thinking Skills.

The ultimate goal of thinking is to be able to make clinical judgements in the practice environment so that all client health, delivery of client care, and the health care system can be optimized. With clinical reasoning and judgement skills, nurses can be strong advocates for their clients. Because clinical judgement is a desired outcome of the thinking process, it is the focus of measurement on the Next Generation NCLEX-RN®, the registration exam required by most provinces and territories in Canada for entry into nursing practice. Therefore, the concept of clinical judgement will be a focus in this textbook.

## What Makes Thinking in Nursing So Challenging?

Everyone has a unique, personal approach to arriving at decisions in their daily lives. For professional nurses, understanding how clients see their own world and make decisions is important for practice. Effective thinking involves seeking a rationale for how and why an action is used in nursing practice, as well as incorporating others' perspectives. This requires professional education.

In all nursing programs, students gain the knowledge they need to practise safely, competently, and ethically and meet provincial and territorial regulatory program approval processes and Canadian accreditation requirements. Students must also *apply* this knowledge to demonstrate safe, competent, and ethical practice. Usually, application involves using the knowledge acquired in nursing and science courses to answer questions or solve clinical issues (in the learning environment or practice setting). Many students find it challenging to effectively apply the content they have learned at the outset, as it may not be entirely clear to them how the content is connected to the real-world setting and because the associated skills take time to develop. Bridging the gap between theory and practice requires the cultivation of critical thinking skills.

> **REFLECTIVE PRACTICE MOMENT**
> **What does "application" of knowledge mean? Ask yourself:**
> *How do I organize all the information I have learned so that I can use the right information to answer a question?*

Working with clinical instructors and preceptors can help nursing students think through ways to address the theory–practice gap. For instance, instructors are able to model their thinking about client care when talking through their thought processes in detail. As well, nurses may be able to provide students with a description of a client's significant clinical manifestations and their meaning in relation to the client's diagnosis. Then they may be able

to talk about different options and why one intervention would be selected over another. You may have had clinical instructors and preceptors who were able to describe their thinking, which then allowed you to compare that thinking with your own.

Sometimes, it is difficult for students to understand the intricate thought processes of clinical instructors and preceptors. Expert nurses may use intuition to sort out information and arrive at a particular decision; that is, they may not have consciously thought through the detailed process of formulating a decision about complex care. Alternatively, they may use different ways of thinking about a client or clinical issue than students are used to, making it more challenging for students to grasp the way in which information was processed. As observers and learners, students cannot always see how nurses think and use all of the relevant information, even though they carefully watch nurses in action.

The big questions student often ask are, "How will I know what to do?" and "How will I know what to do when I am on my own?"

## Factors That Influence Clinical Decisions

What factors influence how a nurse makes clinical decisions? To answer this question, it is helpful to understand the information, resources, tools, and models that are available to begin thinking critically and make decisions as a nurse would.

An extensive literature review, supported in part by the National Council of State Boards of Nursing (NCSBN) in the United States, considered the factors that contribute to clinical decision making in novice nurses (Muntean, 2012). These factors were identified as either individual (i.e., internal) or environmental (i.e., external). Individual factors focus on the decision maker, while environmental factors focus on the decision task (with some overlap between the two categories). A focus on the client is integrated in these factors, such as in communication, consequences, and task complexity. These factors need to be taught, learned, and tested, but as you may suspect, not all of these factors can be explicitly teased out and evaluated (Table 1.5).

This distinction between individual and environmental factors is helpful as you begin to make clinical decisions. It asks you to categorize the influences on a particular decision into two groups: (1) those that relate to *you* and (2) those that relate to the *setting* in which the decision is made. Although important, considering individual and environmental factors provides only one general way to consider the influences on clinical decision making. Specific models of thinking and decision making used in nursing practice will be discussed in Chapter 2.

## TABLE 1.5   Summary of Factors That Influence Decision Making in Nursing

| Individual Factors | Environmental Factors |
|---|---|
| Age and educational level | Task complexity (any part of the task that increases demands on information processing) |
| Experience (personal and work related, knowledge, and cue recognition) | |
| Hypothesis updating (modifying a plan with new information) | Time pressure (time constraints; higher client-to-nurse ratio; greater potential for errors) |
| Communication (intra-, interprofessional, and client; preferences for ways to communicate) | |
| Emotions and perceptions (mental state of the nurse) | Interruptions (by other health care professionals, clients) |
| Confidence | |
| Professional orientation | Area of specialty (unit, workplace or organizational culture, different levels of risk) |
| Consequences (perception of positive and negative consequences) | |
| Personal values (assumptions, biases, cultural perspective, and background) | Professional autonomy (the ability to make unsupervised decisions) |

Muntean, W. (2012). *Nursing clinical decision-making: A literature review.* https://www.ncsbn.org/research-item/nursing-clinical-decisionmaking-a-literature-review.

## SUMMARY

This chapter presented a foundation for understanding thinking as a whole, critical thinking, and thinking in nursing practice. As a process focused on outcomes, thinking will prepare you for further *thinking about thinking* in general and in all areas of nursing practice. The information presented in this first chapter may seem overwhelming. Review the chapter's learning outcomes. Do you have a better understanding of each one?

A number of ways can be used to describe how nurses think. It is important to remember that not everyone will think in the same way. However, the end result of thinking is always client focused, culturally safe, competent, and ethical care. The concepts presented in this chapter will be used throughout this textbook. *Clinical judgement* will be used as a key concept when discussing thinking in later chapters, because it is the model on which measurement is based for the national registration exam (the Next Generation NCLEX-RN®) and is a foundational element of all nursing practice.

## KEY POINTS TO REMEMBER

These are the key points to remember from this chapter.

### About Thinking in General

- Thinking is a process of mentally sorting or sifting through ideas and information.
- Fast thinking, or System 1 thinking, is intuitive, reflexive, and seemingly effortless; and when it is associated with good outcomes, it is often attributed to expertise.
- Slow thinking, or System 2 thinking, is deliberate, effortful, and provides the foundation for System 1 thinking.
- Critical thinking is the purposeful, informed, and self-regulated thinking about connected ideas in order to increase the likelihood of a desired outcome.
- Attitude, knowledge, and thinking skills are combined to think critically.

- An effective critical thinker asks vital questions, gathers and assesses relevant information, communicates effectively, uses logic and evidence-informed reasoning to arrive at conclusions or solutions, and applies systems and models of thought.

### About Critical Thinking Traits and Skills

- The traits of people who have well-developed critical thinking skills include truth seeking, open-mindedness, intellectual humility, persistence, and curiosity.
- Critical thinking skills can be taught, facilitated, practised, and measured.
- General critical thinking skills include information seeking, discriminating, analyzing, transforming knowledge, predicting, applying standards, and logical reasoning.

- The ability to problem solve is needed when there is a barrier between where you are and where you want to be, to overcome the identified barrier.

### About Critical Thinking Skill Development

- Critical thinking skills are developed through learning activities and experiences, educational programs, and through practice and feedback on demonstrated thinking.
- Self-assessment can help identify obstacles to critical thinking such as a lack of foundational knowledge or the inability to break down a complex problem, overconfidence, a biased viewpoint, a lack of evidence, an unwillingness to admit errors in thinking, a desire to conform, being pressured by deadlines or other external pressures, and a lack of self-confidence.
- Self-efficacy is the overall belief in one's ability or competence to manage challenges or changes in life; it is the belief in oneself and the ability to grow and develop as a thinker.
- Self-regulation is the ability to diagnose one's own learning needs, set goals, select useful resources, self-evaluate accomplishments and subsequent development and to change one's own behaviour based on that evaluation.
- Metacognition is the ability to reflect on and become aware of what we know and what we don't know, and to use this understanding when continuing to learn; it is described as thinking about thinking.

### About Thinking in Nursing

- Critical thinking in nursing practice must be applied to caring for clients in complex in dynamic health care environments.
- *Clinical reasoning* is a term that is specific to nursing knowledge, attitude, and practice; it can be described as "critical thinking at the bedside."
- Clinical reasoning is a thinking process that occurs when gathering and analyzing client information so that options can be identified and prioritized, and research and best practices can be applied to make decisions and final judgements about client care.
- Critical thinking and clinical reasoning skills are competencies required by nursing regulatory bodies across Canada.
- Culturally safe care is a form of client advocacy and helps achieve health equity.

### About How Thinking and Decision Making Relate in Nursing

- Decision making in nursing is a process that requires critical thinking and clinical reasoning when selecting the best option from available alternatives.
- Clinical judgement is the final interpretation or decision about a client's care and is the result of critical thinking and clinical reasoning.
- Sometimes, demonstrating thinking processes in nursing is a challenge.
- Both individual and environmental factors influence decision making in nursing.

## CONCLUSION AND THINKING IT THROUGH

Why is all of this background information important to you as a student and learner? Thinking and making decisions in nursing practice must be learned and continually practised. Critical thinking skills, while used by everyone, need to be intentionally adapted by nurses so that the skills can be applied to health care settings to maintain or improve the health of people, families, groups, communities, and populations. How you will adapt these skills will be based on your own background, practice needs, and the clients you serve.

Now you understand part of the big picture—what thinking is and what needs to be included when thinking and making decisions in nursing practice. Chapter 2 presents another part of that big picture: nursing-related critical thinking frameworks and models.

## CLASS ACTIVITIES TO CHECK THINKING

### Think-Aloud Pair Problem Solving (TAPPS)

Form pairs. Decide who will be a problem solver and a listener for Problem A listed below. The *problem solver* reads the problem aloud and talks through the reasoning process in attempting to identify *possible and relevant responses* to the problem. The *listener* encourages the problem solver to think aloud, asks clarification questions, offers encouragement to keep thinking, but refrains from providing answers. Switch roles for Problem B.

- ***Problem A (non-nursing problem):*** The car keys are missing, and you must leave for an appointment.
- ***Problem B (nursing problem):*** The client arrives at a doctor's office for an appointment. The nurse measures the client's blood pressure as part of the initial

assessment and it is 152/98 mm Hg, which the client says is unusually high for them.

When finished, discuss with each other the differences between thinking about a non-nursing and a nursing problem.

## Activities and Discussion Questions

1. Discuss thinking with your peers in a small group. Develop your own definition of *critical thinking*.
2. Explain barriers to critical thinking and what can be done to help overcome these barriers.
3. Identify the importance of improving one's self-efficacy. What does this idea mean for you?

4. Describe self-regulation and how this ability and process relates to personal development and self-improvement.
5. As a student, examine your own skills in metacognition and connect these skills to your own culture, background, past experiences, and education. How do these factors influence your ability to learn? What do you need to further develop your thinking?
6. Reflect on how learning to think and making decisions in a culturally safe manner is a form of advocacy and helps achieve health equity. Share and compare your ideas with a peer.

## CASE STUDY REVIEW

### Scenario

An 88-year-old client lives in a residence for older adults and is known to be independently mobile, friendly, and talkative. The client's current health issues are hypertension, glaucoma, and diabetes mellitus type 2. Today, the visiting nurse enters the client's apartment at 07:15 to find the client in bed, quiet and withdrawn, and incontinent of urine.

Apply metacognitive thinking and clinical reasoning to what you would do next, based on your nursing knowledge and experience.

### Questions

1. Is this similar to a situation you have experienced in the past?
2. When and how would you seek more information?
3. What may be happening in this scenario?
4. What should you do first?
5. How will you know if you are on the right track?
6. If the client is male or female, or if the client is from a different cultural background than your own, would it affect your responses? Explain your thinking.

## EVIDENCE-INFORMED THINKING ACTIVITY

Think about the information presented in Table 1.4. Canadian provincial and territorial regulatory body documents and standards serve as sources of evidence to guide nurses' thinking and performance. These apply to a nurse's work with individual client in an acute care setting or a vulnerable group in a larger community setting. Examine the entry-to-practice competencies or practice standards that apply to your jurisdiction and answer the following questions.
1. Where is the concept of critical thinking included in the documents? Is an alternate term used instead of "critical thinking"? Look up the term that is used to find a definition and compare it to this chapter's definition of "critical thinking."
2. Why do you think the concept of critical thinking is included under specific standards or competencies?
3. Find one journal article that describes why the concept of critical thinking is necessary for a high standard of nursing care. Does the article's rationale support the use of critical thinking in the documents you reviewed?

## QUESTIONS TO ASSESS LEARNING

### Review Questions

1. A nurse assesses a client and observes that the client is short of breath when at rest. This is a new finding. The nurse considers why this change has occurred, what may be causing the shortness of breath in this client right now, and how the client is currently responding. What concept best describes the nurse's thinking process?
   a. Critical thinking
   b. Clinical reasoning
   c. Clinical judgement
   d. Decision making

2. A client is found on the floor, having tripped on a rug in their home. The client is in pain, cannot move on their own, and is cool to the touch. The nurse determines that in this situation, emergency services must be contacted to transfer the client to hospital. What process used by the nurse best summarizes this thinking?
   a. Critical thinking
   b. Clinical reasoning
   c. Clinical judgement
   d. Decision making
3. A student reads new health information on the Internet and tries to determine whether to believe it or not by considering the source of the information, whether the source is reliable, if the statements are supported by evidence, and if the explanations are logical, based on what is currently known. What concept best represents this thinking process?
   a. Critical thinking
   b. Clinical reasoning
   c. Clinical judgement
   d. Decision making

4. A nurse is evaluating a client who has received care to prevent postoperative respiratory complications using deep breathing, coughing and spirometry, early ambulation, and analgesia, as well as considering the client's preferences and personal needs. The nurse establishes that the approach to care prevented complications and so was successful. What concept does the nurse's thinking process best reflect?
   a. Critical thinking
   b. Clinical reasoning
   c. Clinical judgement
   d. Decision making

## ONE LAST THOUGHT

As you wrap up this introductory chapter about thinking, consider the following points. Can you commit to new thinking that leads to:
- Engaging in self-reflection?
- Reviewing your values and beliefs for how they affect your decisions?
- Questioning what you know?
- Opening yourself to new perspectives?
- Changing your behaviours?

Write down one strategy that you will use to meet each of these commitments.

## ONLINE RESOURCES

The Foundation for Critical Thinking. https://www.criticalthinking.org.
*Indigenous cultural safety, cultural humility and anti-racism—Practice standard companion guide* (2022). British Columbia College of Nurses and Midwives. https://www.bccnm.ca/Documents/cultural_safety_humility/ps_companion_guide.pdf.
*Metacognition*—Learn Alberta (2005). https://www.learnalberta.ca/content/kes/pdf/or_ws_tea_elem_04_metacog.pdf.
*Promoting and assessing critical thinking—Centre for Teaching Excellence* (2024). University of Waterloo. https://uwaterloo.ca/centre-for-teaching-excellence/teaching-resources/teaching-tips/developing-assignments/cross-discipline-skills/promoting-assessing-critical-thinking.
*Promoting positive mental health* (2022). Government of Canada. https://www.canada.ca/en/public-health/services/promoting-positive-mental-health.html.

## REFERENCES

Antoine, A., Mason, R., Mason, R., et al. (2018). *Pulling together: A guide for curriculum developers*. BCcampus. https://opentextbc.ca/indigenizationcurriculumdevelopers.
Bartlett, C., Marshall, M., & Marshall, A. (2012). Two-eyed seeing and other lessons learned within a co-learning journey of bringing together indigenous and mainstream knowledges and ways of knowing. *Journal of Environmental Studies and Sciences, 2*, 331–340. https://doi.org/10.1007/s13412-012-0086-8.
Benner, P., Tanner, C., & Chesla, C. (2009). *Expertise in nursing practice: Caring, clinical judgment, and ethics*. Springer Publishing.
British Columbia College of Nurses and Midwives. (2020). *Nurse practitioners and registered nurses professional standards*. https://www.bccnm.ca/Documents/standards_practice/rn/RN_NP_Professional_Standards.pdf.

College of Nurses of Ontario. (2019). *Entry-to-practice competencies for registered nurses.* https://www.cno.org/globalassets/docs/reg/41037-entry-to-practice-competencies-2020.pdf.

College of Registered Nurses of Newfoundland and Labrador. (2019). *Standards of practice for registered nurses and nurse practitioners.* https://crnnl.ca/site/uploads/2021/09/standards-of-practice-for-rns-and-nps.pdf.

Crockett, L. (2018). The 7 most common traits of highly effective critical thinkers. *Focused Learning Network.* http://blog.future-focusedlearning.net/7-characteristics-effective-critical-thinkers.

Curtis, E., Jones, R., Tipene-Leach, D., et al. (2019). Why cultural safety rather than cultural competency is required to achieve health equity: A literature review and recommended definition. *International Journal for Equity in Health, 18*(174). https://doi.org/10.1186/s12939-019-1082-3.

ElAtia, S., Ipperciel, D., Zaiane, O., et al. (2020). Graduate attributes assessment program. *International Journal of Information and Learning Technology, 38*(1), 117–134. doi:10.1108/IJILT-03-2020-0025. https://www.yorku.ca/wp-content/uploads/sites/300/2020/10/Graduate-Attributes-Assessment-Program-2020.pdf.

Elder, L. (2007). *Defining critical thinking.* The Foundation for Critical Thinking. https://www.criticalthinking.org/pages/defining-critical-thinking/766.

Facione, N. C., Facione, P. A., & Sanchez, C. A. (1994). Critical thinking disposition as a measure of competent clinical judgment: The development of the California critical thinking disposition inventory. *Journal of Nursing Education, 33*(8), 345–350.

The Foundation for Critical Thinking. (2021). *Our concept and definition of critical thinking.* https://www.criticalthinking.org.

Halpern, D. (2014). *Thought and knowledge: An introduction to critical thinking* (5th ed.). Psychology Press.

Hart-Wasekeesikaw, F. (2009). *Cultural competence and cultural safety in nursing education: A framework for First Nations, Inuit and Métis nursing.* Aboriginal Nurses Association of Canada.

Kahneman, D. (2011). *Thinking fast and slow.* Canada: Anchor.

Kuiper, R. A., & Pesut, D. J. (2004). Promoting cognitive and metacognitive reflective reasoning skills in nursing practice: Self-regulated learning theory. *Journal of Advanced Nursing, 45,* 381–391.

Muntean, W. (2012). *Nursing clinical decision-making: A literature review.* https://www.ncsbn.org/research-item/nursing-clinical-decisionmaking-a-literature-review.

Nova Scotia College of Nursing. (2017). *Standards of practice for registered nurses.* https://cdn1.nscn.ca/sites/default/files/documents/resources/RN%20Standards%20of%20Practice.pdf.

Paul, R., & Elder, L (2020). *The miniature guide to critical thinking concepts and tools* (8th ed.). The Foundation for Critical Thinking Press.

Registered Nurses Association of the Northwest Territories and Nunavut. (2019). *Standards of practice for registered nurses and nurse practitioners.* https://rnantnu.ca/wp-content/uploads/2019/10/2019-standards-of-practice.pdf.

Saskatchewan Registered Nurses Association. (2019). *Registered nurse practice standards.* https://www.srna.org/wp-content/uploads/2019/09/RN-Practice-Standards-2019.pdf.

Scheffer, B. K., & Rubenfeld, M. G. (2000). A consensus statement on critical thinking in nursing. *Journal of Nursing Education, 39*(8), 352–359.

Simmons, B. (2010). Clinical reasoning: Concept analysis. *Journal of Advanced Nursing, 66*(5), 1151–1158. https://doi.org/10.1111/j.1365-2648.2010.05262.x.

Tanner, C. A. (2006). Thinking like a nurse: A research-based model of clinical judgment in nursing. *Journal of Nursing Education, 45*(6), 204–211.

VARK Learn Limited. (2022). *Research statistics.* https://vark-learn.com/research-statistics/.

Zimmerman, B. J. (1995). Self-regulation involves more than metacognition: A social cognitive perspective. *Educational Psychology, 30,* 217–221.

Zimmerman, B. J. (2002). Becoming a self-regulated learner: An overview. *Theory Into Practice, 41*(2), 64–70.

# 2

# Thinking as a Nurse: Using Models in Nursing Practice

## LEARNING OUTCOMES

*After reading this chapter, you will be able to:*
- Apply the essential thinking and decision-making skills associated with models in nursing practice.
- Describe the four components of the NRCE framework used in this textbook for thinking in nursing practice.
- Explain how each component in the NRCE framework can help with each step in the thinking process.
- Describe various models that can be used for thinking and decision making in nursing practice.
- Identify circumstances in which models for thinking and decision making may be used.

## GLOSSARY

**Framework:** a basic structure that describes (but does not fully explain) a system or concept; it helps connect many big ideas about a topic to a method or process of doing something related to that topic

**Model:** a simplified description of a process that can facilitate its understanding and application to different situations; it is a more concrete representation of an abstract idea (Halpern, 2014)

**Self-reflection:** when the nurse clearly identifies, explores, and analyzes their thinking to develop knowledge and an appreciation of their performance in the context of professional practice learning

This chapter presents approaches to thinking in nursing along with a framework that will help you systematically organize information to think effectively as a nurse. It also examines various evidence-informed models and processes for decision making that are commonly used in Canadian nursing education and practice. As well, it considers professional development (e.g., Novice to Expert Theory) and how it influences thinking in nursing.

The models include details on the characteristics or skills required of "thinkers" (students and nurses). These models are applied to nursing scenarios so that you can see how they can be used in practice. Schematics depicting the main features of each model and how these features work together are also included. At the end of the chapter, a number of models are compared to highlight how they relate to one another as central processes for thinking in nursing practice. A unified process for thinking and decision making is provided to summarize all nursing models and related skills in four basic steps.

As you read, think about the various concepts and components as building blocks for how you can begin to think as a nurse. Remember that the ways in which you incorporate this information will be unique to you and your experiences.

## APPROACHES TO THINKING IN NURSING

Chapter 1 provided a general introduction to thinking—what it is and how it occurs. It emphasized the significance of critical thinking in nursing and its importance in meeting provincial and territorial entry-to-practice competencies and standards of practice.

As you may know, an enormous amount of knowledge is needed to think like a nurse and provide safe, competent, and ethical care to clients. Thinking and decision making in nursing require that the client and their health be the central, professional focus. This emphasis is what distinguishes thinking in nursing from thinking in non–health care professions and everyday life. The nature of thinking in nursing must support the unique holistic view of care and the International Council of Nurses' (ICN) definition of nursing:

> *Nursing encompasses autonomous and collaborative care of individuals of all ages, families, groups and communities, sick or well and in all settings. Nursing includes the promotion of health, prevention of illness, and the care of ill, disabled and dying people. Advocacy, promotion of a safe environment, research, participation in shaping health policy and in patient and health systems management, and education are also key nursing roles.*
>
> **(ICN, 2002)**

In addition to the distinct context of nursing practice (and the internal and external influences on decision making identified in Chapter 1), a nurse must consider a lot of other information when making decisions to help ensure a holistic approach to client care. How can this information be organized to achieve that goal? When making decisions using critical thinking and clinical reasoning in nursing, a general framework can be useful in breaking down complex issues and making them easier to understand and address.

A **framework** is a basic structure that describes (but does not fully explain) a system or concept. A framework helps connect many big ideas about a topic to a method or process of doing something related to that topic. Often, this structure is in a written format that outlines each component and the possible relationships among them. These components can be abstract or more concrete.

A framework can support a systematic and informed approach to thinking and to nursing practice. It can be used to organize information on client care (or health care systems) and identify necessary information so that a nurse can make better decisions. One example, based in philosophy and psychology, is the Paul-Elder Critical Thinking Framework (Paul & Elder, 2020). It provides a useful perspective on critical thinking that applies intellectual standards to the elements of thought to build better intellectual traits (Box 2.1).

In some Indigenous cultures, ways of knowing and thinking are described in the Seven Sacred Teachings on human conduct toward all living things. These Teachings help support thinking with a continuous focus on positive character attributes (Alberta Regional Professional Development Consortia [ARPDC], 2023). The Teachings are practised together and comprise the following:

- To cherish knowledge is to know *wisdom*;
- To know *love* is to know peace;
- To honour all of the Creation is to have *respect*;
- *Bravery* is to face the foe with integrity;

- *Honesty* also means "righteousness," be honest first with yourself—in word and action;
- *Humility* is to know yourself as a sacred part of the Creation; and
- *Truth* is to know all of these things (ARPDC, 2023).

Remember: frameworks are general structures that can describe a concept such as thinking or other behaviours.

You have likely used frameworks to think about a particular topic in the past. One example of a framework is the outline of an essay, which structures the main topic or big idea into key parts that provide a guide for writing and presenting your work. Another is a theoretical framework for a research study, which explains how a research problem will be considered and subsequently investigated. Frameworks put forward by nurse theorists provide a perspective that is specific to nursing as a profession. Nursing frameworks therefore facilitate our thinking about nursing research, education, administration, and practice.

Theoretical frameworks in nursing guide nurses on caring for people, families, communities, and populations. For instance, broad, overarching frameworks in nursing theory direct a nurse's practice to incorporate the concepts of person, environment, health, and nursing (Fawcett, 2017).

Routinely using a framework as a guide to think as a nurse has benefits. Nurses who regularly use a broad lens (to gain an overview of the situation) when approaching a client or a health care issue, and at the same time, notice and analyze smaller details or cues may make better-informed decisions. Nurses who only use a narrow approach (focusing on one aspect of the situation) may miss critical information and jump to an inaccurate decision or conclusion. Therefore, using a framework when thinking can help the nurse think *BIG* and *small* at the same time; this approach is challenging but helpful.

---

**REFLECTIVE PRACTICE MOMENT**

**Think *BIG* and *small* at the same time.**

Think back on a client situation that you recently either read about or were involved in.

While considering details of that client situation, step back and think:

- What was the *main* health concern?
- What was the *primary goal* of the client's care?

---

## The Difference Between Frameworks and Models

You have also heard about models. A **model** is more specific than a framework and provides a simplified description of a process that can facilitate its understanding and application to different situations; it is a more concrete representation of an abstract idea (Halpern, 2014). It is often presented in

## BOX 2.1 Summary of the Paul-Elder Critical Thinking Framework

This framework has three main components for improving an individual's critical thinking: intellectual standards, elements of reasoning, and intellectual traits.

### Intellectual Standards

Good quality *intellectual standards* are necessary for good quality outcomes in thinking. Thinking critically requires having command of the following intellectual standards (sample questions are provided):

- *Clarity*—Can you elaborate, illustrate what you mean, or give an example?
- *Accuracy*—Can you check, verify, or test the truth of that?
- *Precision*—Can you be more specific, offer more detail, or be more exact?
- *Relevance*—How does that relate to the problem at hand? How does that help us with the issue?
- *Logic*—Does this make sense? Does it all fit together? Does this follow from the evidence?
- *Depth*—What factors make this challenging or complex? What problems can be anticipated?
- *Breadth*—Can you look at this issue from another perspective or point of view?
- *Significance*—Is this the priority issue? Which of these facts is the most important?
- *Fairness*—Can you justify your thinking? Are you taking into account others' views? Am I approaching this issue in an unbiased manner?
- *Sufficiency*—Is the information complete, unfair or not representative?

### Elements of Reasoning

*Elements of reasoning* are the parts of thinking that are used to understand the topic at hand. They include:

- *Purpose*—used to define a goal or objective related to a topic

- *Point of view*—the perspective held while thinking about a topic (i.e., business vs ethics)
- *Inferences*—used when drawing ideas or conclusions to give meaning to a topic
- *Attempts*—used when figuring out a problem or addressing a question
- *Assumptions*—used as a foundation for thinking about a topic; must be validated
- *Information*—used to establish what acts are known from data, evidence
- *Concepts*—used to shape thinking about a topic; including theories, models, and definitions
- *Implications*—used to identify where the thinking leads and its consequences

### Intellectual Traits

To consistently apply elements of reasoning, *intellectual traits* must be present. They include:

- *Intellectual humility*—acknowledging conscious and unconscious biases and limitations in thinking
- *Intellectual courage*—daring to question or challenge beliefs in light of new data or evidence
- *Intellectual empathy*—considering others' perspectives and where their views come from
- *Intellectual integrity*—holding yourself to the same standards of thinking to which you hold others
- *Intellectual autonomy*—thinking independently when faced with questions or problems
- *Intellectual perseverance*—embracing uncertainty and confusion to gain understanding
- *Confidence in reason*—trusting the process of thinking and its outcomes
- *Fair-mindedness*—striving for unbiased thinking, without influence from personal views

Adapted from Paul, R., & Elder. L. (2020). *The miniature guide to critical thinking concepts and tools* (8th ed.) (pp. 15–17, 19–26). The Foundation for Critical Thinking Press.

a physical form, schematic, diagram, or graphic format so that it is easier to follow. Because of the way it is presented, it usually does not fully describe the process. If a model is used to make decisions, it often involves arrows to direct thinking along a certain path or cycle in a specific arrangement of steps or levels. Sometimes a model is created to help summarize or communicate the essential elements of a larger framework.

One example is a scientific model of the solar system. It is often shown using different sized balls and wires representing planets, moons, and orbits around the sun, and relative distances. Another is a mathematical model. It uses symbols, equations, and numbers to portray a system and how it functions. Professional practice models are often depicted using an image or graphic, and include components such as practice, governance, values, community, and teamwork. Compare the critical thinking framework in Box 2.1 with the critical thinking model in Figure 2.1. Are similar words and language used? Think about the differences between lists and images that include directions. How are the concepts presented in relation to one another in a framework versus a model?

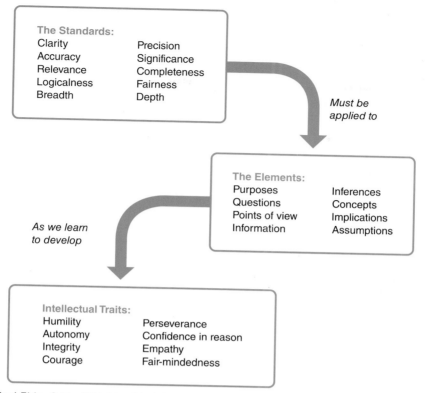

**Fig. 2.1 Paul-Elder Critical Thinking Model.** (Adapted from Paul, R., & Elder. L. (2020). *The miniature guide to critical thinking concepts and tools* (8th ed.). The Foundation for Critical Thinking Press.)

Why is it important to know about thinking and decision-making frameworks and models? Essentially, they help individuals understand and appreciate different ways of thinking. Everyone thinks differently, and it is helpful to know the various evidence-informed approaches to organizing thoughts and information as well as for making decisions.

*It is important to note that some kind of implicit framework is used by every practicing nurse, for we cannot observe, see, or describe, nor can we prescribe anything for which we do not already have some kind of mental image or concept.*

**(Johnson, 1987, p. 195)**

Thinking and decision-making models are more than the diagram shapes, concepts, and relationships (or arrows) depicted; they are based on supporting definitions, assumptions, and theories.

*[W]e all use models to guide our actions, be it the way we conduct our personal lives or the way we nurse.*

**(Kalideen, 1993, p. 4)**

While these quotes are from nurse theorists and researchers from many years ago, they are still relevant today and can be applied to the process of thinking about nursing care and how nurses make decisions in current practice environments.

For the purposes of presenting information in this textbook, a framework to use during every step of the thinking process will be described and illustrated in the following sections.

---

**KNOWLEDGE CHECK-IN**
- A framework is useful because it provides some details about a certain concept or idea and gives the "big picture" of what is involved.
- Models are often used to explain concepts in simpler ways, and with reference to processes or the flow of ideas.
- How do frameworks and models help when thinking about organizing information and decision making?

# THE NRCE FRAMEWORK FOR THINKING IN NURSING PRACTICE

When approaching issues that require thinking and decision making in health care situations, nurses must consider a variety of information. This information can be organized using existing theoretical frameworks, such as a basic nursing metaparadigm of person (human being), environment, health, and nursing (Fawcett, 2017). In current practice environments in Canada and elsewhere, the role of the nurse, according to nursing registration and practice standard requirements, must incorporate thinking frameworks that allow the application of a depth and breadth of knowledge. This is of particular importance because of intraprofessional and interprofessional expectations for collaborative care and an appreciation of the big picture.

The framework used in this textbook identifies the primary components that nurses consider when making decisions about client care and professional nursing practice issues. The components of this framework are as follows:

- **N**ursing knowledge
- Professional **r**oles
- **C**lient context
- Health care **e**nvironment

They are abbreviated as *NRCE* (think "*nurse*"). This "spelling" strategy to remember information will be discussed later in the text book.

$$\boxed{\text{N R C E}}$$

These four components are broad and provide some guidance for remembering the big picture when practising as a nurse. Nurses continuously use all four components *at every step of thinking and decision making*. However, depending on the health issue or problem to be addressed, all components may not be considered with equal weight and importance at a particular step.

The components of the framework are described below in more detail, as are the types of information that are associated with each. This discussion is not meant to form a nursing theory, but it is meant to help you remember the elements that are integral to making holistic decisions when providing nursing care. As you consider the components, think about information you are learning in your nursing program and how that knowledge is associated with each component. This will seem like a summary of your program's content, organized into four areas.

## Nursing Knowledge

Nursing knowledge encompasses science- and nursing-based information about nursing and health care, as well as information from other disciplines. That is a large amount of information. However, the information that you will draw on when making a decision will be guided by the particular health care and client situation you are faced with.

Nursing knowledge includes:

- *Science-based information:* anatomy and physiology, psychology, pharmacology, pathophysiology, biochemistry, statistics, and other scientific information
- *Nursing information:* introductory/foundational skills; advanced practical skills; specialty knowledge (gerontology, mental health, maternal–child, pediatric, rehabilitation, medical–surgical, community and public health, global health); nursing theory and caring; and nursing ethics (as essential knowledge)
- *Memory tools:* mnemonics, acronyms, acrostics, images, etc., to facilitate recall and improve retention of science-based and nursing information
- *Experiential knowledge:* practicum, placement, or clinical learning opportunities that provide other types of less tangible but equally important knowledge

## Professional Roles

The professional requirements and responsibilities that guide a nurse's role within provincial and territorial health care settings are crucial to collaborating and communicating effectively with others. You must be clear not only about your role and scope of practice but also about the role of other health care team members that work with clients.

The professional nursing role includes an understanding of the following:

- Provincial and territorial practice standards
- Entry-to-practice competencies
- Best practices in the particular area of nursing care
- Registered nurse and practical nurse roles and responsibilities or scope of practice
- Safety in therapeutic, relational practice
- Inter-professional roles and related scopes of practice (including nonregistered health care workers)
- Delegation and supervision responsibilities and processes
- Leadership and communication theory
- Growth, professional development, and reflection as a nursing practice responsibility

## Client Context

The "client" is described as a person, family, group, community, or population, according to the area and focus of nursing practice. In this framework, the client is integral to the other components. The nurse–client relationship is professional and therapeutic because it is based on the nurse's understanding of the client's context. Broadly consider the client and their entire context, and then specifically explore those contextual aspects that are most relevant to the client.

An understanding of the client context requires knowledge of the following in relation to the unique client:
- Physical health status
- Personal values and background
- Personal goals and perception of health, and preferences for care
- Past health experiences and interactions in health care settings
- Learning needs, literacy, and related educational theory
- Preferences for information sharing
- Cultural, cultural safety, and sociocultural influences
- Gender-influenced perspectives and care needs
- Determinants of health
- Approaches to achieve equity, diversity, and inclusion
- The effects of colonization that may or may not be experienced by the client

## Health Care Environment

The health care environment comprises the physical setting, the administrative infrastructure, governing laws, regulations, policies and procedures, and the available resources and limitations (i.e., supplies and human resources) that affect how client care is delivered and measured.

An understanding of the health care environment requires knowledge of the following:
- Laws and regulations that relate to the practice environment and profession
- The complexity of care delivered in the identified environment
- Hospital codes and trauma criteria
- Staffing and health care delivery structures
- Distractions and conflicts that occur during care delivery

- Organizational culture and practice conventions in the health care environment
- Systemic inequities and colonial structures
- Current policies and procedures
- Occupational, technological, and physical safety
- Mental health and self-care practice supports
- Quality indicators and evaluative processes and standards

An additional benefit of the NRCE framework is that it can be applied to various established models for thinking and decision making in nursing practice. The nurse situates the four NRCE components within each step of the selected model for thinking and decision making in nursing practice to achieve optimal client care and health (Figure 2.2). No matter the model the nurse prefers to use, the NRCE components help ensure that thinking at every step incorporates current and relevant evidence, the nurse's role (including the nurse's own abilities/experience), the role of involved health care colleagues, and the environment in which the client and/or nurse are situated.

## How the Framework Will Be Used in This Text book

The components of the NRCE framework will be used in this text book to organize the presentation of information. They will also help you to think *BIG* and *small* at the same time. Remember: the components include information that is studied in most nursing programs and is part of required nursing curricula.

The NRCE framework will help you incorporate necessary information when applying any thinking and decision-making model in practice. It can be used at each step of any chosen model. Also, the NRCE framework will help you quickly understand whether all relevant aspects

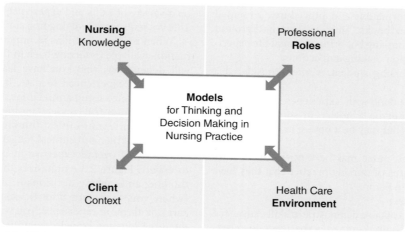

**Fig. 2.2 NRCE Components.** Connecting models of thinking and decision making in nursing.

of a situation where a decision must be made have been included. It will be used in upcoming chapters to examine thinking and decision making.

## A Key Point When Using the Framework: Novice or Expert Practitioner?

It is important to keep in mind that the information you use while applying the NRCE framework will always reflect your current level in the nursing program, or your experiences as a graduate in providing nursing care. What you know depends on whether you are at the start of your nursing program, in your final year, or entering practice. A research-based theory by Dr. Patricia Benner informs the inclusion of this valuable key point, and it is worth reviewing here.

Benner (1982, 1984) proposed that a theory of skills acquisition developed by Dreyfus and Dreyfus (1980) be applied to the development of nursing skills and professional practice. Since then, Benner's Novice to Expert Theory has been a guide to many educators and students as they teach and learn in nursing and as they gain experience in the clinical setting.

To summarize, Benner (2001) stated that nurses develop through five levels as they practice in their careers. This development is usually (but not always) sequential (which means development occurs in order from the least experienced level to the most). It is also important to note that nursing practice experience is context based, which means that how a nurse at each level uses information (e.g., NRCE) when making decisions will depend on the specific client situation and the nurse's past experiences in similar situations.

Benner (2001) describes the five levels of experience as follows:

- *Novice:*
  Novices engage in nursing practice focusing mostly on the "rules" or information and procedures presented in introductory textbooks. They have no background understanding of nursing but bring personal life experience to their decision making and actions.
  - A first-year nursing student is often considered a novice.
  - A first-year student with experience as a nursing assistant will not be a novice in some previously practised skills but may be a novice in other areas of practice.
  - An experienced nurse may be a novice if they are moved to an area of nursing practice that they have never worked in before.
- *Advanced beginner:*
  With minimally acceptable demonstrated skills, advanced beginners have acquired enough experience to recognize "aspects of a situation." This means that they have

enough prior clinical experience to recognize subtle, less measurable signs in client care, such as readiness to learn self-care or signs of withdrawal in a child separated from a parent.
  - A new graduate from a nursing program will perform at the advanced-beginner level.
- *Competent:*
  Competent nurses demonstrate conscious or intentional care planning. In the competent stage, nurses become more efficient because they can more easily recognize which aspects of the situation are more important and which are less relevant to the current and future care of the client.
  - A graduate nurse working in a consistent environment can achieve a competent level.
- *Proficient:*
  Typically, proficient nurses have worked for several years and understand a situation as a whole (i.e., the *BIG* picture) rather than its parts only. These nurses have a deep background understanding of client presentation.
- *Expert:*
  Expert nurses perform most intuitively compared to nurses at other levels based on many similar experiences and the application of not only practical but also theoretical/abstract knowledge to the client situation.

It is important to understand that not all nurses will become experts. There are many reasons why. For example, a nurse who frequently changes practice areas may not develop a profound understanding of one context, environment, or specialty area. Thus, while competent or proficient, this nurse may not become an expert. In another example, a nurse who continues to seek only superficial knowledge in new situations or who does not reflect on their own practice may not have enough opportunities to become proficient or expert. However, all nurses will build on a variety of skills and experience during their practice. This is a requirement of ongoing competency and safety.

When making decisions in nursing practice, the information available (referring back to the NRCE framework) will depend on what you have learned in the nursing program or experienced to date. It will also depend on your experience using a model for thinking and organizing information (i.e., understanding aspects of the situation). In short, your critical thinking, clinical reasoning, decision making, and clinical judgements will depend on your level of overall expertise in nursing—from novice to expert. Figure 2.3 emphasizes that the framework for thinking and making decisions is practitioner dependent (where you, as the practitioner, are part of the context of care). With more experience, you will be able to incorporate more nursing knowledge, understanding of the roles, the client context, and information about the health care

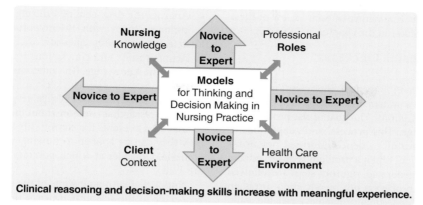

Fig. 2.3  The Influence of Nursing Experience on the use of the NRCE Framework and Components.

environment in what you do. Nurses and the way they think make the difference in whether care is client centred or not.

One last important point must be considered. Because experience and exposure to clinical situations are critical to development as a nurse, it is important to gain them early in the nursing program and to sustain them throughout the learning process. *Early experiences with ways of thinking are also fundamental* to learning. Each nursing program looks different, and curricula are offered in many acceptable forms. The introduction of decision-making models in the first half of the program will allow novice nurses to become familiar with thinking processes early on and give them time to practice and apply these models in clinical settings. If the components of the NRCE framework are used along with nursing models to deepen thinking, then you (with your own views, knowledge of nursing, and growing expertise) will enrich your capacity for decision making.

> **KNOWLEDGE CHECK-IN**
> Why is it important to consider nursing knowledge, professional roles, the client context, and the health care environment in every step of the thinking process?
> • Explain how the use and application of a framework or model will depend on the experiences of the nurse who uses it.

You now understand the *BIG* picture for framing nursing information that includes the types of information that are important to consider, and how your level of expertise affects what you know and how you engage in client care. Next, models for thinking and decision making will be presented. Consider them as your maps, or blueprints, for building knowledge on ways of thinking, and keep in

mind the NRCE components as you explore the following models.

## MODELS FOR THINKING AND DECISION MAKING IN NURSING

Many thinking and decision-making models exist in nursing. The primary models for thinking and making decisions as a nurse help organize information from practice-based experiences in a logical and rational manner so that safe, competent, and ethical care can be delivered. Such models help nurses provide care that is professional, accountable, defendable, and explainable to others. Nurses have an obligation to the public and to their profession to provide safe, competent, and ethical care to clients. The use of a model for thinking and arriving at decisions in practice will support them in these goals.

Several models will be outlined next. You may be familiar with some of them, while others may be new to you. Each of them offers a distinct process through which understanding is achieved. Generally, each model involves identifying reliable information and then, based on that information, making a decision. So, decisions are never made based on no information or evidence. There has to be a reason for a nurse to act or not to act. (Always ask yourself, *If someone asked me why I was performing this particular activity or intervention, what rationale could I give?*) Using a model helps.

Moving from non-nursing to nursing approaches, the models presented are the scientific process, Gibbs's reflective cycle, the nursing process, the clinical reasoning cycle, Tanner's Clinical Judgement Model, and the ethical decision-making model. Examples of nursing applications of these models are also included. As you review these models, notice whether they have similar steps and pay attention to the cyclical nature of each. A few of these models are compared later in the chapter in Table 2.7.

## Scientific and Research Processes

### Scientific Process

Also known as the *scientific method,* the scientific process used by researchers is a systematic and logical approach to seeking answers to questions. The goal of the process is to acquire new knowledge. This process, and adaptations of it, is the foundation for all evidence-informed practice—not just nursing practice. When a problem is observed or a question or an idea is generated, rigorous steps are followed to investigate it. This process is not merely about problem solving; the aim is to experiment to achieve reliable, valid results and (at least somewhat) generalizable results.

The steps of the scientific process are as follows:

- Make an observation, ask a question, or identify an idea and generate a research question.
- Review the available literature to reveal what is currently known about the specific topic.
- Formulate a hypothesis or "educated guess" to answer a focused question, based on the literature.
- Conduct an experiment (or test) to either prove or disprove the hypothesis. This experiment must be as unbiased as possible and involve relevant subjects using appropriate measurement tools and ethical processes.

- Analyze the data obtained during the experiment and compare them with the hypothesis. The researcher determines how the question can be answered.
- Report results and conclusions to develop the body of scientific knowledge. The outcome may generate more questions.

The scientific process is cyclical (Figure 2.4). It continues as long as researchers wonder about the world around them.

Table 2.1 presents the steps in the scientific process and how they can be applied to nursing activities in a clinical scenario. Consider at which point(s) choices or decisions are made.

Notice that, although some of the language in each step is specific to the scientific process, there are general steps that relate to carefully gathering information, analyzing relevant data, and drawing an informed conclusion. These general steps appear in other processes.

### Research Process

The research process, which mirrors the scientific process, includes more specific procedural steps that ensure transparent, ethical, and sustainable activities. Seeking and obtaining funding from donors or organizations and approval from ethics review bodies are important to this process. The research process can be categorized as quantitative and/or qualitative (Singh & Thirsk, 2022, pp. 29–30).

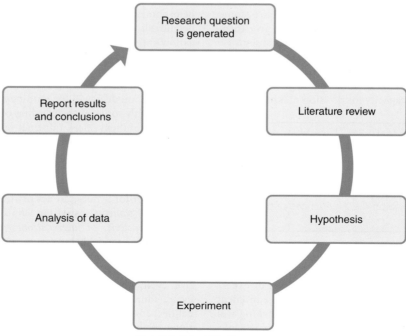

**Fig. 2.4** Scientific Process.

**TABLE 2.1   Application of the Scientific Process**

| Scientific Process Steps | Nursing Activities |
|---|---|
| Observation, question, or idea | A nurse researcher wonders whether clients who listen to music before surgery will experience less pain in the postoperative period. |
| Literature review | A systematic review is conducted of relevant nursing and other peer-reviewed publications; the review revealed that anxiety plays a part in pain. |
| Hypothesis | Clients who listen to music for 1 hour before surgery will report less pain on the pain scale in the 24-hour period after surgery than clients who do not listen to any music. |
| Experiment or testing | With ethics approval, one group of clients is offered their choice of music to listen to before surgery. The other group is not offered music and has the regular preoperative experience. Anxiety is measured preoperatively and pain is measured postoperatively. |
| Analysis of data | Group results on reported pain in the 24-hour period after surgery are compared and analyzed. |
| Report results and conclusions | Results are reported and conclusions formed based on the results. For similar clients scheduled for similar surgeries, music may reduce anxiety and reported severity of pain postoperatively. |

Overall, the logical process aims to organize a research study to best answer the type of research question.

The general research process is as follows:

- Generate an idea, a research purpose, and a question.
- Conduct a literature review and identify a framework to understand what is known, or target a group with knowledge.
- Refine the research question as needed.
- Design and plan a research methodology.
- Create a research proposal.
- Apply for funding as needed.
- Apply for ethics approval.
- Measure the concepts of interest, and collect and analyze data.
- Draw conclusions and summarize and relate the findings. This non-nursing process can be used in nursing practice.

## Reflective Cycle

Reflection in the context of nursing practice involves clearly identifying, exploring, and analyzing thinking and performance to develop knowledge. It is more than just recalling past experiences and the mistakes and successes that occurred. As part of metacognition, reflection contributes to safe practice and professional development from a novice to an expert (Johns, 2022). Reflexivity—which involves an awareness and examination of our existence, thoughts, and behaviours—also requires reflective skills. Reflexivity is concerned with how a person is in relation to others; that is, how one's own ways of knowing, being, and doing shape their interpretation of, and behaviour toward, other people (Dawson et al., 2022).

According to Boud et al. (1985), reflection involves three key stages: returning to the experience; attending to feelings that arose during that experience; and re-evaluating the experience in light of its purpose. These stages enable the integration of knowledge with existing knowledge, and the use of new knowledge in future actions. Alternatively, Gibbs (1988) describes a cyclical model of reflection that begins with description (What happened?) and moves through feelings (What were you thinking and feeling?), evaluation (What was good/bad about what happened?), analysis (What sense can you make of what happened?), conclusion (What else could have been done?), and an action plan (If this happens again, what would you do?) (Figure 2.5). The aim of this reflective process is to identify what went well and did not go well to improve future practice.

As a cyclical process used in nursing practice, Gibbs's reflective cycle is designed to offer opportunities to engage in ongoing performance improvement. Implementing an action plan in future nursing practice requires a description of the new situation and application of previous learning. Then, using the information that is collected and analyzed on the new experience, a conclusion is drawn, a new action plan is generated, and the cycle continues. This process typically happens after an event has occurred. Table 2.2 presents the steps in Gibbs's reflective cycle and how they can be applied to nursing activities in a clinical scenario.

Note the use of the word *evaluation* in the middle of this cycle and how it is similar to *analysis*. Did the placement of *evaluation* in the middle of the cycle surprise you? If so, remember to think *BIG* picture, and that an evaluation

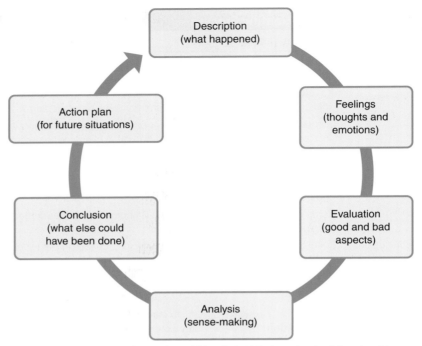

**Fig. 2.5** Gibbs's Reflective Cycle. (Adapted from Gibbs, G. (1988). *Learning by doing: A guide to teaching and learning methods.* Further Education Unit, Oxford Polytechnic.)

### TABLE 2.2    Application of Gibbs's Reflective Cycle

| Reflective Cycle Steps | Nursing Activities |
| --- | --- |
| Description | A nurse incorrectly administered daily medication, and the client received a higher dose than what was prescribed. After reporting the error, monitoring the client, and communicating to others, the client experienced no adverse effects. |
| Feelings | The nurse felt devastated and embarrassed. The nurse was overly tired while working an extra shift, and was distracted by call bells while checking the medication. |
| Evaluation | The client recovered. The nurse manager expressed support for the nurse's self-report of the incident. |
| Analysis | The nurse's confidence was shaken, as this had been the first medication error. A series of events—internal and external—contributed to this error. Clients are dependent on nurses to provide care accurately and safely. |
| Conclusion | The client was made aware of the error and was not harmed. If the client had been harmed, the nurse would have felt unable to continue working. Various steps could have been taken to reduce the chance of error. |
| Action plan | The nurse reviewed medication administration processes and the dosages of common drugs prescribed on the unit. Mindfulness techniques and self-care were practised to ensure focused care while on shift. A quiet area for preparing medications was established. |

Gibbs, G. (1988). *Learning by doing: A guide to teaching and learning methods.* Further Education Unit, Oxford Polytechnic.

means asking, What is occurring with your thinking at that point in time?

Reflection occurs all the time in nursing practice. As you read this text book, you will notice that reflection is part of other nursing models and thinking processes. Nurses continually reflect before, during, and after their actions, as well as after each day of practice. This self-reflection is facilitated by applying a reflection model and helps each nurse clearly identify, explore, and analyze their thinking. Self-reflection helps to develop knowledge and an appreciation of one's performance in the context of continual professional practice learning. Using the questions associated with Gibbs's reflective cycle is a good place to start your reflective practice.

The scientific process and the reflective cycle are comparable in structure. Processes that are specific to nursing follow similar structures, and in fact incorporate science-based and reflective concepts. When reading, see if you can identify similarities and differences in the following processes and models that will be presented (note that doing so uses critical thinking skills).

## Nursing Process

The nursing process is a fundamental way of thinking about client health issues and how nurses can support a client's optimal health. It is an intellectual process of reasoning in practice that is essential to understand and be able to apply.

Each step of the nursing process involves a number of details and considerations that support a holistic and comprehensive approach to practice (think about applying the NRCE framework to each step). The nursing process involves *a*ssessment, *a*nalysis, *p*lanning, *i*mplementation, and *e*valuation, or *AAPIE* (Astle & Duggleby, 2024).

The nursing process is a cycle where movement from one step to the next is not necessarily linear or sequential but iterative (you can go back and forth between steps) and continuous. As such, a model of the nursing process would look like the one depicted in Figure 2.6.

The second step, "analysis," is sometimes named "diagnosis" in other nursing textbooks because it can involve making a formal nursing diagnosis. This is one way of framing client issues within nursing practice. Not all nurses formulate nursing diagnoses, and not all employers require diagnoses when creating client care plans or critical pathways. What is important here is that analysis of the information gained during assessment is interpreted in context, in an unbiased and client-centred manner, and weighed and prioritized so that a plan can be effectively proposed.

Like other models, the nursing process is cyclical: information is collected, interpreted, and analyzed; an informed decision on an action is implemented; and outcomes are evaluated for how the results may be used in future nursing care and practice. Students may struggle with applying this model (and others) in the live clinical setting and are

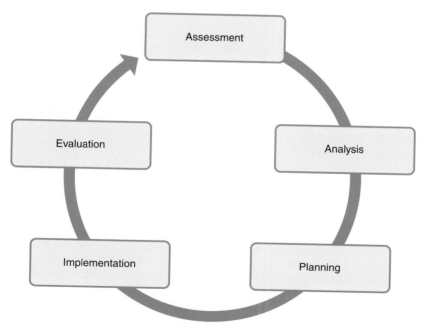

Fig. 2.6 Nursing Process.

**TABLE 2.3  Application of the Nursing Process**

| Steps in the Nursing Process | Nursing Activities |
|---|---|
| Assessment | A 58-year-old client, who experienced recent surgery reports discomfort, is not able to move without grimacing, and refuses food. Collect other data, including the client's culture and perceptions of pain. |
| Analysis | The data indicate that untreated surgical pain can lead to anxiety, respiratory infection, and poor nutrition for wound healing. Verify pain with client as needed. |
| Planning | Measurable and achievable goals that recognize culture and preferences are set with the client, such as administration of adequate medication based on pain levels, moving to a chair at least three times per day, and eating smaller, frequent meals each day. |
| Implementation | Care is delivered according to the plan for addressing the highest priorities. Continuity is ensured through documentation, communication, and preparation for discharge. |
| Evaluation | The client's pain experience is monitored and reassessed for how goals were met and whether the plan should be modified. |

tempted to implement care without an appropriate or complete assessment. Table 2.3 presents the steps in the nursing process and how they can be applied to nursing activities in a clinical scenario. Review your health assessment course and consider other activities that could be conducted in the scenario provided. Considering all of the nursing actions in the nursing process cycle can assist with *BIG* picture thinking, while attending to the details of a specific client situation.

At this point, it is important for you to recall that *critical thinking* and *clinical reasoning* skills in the client and health care context are necessary in the application of the nursing process (and the scientific process, the reflective cycle, and the next few models you will read about). For example, you may remember from Chapter 1 that "information seeking" is a critical thinking skill that involves searching for evidence, facts, and knowledge using relevant sources and appropriate data. The information-seeking skill is used during the assessment step of the nursing process. The critical thinking skill "applying standards" (judging according to approved professional or social rules/criteria, or identified personal values) would be used when analyzing the information collected and when planning client care to ensure competent health care delivery.

Working through this thinking process facilitates decision making for the nurse and the client. When looking at the nursing process, you may be thinking that reflection and decision making actually occur at each step. That is correct. While assessing a client or health care situation, the nurse is deciding whether the assessment is appropriate for the identified issue, anything is being overlooked, and more assessment is needed. Part of this process is analysis, but a definitive analysis cannot be conducted until all necessary

and available assessment data are gathered. While implementing care, the nurse is reflecting (in the moment) on whether their actions are competent and safe, and whether the care being provided is effective for addressing the client issue. Consider all of these points as you read about the clinical reasoning and clinical judgement models.

## Clinical Reasoning Cycle

The research-informed clinical reasoning cycle (CRC) was developed by Levett-Jones et al. (2009) and is a systematic process for guiding clinical decision making in practice settings. The level of detail offered in this process makes it valuable to nurses who are providing care in unpredictable and complex health care situations as well as less complex situations. The CRC describes nursing actions in eight steps: consider the client situation, collect cues/information, process information, identify problems/issues, establish goal(s), take action, evaluate outcomes, and reflect on process and new learning (Figure 2.7).

When compared with the nursing process, the CRC is more detailed and offers an expanded view of assessment, analysis, planning, implementation, and evaluation. Table 2.4 presents the steps in the CRC and how they can be applied to nursing activities in a clinical scenario.

The CRC is a full and continuous process. Like other cycles, in reality, there is no clear delineation between each step: each step blends into the next, and the nurse may find themselves going backward at times. This is expected if reflection prompts the nurse to rethink and return to a previous step.

During the CRC process, the nurse uses critical thinking skills at each step. These skills ensure that the model is applied in a logical and rational manner so that the thinking process can be explained to and understood by others.

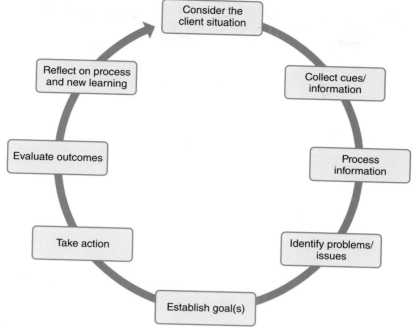

**Fig. 2.7 Clinical Reasoning Cycle.** (Levett-Jones, T., Hoffman, K., Dempsey, J., et al. (2009). The "five rights" of clinical reasoning: An educational model to enhance nursing students' ability to identify and manage clinically "at risk" clients. *Nurse Education Today, 30*(6), 515–520.)

If a nurse must collaborate with other professionals, share health care plans, or provide a handover report, clear thinking must be apparent.

## Clinical Judgement Model

The Clinical Judgement Model by Tanner (2006) is another thinking and decision-making model that you, as a skill builder, can use with the available nursing information and the NRCE framework when addressing client health issues. This research-based approach to thinking uses language that describes how nurses think when they provide care in complex situations that require judgement. The model has four aspects, as follows (Figure 2.8):

- *Noticing*: the perception, expectations, and initial grasp of the client and health care situation at hand; it is based on experience, knowledge of the client, and textbook knowledge
- *Interpreting*: the development of a sufficient understanding of the client situation to respond safely, competently, and ethically; clinical reasoning is involved in determining a course of action
- *Responding*: the ability to decide on an appropriate course of action for the situation, and to act (it includes "do nothing right now")

- *Reflecting*: attention to the client's response to nursing actions and a review of the outcomes related to nursing actions and other aspects of the situation as a whole

Tanner (2006) described this process as a cycle that starts with noticing what is happening with the client and situating the client issue, and where reflection "completes the cycle; showing what nurses gain from their experience contributes to their ongoing clinical knowledge development and their capacity for clinical judgement in future situations" (p. 209). Refer again to Figure 2.8. You will notice that reflection is an important part of the model and that it refers to both *reflection-in-action* and *reflection-on-action* (Schön, 1983):

- Reflection-*in*-action occurs during "responding," when the nurse is observing client responses to interventions in the moment they are happening *and* is able to modify the interventions based on the interpretation of those observed responses. You may find that this type of reflection happens unconsciously when providing care (unless outcomes are not met, and you notice that you missed something!).
- Reflection-*on*-action occurs during "reflecting," at the end of the cycle, when the nurse is looking back on what knowledge was gained from the clinical experience. You

## TABLE 2.4    Application of the Clinical Reasoning Cycle

| Clinical Reasoning Steps | Nursing Activities |
| --- | --- |
| **Consider the client situation:**<br>• Describe facts, contexts, situations, and people. | • A 6-year-old client is admitted to hospital because of an anaphylactic reaction. |
| **Collect cues/information:**<br>• Review available information from handover reports, history and charts, and previous medical and nursing assessments.<br>• Gather new information.<br><br>• Recall knowledge from the sciences, pharmacology, nursing therapeutics, scope of practice, client learning, and the health care environment. | • The client is allergic to nuts and has a prescription for a single-use, epinephrine injectable. This is the third admission this year. Emergency treatment was given.<br>• Current oxygen saturation is normal; client and parent share that they don't usually carry medication with them.<br>• Epinephrine in self-inject/single-use delivery is the drug of choice for acute anaphylaxis.<br>• The client and parent should be included in teaching sessions.<br>• Exploring client lifestyle and preferences/needs will guide priorities for teaching and learning. |
| **Process information:**<br>• *Interpret*—Analyze data (compare normal versus abnormal).<br>• *Discriminate*—Recognize inconsistencies, eliminate irrelevant data, focus on priorities, and identify gaps in the information collected.<br>• *Relate*—Find patterns and group similar data.<br>• *Infer*—Weigh options and form a logical conclusion based on data.<br>• *Match*—Compare the situation to similar past experiences.<br>• *Predict*—Anticipate an outcome. | • Vital signs are now within normal range.<br>• The client and parent's understanding of the necessity of epinephrine seems accurate, yet they do not keep it available.<br><br><br>• Readmissions may be related to lack of education.<br>• There may be lifestyle or habits which do not facilitate carrying the medication.<br>• Other clients with similar self-care gaps have responded well to one-on-one teaching.<br>• If education and specific needs are not addressed, another reaction is possible. |
| **Identify problems/issues:**<br>• Synthesize all available information to focus on the main client health issue. | • The client and parent require teaching about the importance of carrying epinephrine and how it is used. |
| **Establish goal(s):**<br>• Describe the preferred outcome and a time frame. | • The client and parent will correctly describe the importance and use of epinephrine during an identified asthma experience before discharge, and they will have a plan for carrying it at all times. |
| **Take action:**<br>• Select a course of action from the available options. | • Teach the client and parent about epinephrine, based on a needs assessment and starting with client-prioritized questions and identified solutions. |
| **Evaluate outcomes:**<br>• Evaluate the effectiveness of outcomes and whether improvements have been made. | • The client and parent demonstrate an understanding of the necessity of medication for asthma and can give examples of how epinephrine can be carried at all times, before discharge. |
| **Reflect on process and learning:**<br>• Contemplate learning and areas for improvement. | • I think next time I should . . .<br>• I have more knowledge about . . .<br>• If I had only . . . |

Adapted from School of Nursing and Midwifery, Faculty of Health, University of Newcastle. (2009). *Clinical reasoning instructor resources.* https://www.utas.edu.au/__data/assets/pdf_file/0003/263487/Clinical-Reasoning-Instructor-Resources.pdf.

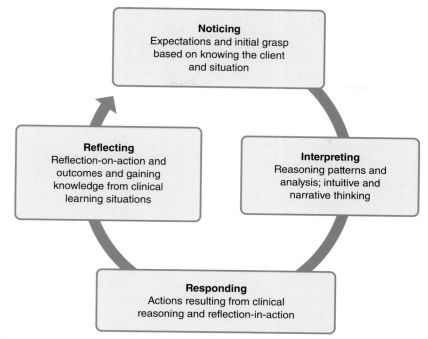

**Fig. 2.8** Tanner's Clinical Judgement Model. (Adapted from Tanner, C. A. (2006). Thinking like a nurse: A research-based model of clinical judgement in nursing. *Journal of Nursing Education, 45*(6), 204–211.)

### TABLE 2.5 Application of Tanner's Clinical Judgement Model

| Clinical Judgement Aspects | Nursing Activities |
| --- | --- |
| Noticing | The nurse observes that an older client living with diabetes has experienced a stroke and has very limited mobility. The client is frequently incontinent of urine. The client shares with the nurse that the incontinence affects their dignity. |
| Interpreting | The nurse analyzes the situation and determines that the client may be at risk for pressure injuries or ulcers due to physiological and environmental circumstances. The nurse considers options and possible goals with the client. |
| Responding | The nurse intervenes and communicates a plan for frequent position changes, toileting, and hygiene to other health care workers. The nurse collaborates with the client on a plan in a reassuring manner and involves family members as appropriate. |
| Reflecting | The nurse evaluates the client to identify whether goals (such as zero pressure injuries) have been achieved and how the client feels about their care. The nurse self-evaluates their nursing performance. |

Tanner, C. A. (2006). Thinking like a nurse: A research-based model of clinical judgment in nursing. *Journal of Nursing Education, 45*(6), 204–211.

must have a sense of professional responsibility for this level of reflection, and you must have the ability to connect your actions with client outcomes and future practice.

Table 2.5 presents the aspects of this model of clinical judgement and how they (and the different levels of reflection) relate to nursing activities in a clinical situation.

In 2007, Lasater created a rubric (a scoring guide) to measure students' skill performance in clinical judgement. The Lasater Clinical Judgment Rubric describes four levels of achievement (beginning, developing, accomplished, and exemplary) and breaks down the phases of noticing, interpreting, responding, and reflecting into a total of 11 dimensions (see Table 2.7, later in the chapter). Although recent revisions of the original Tanner model have emphasized the role of the client in the decision-making process and underscored challenges with fully measuring clinical judgement (Lasater & Nielsen, 2024), this sort of rubric is a useful way to gauge the development of clinical judgement skills across a program.

The National Council of State Boards of Nursing (NCSBN) has adopted the concept of clinical judgement to measure competence in the provincial and territorial registration exams across Canada (and in the United States), so it is important to be familiar with this model.

## Ethical Decision-Making Model

*"Thinking like a nurse" is a form of engaged moral reasoning. Educational practices must help students engage with patients with a deep concern for their well being.*
**(Tanner, 2006, p. 209)**

In Canada, ethical practice is just as important as safety and competency in nursing. In fact, ethical practice is safe and competent practice. Nurses deal with ethical issues on a daily basis. An ethical decision-making framework or model can help guide nurses to make informed decisions and evaluate the outcomes of their actions. Because it is familiar to students and nurses, the nursing process provides a useful foundation for examining situations that involve ethical values (College of Nurses of Ontario, 2019). These situations can include ethical uncertainties, distress, or conflicts and dilemmas that pertain to the client, health care, or the health care system.

Clinicians prefer approaches to ethical decision making that include a step-by-step process, as clinicians are generally not well trained in complex medical ethics and find the practical guidance of a step-by-step plan helpful (van Bruchem-Visser et al., 2020). One such approach is the Oberle and Raffin model, which is included in the Canadian Nurses Association (CNA) (2017) code of ethics. Typically, this ethical decision-making model and others like it are meant to be applied along with a professional code of ethics for nurses and other thinking and decision-making models. In complex clinical situations, such as those made more challenging by a pandemic, for instance, using more than one decision-making model may be necessary when fully considering challenging decisions.

The Oberle and Raffin model may be applied to all kinds of ethical situations and comprises the following steps (CNA, 2017, pp. 29–30):

- **Assessing:**
  Identify what is known about the ethical situation and issue, what is not known, and who should be included in the decision making, with the aim to clarify goals and focus the decision. (e.g., What are the beliefs and values of *all* involved? What are the goals of care? What codes of ethics apply? What are the relationships in this situation? Do the individuals involved have conflicting values?)

- **Reflecting on and reviewing potential actions:**
  Find all available options for addressing the ethical issue, and how any choices may be perceived, valued, and implemented. (e.g., What actions would do the most good? What actions would cause the least distress? What risks are involved with choosing or not choosing each option? What is the impact of each option on those involved? Are there legal implications?)

- **Selecting an ethical action (maximizing good):**
  Acknowledge your professional obligations when selecting an action. (e.g., What would be the best action? Is that action supported by nursing policies, standards, experience, and professional judgement? Can you support the client's choice? Do you have the knowledge and skills required to act? Do you have the virtues and courage required to act?)

- **Engaging in ethical action:**
  Proceed with the best alternative as selected, using a clear and rational implementation plan, and involving all relevant participants. (e.g., Are you acting according to a code of ethics and in a reasonable, prudent, collaborative, caring, and compassionate manner? Are you meeting professional and institutional expectations in this action?)

- **Reflecting on and reviewing the ethical action:**
  Consult with those involved to obtain feedback on the process and how they were affected. Debrief and reflect on the decisions made and actions taken. (e.g., Were the outcomes acceptable? Was the action reported and documented appropriately? What can you learn from actions that were acceptable and valuable? What could have been done differently?)

As Figure 2.9 shows, the ethical decision-making model (like other models discussed in this chapter) is cyclical. Ultimately, the learning gained from the experience and evaluation is meant to carry over into future situations. The new knowledge will be applied to the next assessment activity, leading to greater expertise. It is important to note that if the new learning is not applied, expertise may not be developed. Table 2.6 presents the steps in the ethical decision-making model and how they are demonstrated by nursing activities in a clinical scenario.

At this point, you may be wondering why there are so many models. Some of them were developed out of previously published models or from other nursing or interprofessional research and knowledge sources. The models that are specific to nursing offer a unique way of looking at decision making and thinking like a nurse.

The models have been adapted slightly from their originally published formats and intentionally presented as the cycles that they demonstrate. As a result, you can observe how they are alike. Look carefully at other similarities between them. Can you see that the same critical thinking skills are required for each process?

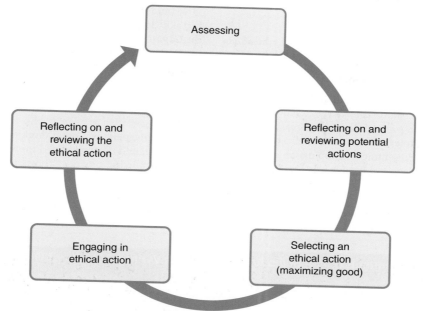

**Fig. 2.9** **Ethical Decision-Making Model.** (Canadian Nurses Association. (2017). *Code of ethics for registered nurses.* https://www.cna-aiic.ca/en/nursing/regulated-nursing-in-canada/nursing-ethics.)

| TABLE 2.6 **Application of the Ethical Decision-Making Model** | |
|---|---|
| **Ethical Decision-Making Steps** | **Nursing Activities** |
| Assessing | A nurse determines that a client experiencing a terminal illness wants to die at home, in surroundings that are familiar and comforting to them. The family is concerned that this will be unduly stressful for all other family members. The nurse is cognizant of the professional code of ethics and professional commitments to client care. The nurse caring for the client is asked by the palliative care team to "convince" the family to take the client home, which the nurse is uncomfortable doing. |
| Reflecting on and reviewing potential actions | The nurse considers client needs and wishes, and that these conflict with those of the family and their expectations for where care will be delivered. Supports and resources within the palliative care team are identified that would enable the client to return home. The nurse identifies their own values and beliefs and any obstacles to meeting obligations and taking appropriate action. |
| Selecting an ethical action (maximizing good) | Maintaining quality care and client safety is a priority. The nurse decides that they have the skill, capacity, and relationship with the family and client to engage in open discussion about solutions. |
| Engaging in ethical action | Knowledgeable, client-centred care is provided. Caring and compassion are evident when arranging for the client to be transferred home. Family needs for mental health support are addressed. |
| Reflecting on and reviewing the ethical action | The process of how all views were acknowledged or excluded is considered. The palliative care team involvement is examined, and procedures are reviewed. The nurse reflects on how the client is affected by the action, and how the family is feeling. The nurse engages in self-reflection and how decisions can be made in the future that will reduce distress for all participants. |

## SUMMATIVE APPROACHES

Over the last two decades, nursing authors and educators have combined a number of models and ways of thinking in nursing. For example, Dr. Rosalinda Alfaro-Lefevre has published textbooks that incorporate critical thinking, clinical reasoning, and clinical judgement in nursing. Focusing on practice readiness, Alfaro-Lefevre (2020) covered critical thinking, becoming a critical thinker, reasoning and decision making, the role of ethics and evidence, and clinical reasoning skills. Presenting a combination of models helps emphasize a holistic and flexible way of thinking.

Dr. Linda Caputi has published content that supports the development of both critical thinking and judgement skills in nursing. Caputi (2022) integrated critical thinking skills and strategies with Tanner's Clinical Judgement Model

(2006) and Benner's Novice to Expert Theory (2001) to support skill development in clinical reasoning and judgement. The *Caputi Clinical Judgment Framework* (2022) was developed, along with a related handbook adapted for Canadian learners, to support students' thinking skills.

## A COMPARISON OF THE VARIOUS NURSING MODELS

General agreement exists that thinking and decision-making skills should be emphasized in nursing education and applied to nursing practice. The skills in various nursing models presented in this chapter are compared in Table 2.7.

As you look at Table 2.7, note the similarities among the *BIG* skills (the bolded headings) aligned across the columns and among the *smaller* skills listed below them.

**TABLE 2.7    Comparison of the Skills Associated With Various Models of Thinking and Decision Making**

| Nursing Process[a] | Clinical Reasoning Cycle[b] | Tanner's Clinical Judgement Model[c] | Lasater Clinical Judgement Rubric[d] | Caputi Clinical Judgement Framework[e] | Skills for Clinical Reasoning[f] |
|---|---|---|---|---|---|
| **Assessment** | **Consider the client situation:** | **Notice** | **Noticing:** | **Getting the information:** | |
| | • Describe facts, context, situations, and people. | | • Focused observation | • Determining important information to collect | • Identifying assumptions |
| | **Collect cues/ information:** | | | | |
| | • Review available information. | | • Recognizing deviations from expected patterns | • Scanning the environment | • Assessing systematically and comprehensively |
| | • Gather new information. | | • Information seeking | • Identifying signs and symptoms | • Checking accuracy and reliability (validating data) |
| | • Recall knowledge. | | | • Assessing systematically and comprehensively | • Distinguishing normal from abnormal—detecting signs and symptoms (cues) |
| | | | | • Ensuring accurate information | • Making inferences (drawing valid conclusions) |

**TABLE 2.7   Comparison of the Skills Associated With Various Models of Thinking and Decision Making—cont'd**

| Nursing Process[a] | Clinical Reasoning Cycle[b] | Tanner's Clinical Judgement Model[c] | Lasater Clinical Judgement Rubric[d] | Caputi Clinical Judgement Frame-Work[e] | Skills for Clinical Reasoning[f] |
|---|---|---|---|---|---|
| Analysis | **Process information:** | Interpret | **Interpreting:** | **Making meaning of the information:** | |
| | • *Interpret*—Analyze data and compare normal versus abnormal. | | • Prioritizing data | • Clustering related information | • Clustering related signs and symptoms |
| | • *Discriminate*—Recognize inconsistencies and eliminate irrelevant data. | | • Making sense of data | • Identifying assumptions | • Identifying patterns |
| | • *Relate*—Find patterns and group similar data. | | | • Recognizing inconsistencies<br>• Distinguishing relevant from irrelevant information | • Recognizing inconsistencies<br>• Distinguishing relevant from irrelevant data |
| | • *Infer*—Weigh options and form a logical conclusion based on data. | | | • Judging how much ambiguity is acceptable | |
| | • *Match*—Compare the situation to past experiences. | | | • Comparing and contrasting | • Identifying missing information |
| | • *Predict*—Anticipate an outcome. | | | • Predicting potential complications | • Managing risk factors and promoting health |
| | | | | • Collaborating with health care team members | • Diagnosing actual and potential health problems |
| | | | | • Determining client care needs/ health care environment issues | |
| Planning | **Identify problems/ issues:** | | | **Determining actions to take:** | |
| | • Synthesize all available information. | | | • Setting priorities<br>• Managing potential complications | Setting priorities |

*Continued*

**TABLE 2.7   Comparison of the Skills Associated With Various Models of Thinking and Decision Making—cont'd**

| Nursing Process[a] | Clinical Reasoning Cycle[b] | Tanner's Clinical Judgement Model[c] | Lasater Clinical Judgement Rubric[d] | Caputi Clinical Judgement Framework[e] | Skills for Clinical Reasoning[f] |
|---|---|---|---|---|---|
| | **Establish goal(s):** | | | • Selecting interventions | • Determining client-centred outcomes |
| | • Describe the preferred outcome and a time frame. | | | | |
| **Implementation** | **Take action:** | **Respond** | **Responding:** | **Taking action:** | |
| | • Select a course of action from the available options. | | • Calm, confident manner | • Determining how to implement the planned interventions | • Determining individualized interventions |
| | | | • Clear communication | • Communicating | |
| | | | • Well-planned intervention/ flexibility | • Teaching others | |
| | | | • Being skillful | • Assigning | |
| **Evaluation** | **Evaluate outcomes:** | **Reflect** | **Reflecting:** | **Evaluating outcomes and your thinking:** | |
| | • Evaluate the effectiveness of outcomes. | | • Evaluation/ self-analysis | • Evaluating data | • Evaluating and correcting thinking (self-regulation) |
| | **Reflect on process and new learning:** | | | | |
| | • Contemplate learning and areas for improvement. | | • Evaluation and self-reflection<br>• Commitment to improvement | • Evaluating and correcting thinking | • Determining a comprehensive plan/evaluating and updating the plan |

[a]Astle, B., & Duggleby, W. (2024). *Potter and Perry's Canadian fundamentals of nursing* (7th ed.). Elsevier.
[b]Levett-Jones, T., Hoffman, K., Dempsey, J., et al. (2009). The "five rights" of clinical reasoning: An educational model to enhance nursing students' ability to identify and manage clinically "at risk" clients. *Nurse Education Today, 30*(6), 515–520.
[c]Tanner, C. A. (2006). Thinking like a nurse: A research-based model of clinical judgement in nursing. *Journal of Nursing Education, 45*(6), 204–211.
[d]Lasater, K. (2007). Clinical judgement development: Using simulation to create an assessment rubric. *Journal of Nursing Education, 46*(11), 496–503.
[e]Caputi, L. (2022). *Think like a nurse: The Caputi method for learning clinical judgement* (Cdn. ed.). Windy City Publishers.
[f]Alfaro-Lefevre, R. (2020). *Critical thinking, clinical reasoning, and clinical judgement: A practical approach* (7th ed.). Elsevier.

Similar actions and thinking skills are recommended by all of the models, which means that it is important to master them.

---

**REFLECTIVE PRACTICE MOMENT**

**Think *BIG* and *small* when thinking about frameworks and models in nursing practice.**

Look closely at Table 2.7. What do you notice about the skills that leaders in nursing education consider necessary to "think like a nurse"?

---

These thinking and decision-making models involve four common steps: *finding* information; *deciding* what to do; *acting* on the decision; and *reviewing* the action and decision outcomes. While individual nursing models use slightly different terms to describe how thinking and decision making occur, these are the essential four steps.

Figure 2.10 unifies these general steps into a common process. The blue centre areas summarize the models' common steps. In the next few chapters, examples of specific models will be inserted in the blue areas. You can also insert details on your preferred model as you develop your thinking and decision-making skills. This figure also presents cognitive and other skills in the outer four boxes that are useful to learners as they apply any model and develop proficiency in each of the steps. These skills will be expanded on in the next few chapters. In evidence-informed practice, it is important to apply research-based models that are understood by professional nurses.

## A FINAL MODEL TO CONSIDER: THE NCLEX CLINICAL JUDGEMENT MEASUREMENT MODEL

The NCSBN (2022), which develops and maintains the national nursing registration exam, conducted research and testing on new questions that were included in the exam in 2023. These "next generation NCLEX" (or NGN) question types involve more complex, context-based scenarios that present more realistic client information to exam writers. Case studies and stand-alone questions evaluate clinical judgement skills using the NCLEX-RN® Clinical Judgement Measurement Model (NCJMM). The NCSBN NCJMM *was* *not designed to assist with making decisions in practice but is used to measure the clinical judgement and thinking skills that are demonstrated when nurses engage in making decisions on the registration exam.*

The following six cognitive steps are tested on the exam:

1. *Recognize cues:* Identify relevant data in a clinical situation that will require the nurse's attention. This action incorporates assessment activities and thinking about which aspects of assessment are directly related to the client's main issues or concerns. Ask yourself, *What cues matter most?*
2. *Analyze cues:* Organize and link the recognized cues to the clinical situation. Consider the context or background of the client. Determine why certain information is more concerning than another. Ask yourself, *What could this cue mean?*
3. *Prioritize hypotheses:* Weigh and rank hypotheses according to priority (e.g., urgency, likelihood, risk). Think about which explanations are most likely or which are most serious. Ask yourself, *Where do I start?*
4. *Generate solutions:* Identify expected outcomes and use hypotheses to determine interventions to meet those expected outcomes. Plan possible actions with the associated rationale and reject any that should be avoided or are contraindicated. Ask yourself, *What can I do?*
5. *Take actions:* Implement the interventions that address the highest priorities and determine the order in which they will be performed. Ask yourself, *What will I do?*
6. *Evaluate outcomes:* Compare observed outcomes with expected outcomes. Establish how improvement or continued deterioration will be determined, using which client findings. Decide what interventions were effective, or not. Ask yourself, *Did it help?*

These cognitive steps should not be that new to you now, because you have already encountered them in the practice-based models that we have examined in this chapter. Compare Tanner's Clinical Judgement Model with the nursing process and these steps, and then refer to Figure 2.11.

The provincial or territorial registration or licensing exam tests these cognitive steps and the skills associated with them, *no matter which nursing model and decision making process you have been exposed to and practised.*

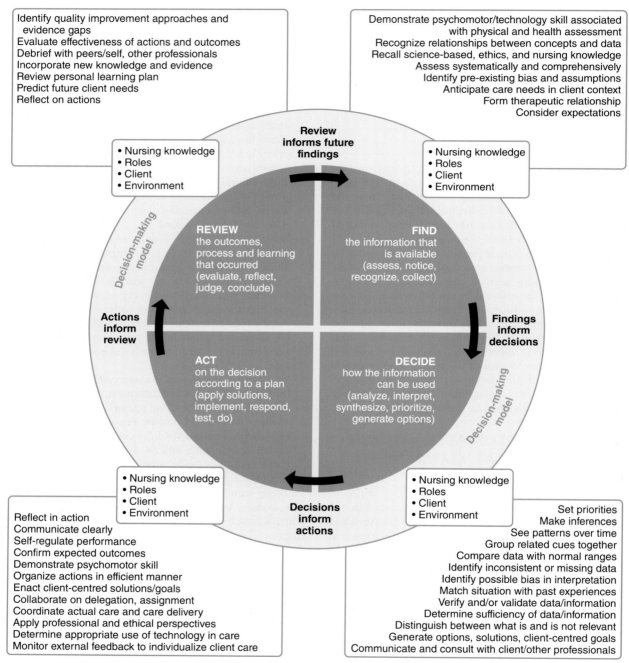

Identify quality improvement approaches and
  evidence gaps
Evaluate effectiveness of actions and outcomes
Debrief with peers/self, other professionals
Incorporate new knowledge and evidence
Review personal learning plan
Predict future client needs
Reflect on actions

Demonstrate psychomotor/technology skill associated
  with physical and health assessment
Recognize relationships between concepts and data
Recall science-based, ethics, and nursing knowledge
Assess systematically and comprehensively
Identify pre-existing bias and assumptions
Anticipate care needs in client context
Form therapeutic relationship
Consider expectations

- Nursing knowledge
- Roles
- Client
- Environment

- Nursing knowledge
- Roles
- Client
- Environment

**Review
informs future
findings**

**REVIEW**
the outcomes,
process and learning
that occurred
(evaluate, reflect,
judge, conclude)

**FIND**
the information that
is available
(assess, notice,
recognize, collect)

Decision-making
model

**Actions
inform
review**

**Findings
inform
decisions**

**ACT**
on the decision
according to a plan
(apply solutions,
implement, respond,
test, do)

**DECIDE**
how the information
can be used
(analyze, interpret,
synthesize, prioritize,
generate options)

Decision-making
model

- Nursing knowledge
- Roles
- Client
- Environment

- Nursing knowledge
- Roles
- Client
- Environment

**Decisions
inform
actions**

Reflect in action
Communicate clearly
Self-regulate performance
Confirm expected outcomes
Demonstrate psychomotor skill
Organize actions in efficient manner
Enact client-centred solutions/goals
Collaborate on delegation, assignment
Coordinate actual care and care delivery
Apply professional and ethical perspectives
Determine appropriate use of technology in care
Monitor external feedback to individualize client care

Set priorities
Make inferences
See patterns over time
Group related cues together
Compare data with normal ranges
Identify inconsistent or missing data
Identify possible bias in interpretation
Match situation with past experiences
Verify and/or validate data/information
Determine sufficiency of data/information
Distinguish between what is and is not relevant
Generate options, solutions, client-centred goals
Communicate and consult with client/other professionals

**Fig. 2.10  Unified Process for Thinking and Decision Making.** This figure shows connections between
decision-making models, the four common steps associated with thinking processes, and related nursing
skills. The nurse may select any given model for thinking and decision making in nursing (such as the nursing
process, the clinical reasoning cycle, or Tanner's Clinical Judgement Model) and insert it in this diagram.

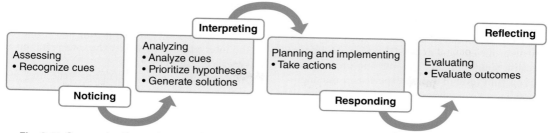

**Fig. 2.11** Comparing Tanner's Clinical Judgement Model with the Nursing Process and the NCJMM Cognitive Steps.

## SUMMARY

This chapter has provided an introduction to various structures that may be used for thinking as a nurse in practice. It has built on Chapter 1 and elaborated on the importance of critical thinking, clinical reasoning, and clinical judgement, and emphasized the use of these skills during specific processes for thinking as a nurse in professional practice settings. While many models have been described, they share similarities such as collecting sufficient information, sorting data, choosing what to do next, and evaluating outcomes. A broad framework for organizing thinking in nursing—NRCE—was introduced, which will be referenced throughout this textbook.

## KEY POINTS TO REMEMBER

These are the key points to remember from this chapter.

### About Approaches to Thinking in Nursing

- A framework is a basic structure that describes (but does not explain) a system or concept; it helps connect many big ideas about a topic to a method or process of doing something related to that topic.
- Frameworks are often in a written format that outlines each component and the possible relationships between them.
- A framework can support a systematic and informed approach to thinking and to nursing practice; frameworks can come from other disciplines and cultures.
- A model is more specific than a framework and provides a simplified description of a process that can facilitate its understanding and application to different situations.
- A model is often presented in a physical form, a schematic, or in a diagrammatic or graphic format, so that it is easier to follow.
- The Paul-Elder Critical Thinking Framework (Paul & Elder, 2020) describes components for improving one's critical thinking skills and can also be depicted as a model.

### About the NRCE Framework for Thinking in Nursing

- For the purposes of organizing information in this textbook, particularly in Chapters 3, 4, 5, and 6, the NRCE framework will be used; it is also depicted as a model (in diagrammatic form) and can be remembered by reading it as "nurse."
- The NRCE framework can be used and adapted to every instance where a nurse needs to recall information, analyze information, engage in action, and reflect on the action and areas for improvement.
  - *N* is for "*n*ursing knowledge" and prompts the nurse to recall relevant nursing knowledge and science, nursing theory, ethics, and ways to remember more detailed information.
  - *R* is for "professional *r*oles" and prompts the nurse to consider roles and scopes of practice for nursing and other health care professionals, as well as provincial and territorial practice standards, competencies, safety, best practices, delegation, leadership and communication theory, and professional growth.
  - *C* is for "*c*lient context" and prompts the nurse to focus on the client's past health experiences, personal goals and needs, and effects of colonization, and to respect and incorporate culture, cultural safety, gender, equity, diversity, and inclusion in thinking and action.
  - *E* is for "health care *e*nvironment" and prompts the nurse to incorporate the physical health care setting, the administrative infrastructure, governing law, regulations, policies and procedures, and the available resources and limitations that are relevant to health care.

- Benner's Novice to Expert Theory (2001) states that nurses develop through the following five levels of experience during their careers: novice, advanced beginner, competent, proficient, and expert. This theory is important because your thinking, as a nursing professional, depends on your level of overall expertise in nursing—which is as a novice or advanced beginner, most likely, if you are a student.
- Your thinking, when using the NRCE framework, will be influenced by your level of expertise.

## About Models for Thinking and Decision Making in Nursing

- The scientific process involves the general steps of carefully gathering information, analyzing relevant data, and drawing a conclusion.
- The research process, which mirrors the scientific process, is a systematic and logical approach for seeking answers to questions that includes observation, hypothesis generation, a literature review, experimentation and testing, analysis of data, and sharing results and conclusions.
- Gibbs's reflective cycle is used by nurses and describes a cyclical process for returning to an experience, attending to feelings, and re-evaluating the experience in light of its purpose; it involves description, feelings, evaluation, analysis, a conclusion, and an action plan.
- The nursing process involves *assessment, analysis, planning, implementation,* and *evaluation,* or *AAPIE.*
- Critical thinking skills and clinical reasoning in the client and health care context are necessary in the application of the nursing models.
- The clinical reasoning cycle (CRC) describes nursing actions in eight steps: consider the client situation, collect cues/information, process information, identify problems/issues, establish goal(s), take action, evaluate outcomes, and reflect on process and learning.
- Tanner's Clinical Judgement Model (2006) is a research-based approach to thinking and uses language that describes how nurses think when they provide care in complex situations that require judgement and has four aspects: noticing, interpreting, responding, and reflecting.

- Reflection-*in*-action occurs during "responding," when the nurse is observing client responses to interventions in the moment they are happening *and* is able to modify the interventions based on the interpretation of those observed responses.
- Reflection-*on*-action occurs during "reflecting," at the end of the cycle, when the nurse is looking back on what knowledge was gained from the clinical experience.
- Ethical decision-making frameworks and models provide nurses and other health care providers with a useful foundation for examining and resolving situations involving ethical values.
- The models used by nurses when thinking about client care and issues relating to health care systems are cyclical.
- Some of these models were developed from previously published models or from other nursing or interprofessional research and knowledge.

### About Summative Approaches

- Nursing authors have incorporated various approaches to develop skills for thinking like a nurse.
- Combining models or frameworks helps emphasize holistic and flexible ways of thinking in nursing.

### About the Similarities Among the Nursing Models

- A summary of the models (see Figure 2.10) shows *BIG,* common steps in thinking and decision making seen in many of the models described in this chapter and presents a unified process; it also shows similar *smaller* critical thinking and clinical reasoning skills.
- The thinking and decision-making models are summarized in four common steps: *find* the information that is available; *decide* how the information can be used; *act* on the decision according to a plan; and *review* the actions, outcomes, processes, and learning that occurred.

### About the NCLEX Clinical Judgement Measurement Model

- The NCSBN uses the NCJMM, a way to measure clinical judgement, when evaluating writers' competence during the national nursing registration exam.

## CONCLUSION AND THINKING IT THROUGH

Part A of this textbook has introduced you to different approaches to thinking and various structures for thinking in nursing practice. Now that you know that thinking and decision making in nursing can be framed and organized in a methodical way, you will have the chance to further

learn about ways in which the associated processes can be applied in practice.

Part B explores the four steps that are common to thinking and decision-making models: *find* the information that is available; *decide* how to use the information; *act* on the decision according to a plan; and *review* the actions, outcomes, process, and learning that occurred. The NRCE framework will be applied to each of these steps. As well, examples of nursing models and simple clinical situations will be provided so that the application of ways to think it through will be apparent.

## CLASS ACTIVITIES TO CHECK THINKING

### Think-Aloud Pair Problem Solve (TAPPS)

Form pairs. Decide who will be a problem solver and listener for Problem A. The problem solver reads the problem aloud and talks through a response to the problem, while the listener reminds the problem solver to think aloud, asks clarification questions, offers encouragement to keep thinking, but refrains from providing possible answers. Switch roles for Problem B.

For each of these problems, apply the identified process.

- **Problem A (apply the research process):** A nurse working in a rural community health centre observes that over the last 6 months some clients receive treatment more quickly for the same health problems than other clients.
- **Problem B (apply the reflective cycle):** A nurse is assigned to provide pre-operative information to a client scheduled for surgery tomorrow. The client does not speak English and a family member volunteers to translate what the nurse says. Afterwards, the nurse is unsure that the information was accurately conveyed to the client.

When finished, discuss with each other how easy or difficult it was to apply the identified process.

### Activities and Discussion Questions

1. Describe how the NRCE framework can be used in each part of the nursing process.
2. Draw a picture or create a diagram to show how you visualize Tanner's Clinical Judgement Model.
3. Compare and contrast the nursing process and the clinical reasoning cycle.
4. Discuss in a small group how using an ethical decision-making process can help challenging clinical situations.
5. Make a list of what you like and don't like about each of the following: the nursing process, Tanner's Clinical Judgement Model, and clinical reasoning cycle. Jot down your rationale.
6. Look at the skills listed in Table 2.7, as described by Caputi and Alfaro-Lefevre. In small groups, discuss how these skills are similar. How can these skills be developed in your nursing practice?

## CASE STUDY REVIEW

### Scenario

A registered nurse observes a client, who had surgery 3 days ago to repair a fractured femur, as alert and oriented to time, place, and person but slow to respond to questions. The dressing had been removed, and the incision was well approximated, dry and intact, with no drainage. The client stated that the leg pain is 4/10 on a 1 to 10 pain intensity scale. The client reports dyspnea accompanied by increased anxiety, which started 1 hour ago. A dry cough and crackles in the left side of the chest are noted. Chest pain is reported with deep breaths. Vital signs: T: 37.6°C (99.68°F); P: 96; R: 32; BP: 110/90 mm Hg; SpO$_2$: 88% on room air.

Before answering the following questions: Choose a specific nursing model to apply to your thinking (nursing process, clinical reasoning cycle, Tanner's Clinical Judgement Model, or another). Refer to the description of the model and its steps or stages as you answer the questions.

### Questions

1. Describe the client situation.
2. How can this situation be understood? Do you need more information?
3. What will you do next and why?
4. How will you know if what you have planned and acted on will help the client?

### Reflect

- How did you apply the model to this scenario?
- Did it help you to provide answers?

## EVIDENCE-INFORMED THINKING ACTIVITY

Consult the chapter's online resource section and review the information on the Next Generation NCLEX registration exam's NCSBN Clinical Judgment Measurement Model (NCJMM). Review the model and the graphic that shows Layers 0 to 4 and then compare the model components to those from the nursing models in this chapter.

1. How has the National Council of State Boards of Nursing (NCSBN) adapted existing nursing models such as the nursing process to measure thinking?
2. What research did the NCSBN use to create the NCJMM? Find one source.
3. Describe how the 6 evidence-informed cognitive steps in the model will help you prepare for the registration exam.

## QUESTIONS TO ASSESS LEARNING

### Review Questions

1. Which topic relates most directly to *nursing knowledge* of clinical intervention options?
   a. Mnemonics to facilitate recall of nursing clinical information
   b. Leadership and communication theory
   c. Client's past experiences in the health care system
   d. Self-care practices and supports
2. What aspect of the *health care environment* does the nurse consider most likely to affect the decision-making process?
   a. Nursing theory and caring
   b. Entry-to-practice competencies
   c. Cultural preferences of the client
   d. Available policies and procedures
3. What statement by the nurse indicates they are incorporating the *client context* in decision making?
   a. "The distractions in this setting should be identified before providing client care."
   b. "I should find out what the client's goals are for their own overall health."
   c. "The best practices for managing wound care will be reviewed carefully."
   d. "I will use the most current evidence when caring for the client."
4. What aspect relating to *professional roles* will a nurse consider when making decisions in practice?
   a. Knowledge required for performing advanced clinical skills
   b. Scope of practice of other health care professionals
   c. Approaches to achieve inclusive client care
   d. Policy descriptions of responses to hospital codes

## ONE LAST THOUGHT

Reflect on the decision-making processes that are supported by the various nursing models in this chapter. How will you remember the details of each model? Is there a way for you to recall the processes more easily? Make a note of how you can begin to think this through.

## ONLINE RESOURCES

*Clinical Judgement Model*—Tanner, C. A. (2006). Thinking like a nurse: A research-based model of clinical judgment in nursing. *Journal of Nursing Education, 45*(6), 204–211. https://www.mccc.edu/nursing/documents/Thinking_Like_A_Nurse_Tanner.pdf.

*Clinical reasoning: Instructor resources* (2009). School of Nursing and Midwifery, Faculty of Health, University of Newcastle. https://www.utas.edu.au/__data/assets/pdf_file/0003/263487/Clinical-Reasoning-Instructor-Resources.pdf.

*Next Generation NCLEX Clinical Judgment Measurement Model* (2024). National Council of State Boards of Nursing. https://www.nclex.com/clinical-judgment-measurement-model.page.

## REFERENCES

Alberta Regional Professional Development Consortia. (2023). *Seven Sacred Teachings.* https://empoweringthespirit.ca/cultures-of-belonging/seven-grandfathers-teachings/.

Alfaro-Lefevre, R. (2020). *Critical thinking, clinical reasoning, and clinical judgement: A practical approach* (7th ed.). Elsevier.

Astle, B., & Duggleby, W. (2024). *Potter and Perry's Canadian fundamentals of nursing* (7th ed.). Elsevier.

Benner, P. (1982). From novice to expert. *American Journal of Nursing, 82*(3), 402–407.

Benner, P. (1984). *From novice to expert: Excellence and power in clinical nursing practice.* Addison-Wesley Publishing Company.

Benner, P. (2001). *From novice to expert: Excellence and power in clinical nursing practice.* Prentice Hall.

Boud, D., Keogh, R., & Walker, D. (1985). Promoting reflection in learning: A model. In Boud, D., Keogh, R., & Walter, D. (Eds.), *Reflection: Turning experience into learning* (pp. 18–40). RoutledgeFalmer.

Canadian Nurses Association. (2017). *Code of ethics for registered nurses.* https://www.cna-aiic.ca/en/nursing/regulated-nursing-in-canada/nursing-ethics.

Caputi, L. (2022). *Think like a nurse: The Caputi method for learning clinical judgment* (Cdn. ed.). Windy City Publishers.

College of Nurses of Ontario. (2019). *Ethics*. https://www.cno.org/globalassets/docs/prac/41034_ethics.pdf.

Dawson, J., Laccos-Barrett, K., Hammond, C., et al. (2022). Reflexive practice as an approach to improve healthcare delivery for Indigenous peoples: A systematic critical synthesis and exploration of the cultural safety education literature. *International Journal of Environmental Research and Public Health, 19*(11), 6691. doi:10.3390/ijerph19116691.

Dreyfus, S., & Dreyfus, H. (1980). *A five-stage model of the mental activities involved in directed skill acquisition [Unpublished manuscript]*. U.S. Air Force, Office of Scientific Research [AFSC] under contract F49620-C-0063 with the University of California Berkeley.

Fawcett, J. (2017). *Applying conceptual models of nursing: Quality improvement, research, and practice*. Springer Publishing.

Gibbs, G. (1988). *Learning by doing: A guide to teaching and learning methods*. Further Education Unit, Oxford Polytechnic.

Halpern, D. (2014). *Thought and knowledge: An introduction to critical thinking* (5th ed.). Psychology Press.

International Council of Nurses. (2002). *Nursing definitions*. https://www.icn.ch/nursing-policy/nursing-definitions.

Johns, C. (2022). *Becoming a reflective practitioner* (6th ed.). Wiley-Blackwell.

Johnson, D. E. (1987). Guest editorial: Evaluating conceptual models for use in critical care nursing practice. *Dimensions of Critical Care Nursing, 6*, 195–197.

Kalideen, D. (1993). Is there a place for nursing models in theatre nursing? *British Journal of Theatre Nursing, 3*(5), 4–6.

Lasater, K. (2007). Clinical judgement development: Using simulation to create an assessment rubric. *Journal of Nursing Education, 46*(11), 496–503.

Lasater, K., & Nielsen, A. (2024). The Lasater Clinical Judgment Rubric: 17 years later. *Journal of Nursing Education, 63*(3), 149–155. doi:10.3928/01484834-20240108-05.

Levett-Jones, T., Hoffman, K., Dempsey, J., et al. (2009). The "five rights" of clinical reasoning: An educational model to enhance nursing students' ability to identify and manage clinically "at risk" clients. *Nurse Education Today, 30*(6), 515–520.

National Council of State Boards of Nursing. (2022). *Next Generation NCLEX—The NGN project*. https://www.ncsbn.org/next-generation-nclex.htm.

Paul, R., & Elder, L (2020). *The miniature guide to critical thinking concepts and tools* (8th ed.). The Foundation for Critical Thinking Press.

Schön, D. A. (1983). *The reflective practitioner: How professionals think in action*. Basic Books.

School of Nursing and Midwifery, Faculty of Health, University of Newcastle. (2009). *Clinical reasoning: Instructor resources*. https://www.utas.edu.au/__data/assets/pdf_file/0003/263487/Clinical-Reasoning-Instructor-Resources.pdf.

Singh, M., & Thirsk, L. (2022). *LoBiondo-Wood and Haber's nursing research in Canada* (5th ed.). Elsevier.

Tanner, C. A. (2006). Thinking like a nurse: A research-based model of clinical judgment in nursing. *Journal of Nursing Education, 45*(6), 204–211.

van Bruchem-Visser, R. L., van Dijk, G., de Beaufort, I., et al. (2020). Ethical frameworks for complex medical decision making in older patients: A narrative review. *Archives of Gerontology and Geriatrics, 90*. https://doi.org/10.1016/j.archger.2020.104160.

# The Processes of Clinical Reasoning, Decision Making, and Clinical Judgement

This second section of the textbook is the largest and includes the next four chapters. It provides you with an overview of the basic four steps in thinking it through in nursing practice – *finding information, deciding what to do, acting on decisions,* and *reviewing actions.* These steps may seem discrete and linear but overlap and are integrated and cyclical. These steps also give you the impression that there is only one decision to make during the thinking process but there are many decisions for the nurse to make when providing care. To illustrate thinking it through, the four steps of the unified process for thinking and decision making are highlighted in each of the chapters. Various nursing models are applied to this unified process to illustrate the similarities of the models.

Chapter 3 presents the first step – finding information. This is an important initial aspect of thinking which must be completed reasonably and accurately to form a reliable basis for the steps that follow. Chapter 4 describes the step of deciding what to do. Decisions involve several cognitive activities; analysis, interpretation, synthesis, and prioritization are identified and described. Chapter 5 explains the step of acting on decisions. Building on the previous chapter information, the actions of planning based on what has been decided and implementing the plan are described. Chapter 6 looks at what is involved in reviewing actions. This is the last step in the 4-step process of thinking it through. However, reviewing actions is not an end point; instead, it is the beginning of a new cycle of thinking. Even if care has been completed for an individual client, your reflection on what you have done will be used in your future practice. Approaches for looking back on nursing actions and evaluating clinical judgements that have been made are presented.

In every chapter, certain clinical reasoning skills are presented. Barriers encountered during each step and strategies to overcome these challenges are discussed. A detailed outline of what you need to consider when thinking at each step is provided using the NRCE framework. Case studies are used to illustrate thinking at every step.

**Part B will help you answer the questions,** *what are the steps in thinking through a client or nursing practice issue and at what points do I need to make decisions in the thinking process*?

# Finding Information

## LEARNING OUTCOMES

*After reading this chapter, you will be able to:*

- Explain the influence of evidence, nursing theories, and client-centred care perspectives when finding information.
- Identify the clinical reasoning skills used when finding information.
- Provide examples of potential barriers to finding information.
- Describe how methods for remembering nursing assessment strategies will assist with collecting information in client care situations.

- Identify different health care professional roles that can potentially contribute to the full assessment picture of the client.
- Incorporate aspects of the client situation that are needed to plan for holistic care.
- Describe elements in the health care environment that may affect how client information and clinical data are collected.

## GLOSSARY

**Acronym:** a word, pronounced as such, that is created from the initial letters of other words; it is used to describe something in an abbreviated way; a type of mnemonic

**Acrostic:** a saying, phrase, rhyme, or some other composition taken from letters in a group of words in order used to improve recall; a type of mnemonic

**Anticipatory reflection:** a future-focused reflection; consideration of what may occur next, based on past experiences and learning

**Assessment:** the first step of the nursing process, which involves comprehensive data collection; recognition of the client's status, situation, and environment; and of the nurse's and others' knowledge and role

**Mnemonic:** a device—such as a pattern of letters, ideas, or associations—for remembering facts and information more easily

**Situation awareness:** being aware of what is happening around you and understanding what that information means, now and in the future (Endsley & Jones, 2012); the focus or context of awareness is related to the specific purpose of the activity, such as caring for a client

**Unconscious bias:** also called *implicit bias*, it refers to unrecognized stereotypes and ideas that one has about cultures or people that influence one's decision making and behaviours; occurs outside of conscious awareness

---

This chapter and the three that follow explore the four common steps in thinking and decision making: finding information; deciding what to do; acting on the decision; and reviewing the action and decision outcomes. This chapter addresses the first step of *finding information*. In the models presented in Chapter 2, this first step was also described as *assessing, noticing, recognizing,* and *collecting.* For each step, the NRCE (*nursing* knowledge, professional *roles, client* context, and the health care *environment*) framework will be used as a basis for demonstrating ways to think it through.

Later in this chapter, the clinical reasoning cycle (Levett-Jones et al., 2010) is applied to a case study that shows how solid nursing knowledge and evidence, an understanding of the scope of professional health care roles, and knowledge of the client and the health care environment are all essential to providing a foundation for nursing care. Applying the concepts in this chapter will help answer the question, *What am I missing?* when finding information.

## THE IMPORTANCE OF FINDING INFORMATION AS A FIRST STEP

The first step in *thinking it through* is understanding the client or health care–related situation that requires a nursing decision or action. This step is grounded in having the most appropriate information, which includes data, evidence, and resources on which to base thinking to support optimal care. Having the necessary information on which to base a decision is not only important for thinking in daily life but also critical for working with clients in a professional health care setting.

How do nurses know what information to gather? How do they ensure that they have considered what is necessary for the next steps in thinking about care? Guidance is available for nurses who engage in thinking and decision making in nursing practice from many areas. Science and acquired nursing knowledge are immediately obvious sources that can guide nurses seeking information. Although perhaps less obvious, others are nursing theory, client-centred values and culture, and best practice guidelines. Discipline-specific knowledge and a theoretical base are part of what defines nursing as a profession and guides nurses' thinking processes, including how they seek information. All of these sources are studied during basic nursing and continuing education programs for the purpose of supporting fundamental thinking in nursing practice.

In nursing practice, finding information is integral to participating in shared safe, ethical, and competent decision making. Correctly applying this first step is fundamental to client advocacy and meeting client needs and goals for health. When finding information, consider the value of incorporating the following factors.

### Evidence-Informed Sources of Information

Research evidence is a basis for professional and efficient decision making in practice (Melnyk & Fineout-Overholt, 2015). It guides the information collected during the first step of care. Statistical information gathered by federal government or provincial and territorial agencies on populations, groups, and communities can offer guidance on who is most in need of what health care services and which clients may be at risk for certain health concerns.

When seeking information, the nurse draws on various sources of knowledge from different scientific disciplines. In nursing practice, finding information is often referred to as assessment, which involves comprehensive data collection, recognition of the client's status, situation, and environment, and of the nurse's and others' knowledge and roles. For example, to conduct physical and other assessments as needed, and to recall facts about normal biological functioning, the nurse must understand anatomy and physiology. Knowledge of the respiratory system and how it functions form a basis for an accurate health assessment, which includes observation of respiratory rate, auscultation of breath sounds, determination of shortness of breath, and examination for cyanosis. The nurse must also draw on their own knowledge and ability to perform the required assessments.

Research and evidence guide the nurse when finding information and conducting an assessment. For example, the nurse must know that when assessing mental health and psychological well-being, there may be associated physical health issues. This evidence-informed approach is based on additional research from disciplines such as psychology and social work. Evidence-informed linkages between different health topics influence what a nurse may further assess when finding information. For instance, the nurse caring for a client who is reporting physical pain will conduct a physiological assessment and gather information on the potential psychological impact of pain, as well as the client's personal and culturally influenced views of pain. Research-informed practices dictate that such assessments go together (Table 3.1).

Often, assumptions are made when using science- or research-based evidence. Those assumptions are that the evidence is valid, relevant, and appropriate to the context of client care. However, when a nurse uses evidence, any assumption about that evidence should be verified. The research process, described in Chapter 2, will have been applied to any peer-reviewed study that forms a basis for clinical care. Choosing sources of information that come from reputable professional groups, associations, and publications, where the information is peer reviewed and widely used, can help the nurse confirm the validity of evidence.

Knowledge of evidence-informed practices ensures that nurses stay abreast of new approaches and scientific advances that optimize the delivery of nursing care. This knowledge helps reduce ritual and unsystematic clinical care and emphasizes the use of the consensus of recognized experts and research from nursing and other disciplines. The application of evidence supports safe, competent, and effective health care practices.

| TABLE 3.1 | Examples of Physical Assessments and Associated Resources | |
|---|---|---|
| Physical Assessment | Related Assessment Examples | Evidence-Informed Resources/Best Practice Guideline Examples |
| Pain | *Physical:* nursing knowledge, measurement<br>*Psychological:* fear, denial<br>*Cultural:* stoicism, beliefs about tolerance<br>*Social:* others' reactions, perception about medication use | *Evidence-informed pain scales:* Wong-Baker FACES scale; Northern Pain Scale[a]<br>*Best practice guideline:* Registered Nurses' Association of Ontario. (2013). *Assessment and management of pain.* https://rnao.ca/sites/rnao-ca/files/AssessAndManagementOfPain_15_WEB-_FINAL_DEC_2.pdf |
| Blood pressure | *Physical:* nursing knwowledge, measurement<br>*Psychological:* anxiety, health care professional presence/white coat syndrome, denial<br>*Cultural:* perception of health and need for treatment, medication<br>*Social:* dietary habits, other lifestyle activities | *Evidence-informed client information:*<br>observed, documented trends in blood pressure readings<br>*Best practice guideline:* Canadian Cardiovascular Society. (2020). Hypertension Canada's 2020 comprehensive guidelines for the prevention, diagnosis, risk assessment, and treatment of hypertension in adults and children. https://doi.org/10.1016/j.cjca.2020.02.086 |
| Pressure injury | *Physical:* nursing knowledge, measurement, body mass index (BMI), pain<br>Psychological: dementia<br>*Cultural:* need for treatment, medication<br>*Social:* dietary habits, other influences, understanding of health are team | *Evidence-informed resource:* Braden Scale for predicting pressure ulcer risk[b]<br>*Best practice guideline:* Registered Nurses' Association of Ontario. (2016). *Assessment and management of pressure injuries for the interprofessional team.* https://rnao.ca/sites/rnao-ca/files/Pressure_Injuries_BPG.pdf |

[a]Ellis, J. A., Ootoova, A., Blouin, R., et al. (2011). Establishing the psychometric properties and preferences for the Northern Pain Scale. *International Journal of Circumpolar Health, 70*(3), 274–285. The Wong-Baker FACES scale is an adapted version of the Wong/Baker FACES Pain Rating Scale from Hockenberry, M. J., & Wilson, D. (2006). *Wong's nursing care of infants and children* (8th ed.) (p. 1876). Elsevier Mosby.

[b]Orsted, H., Keast, D., Foret-Lalande, L., et al. (2018). *Best practice recommendations for the prevention and management of wounds.* Wounds Canada. https://www.woundscanada.ca/docman/public/healthcare-professional/165-wc-bpr-prevention-and-management-of-wounds/file.

---

**REFLECTIVE PRACTICE MOMENT**

How do statistical databases and demographic information on a particular group influence your assessment?

Identify a marginalized or vulnerable group in your practice area and consider:

- What would be important to assess in a client who identified as a member of that group?
- Why do you think that?
- Is your rationale based on evidence, your own observations, or past knowledge?
- Check the evidence. Access an online government database or current literature to confirm your understanding of how and when the data was gathered and any potential biases.

Statistical databases are important resources for finding information; however, the data obtained may not always apply to the individual client.

## Nursing Theories

In addition to knowledge of the sciences—which informs areas such as anatomy, pathophysiology, psychology, and sociocultural influences—nurses must have a deep understanding of the holistic nature of a client's health concerns. This understanding is drawn from nursing theories and is a form of evidence.

Theories are slightly different from models. Where models are simple and more concrete representations or descriptions of how things work, theories aim to present sets of assumptions or propositions that link concepts of concern and interest. Nursing theories help provide a systematic view of nursing phenomena so that the phenomena can be explained or predicted. These theories, of which there are many, represent one aspect of overall nursing disciplinary knowledge that influences care and inquiry within the discipline. Nursing theories are a significant influence on how nurses think and, specifically, how they find information and decide on what is useful for care.

There are different ways in which nursing is conceptualized. Nursing, health, client or person, and environment are overarching and consistent concepts that are embedded in nursing theories and therefore shape nurses' thinking and professional work. Fawcett (1995) referred to these as *metaparadigm concepts*. Descriptions of how nurses come to know or understand information are referred to as *ways of knowing* (Carper, 1978). Ways of knowing clarify that nurses use multiple lenses and types of knowledge— empirical, ethical, personal, and aesthetic—to interpret complex phenomena. Sociopolitical and emancipatory knowing, which further capture the holistic vision of nursing, were later added to these ways of knowing (Chinn et al., 2022; White, 1995). Each of these ideas about nursing inform how nurses think and what they do.

Many Canadian nursing texts provide thorough descriptions of major nursing theories that have been applied in the past and those that are currently in use. Nursing theories have changed over time to align with not only observations and experiences of nurses and clients in health care settings but also health care trends. A nursing theory always provides a lens and guide with which to think about and view the information that is available in the health care setting and that is salient to client care.

Based on their knowledge of nursing theories, nurses learn to focus on the client's particular presentation and to understand the number and complexity of the client's needs and preferences when finding information.

## Client-Centred Care Perspectives

Nursing theories often place clients at the centre of care and provide perspectives on nursing practice. When finding information as part of the process of thinking like a nurse, the client is at the core. Remember that the client can be described as a person, family, defined group, community, or population, depending on the area and focus of nursing practice. Client-centred care (sometimes called *patient-centred care* or *person-centred care*) requires attitudes and behaviours that reflect the importance of knowing the whole client (i.e., biopsychosocial, cultural, and spiritual aspects).

When assessing the client's condition or when seeking and gathering information, nurses attend to what is most relevant to the client's situation (Registered Nurses' Association of Ontario, 2015). For example, a client who has newly immigrated to Canada may need person- or family-specific support related to potential challenges or barriers in accessing health care (Pandey et al., 2022). Similarly, a racialized person will need to have their experiences, needs, and viewpoints incorporated in care. Noticing and acknowledging what is most important to the client is part of client advocacy and culturally safe care.

If the focus of a nurse's concern relates to nonclient issues such as workload, occupational health, or health policy, the impacts of addressing or not addressing those issues can indirectly affect the client or clients that the nurse works with. Therefore, it is important to maintain a client-centred perspective no matter the assessment area— whether in direct client care, administration, education, or research, or whether the client is an individual in an acute care bed or a larger population cohort.

## Situation Awareness

The nurse's assessment of a client or clinical situation requires attention to many aspects of the presenting circumstance. Situation awareness is being cognizant of what is happening around you and understanding what that information means, now and in the future (Endsley & Jones, 2012). This type of awareness is critical in professional activities, including nursing practice (Stubbings et al., 2012; Tower et al., 2019).

Current happenings influence future happenings and any clinical decisions that need to be made. Therefore, undertaking a reasonably comprehensive initial assessment of the situation is key. To do this, the nurse needs to identify appropriate cues and have a sense of what is most important. It is helpful to pay attention to not only the client but also what is going on around the client. For instance, this may include an awareness of a client's determinants of health (e.g., poverty, food insecurity, and level of education) as well as their current physical health.

There are three levels of situation awareness:
1. Perception of elements in the environment
2. Comprehension of the current situation
3. Projection of future status

In situation awareness, each level is dependent on the previous one. In other words, reaching the higher levels of awareness is dependent on achieving the lower levels. Perception of elements in the environment, the first level in situation awareness, involves assessment in a holistic manner to produce optimal results in future decision making. Becoming fully situationally aware is essential; if cues are missed or the client has not been assessed completely, elements that could affect decision making and outcomes may be omitted. Although overlooking certain elements could still result in a minimally acceptable outcome, optimal care may not be achieved. Therefore, the first level of noticing elements in the environment is the foundation to success when finding information. Table 3.2 summarizes the levels of situation awareness.

You cannot make appropriate choices during a nursing activity and the decision-making process if you do not have *essential* information about what is occurring from your perspective, the perspective of the client and others, and in the environment where you are working as a professional. It

## TABLE 3.2  Levels of Situation Awareness and Examples

| Levels of Situation Awareness (SA) | Description | Examples of SA Actions |
|---|---|---|
| **Level 1 SA** Perception of elements in the environment | This level involves the perception of the status, attributes, and dynamics of relevant aspects of the situation through monitoring; gathering auditory, visual, olfactory, tactile, or other verbal and non-verbal cues; and simple recognition. Errors may occur if information is not readily available or apparent. | Monitor vital signs. Note cues that may indicate complications. For example, postoperatively these may include blood pressure, low oxygen saturation, and elevated temperature. Recognize normal versus abnormal cues. |
| **Level 2 SA** Comprehension of the current situation | This level involves the interpretation and synthesis of information and cues from level 1 in terms of their significance and how they will affect the overall goals (i.e., to improve health) of the situation. It can be influenced by mental models. A lack of adequate knowledge base or information may contribute to errors. | Interpret changes or trends in vital signs. For example, postoperatively, progressive hypotension may indicate postoperative hemorrhage. Analyze the impact of action versus inaction. |
| **Level 3 SA** Projection of future status | This level involves the ability to predict how elements will change and affect the situation in the future. It is achieved through knowledge gained from levels 1 and 2. It may take time to achieve. This level assists with the development of strategies and responses to future events. Errors can occur with information overload or assuming that trends will continue. | Predict the specific therapy that will be needed to address deteriorating status in a particular situation. For example, postoperative hemorrhage may require reoperation to repair bleeding, a blood transfusion, and/or medication. Prepare for immediate or future changes in care. |

Adapted from Endsley, M. R. & Jones, D. (2012). Designing for situation awareness: An approach to user-centred design. CRC Press.

is important to understand that even if all the information that was possible to know were available, not all of it may be needed to make a good decision. You can, however, gather the information that is *reasonably* available and *reasonable* to consider at the time and in the particular context of care.

> **KNOWLEDGE CHECK-IN**
> - How do you know whether a source of information is valid or reliable?
> - Explain how nursing theory can inform how nurses find information when trying to make decisions.
> - Describe the value of client perspectives when finding and gathering information.
> - What does it mean to be situationally aware?

## SKILLS USED WHEN FINDING INFORMATION

The competent nurse uses critical thinking and clinical reasoning skills, no matter which thinking and decision-making model or framework is adopted. Figure 3.1 presents a unified process for thinking and decision making. In this chapter, the unified process incorporates the clinical reasoning cycle (CRC) (Levett-Jones et al., 2010),

discussed in Chapter 2, as an example of a model that can be adopted when thinking through nursing care. The blue centre areas summarize the steps and key actions involved in the CRC process. The grey-shaded area highlights the skills needed when finding information. In the CRC process, finding information is referred to as considering the client situation and collecting cues/information. The CRC will be applied to a case study that focuses on finding information, later in this chapter.

### Clinical Reasoning and Other Skills Used When Finding Information

Clinical reasoning skills are needed for finding information and addressing a particular client issue. Many of these skills are thinking or cognitive skills. They can be applied to any thinking and decision-making model or framework. However, when assessing clients, the use of psychomotor skills and being able to competently conduct a physical assessment are also very important. Think of these additional skills as action-based extensions of your clinical reasoning skills. Clinical reasoning skills can be applied in many situations and with many nursing models and are not only used in the CRC described by Levett-Jones et al. (2010).

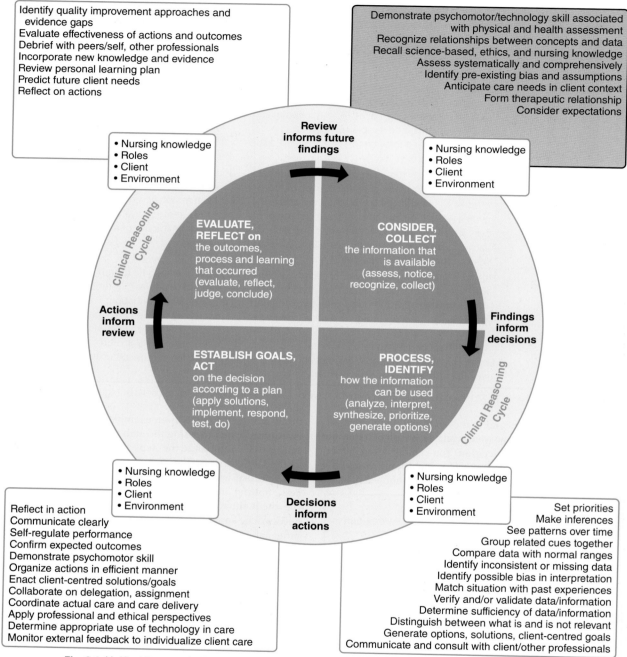

Identify quality improvement approaches and evidence gaps
Evaluate effectiveness of actions and outcomes
Debrief with peers/self, other professionals
Incorporate new knowledge and evidence
Review personal learning plan
Predict future client needs
Reflect on actions

Demonstrate psychomotor/technology skill associated with physical and health assessment
Recognize relationships between concepts and data
Recall science-based, ethics, and nursing knowledge
Assess systematically and comprehensively
Identify pre-existing bias and assumptions
Anticipate care needs in client context
Form therapeutic relationship
Consider expectations

• Nursing knowledge
• Roles
• Client
• Environment

Review informs future findings

• Nursing knowledge
• Roles
• Client
• Environment

Clinical Reasoning Cycle

EVALUATE, REFLECT on
the outcomes, process and learning that occurred (evaluate, reflect, judge, conclude)

CONSIDER, COLLECT
the information that is available (assess, notice, recognize, collect)

Actions inform review

Findings inform decisions

ESTABLISH GOALS, ACT
on the decision according to a plan (apply solutions, implement, respond, test, do)

PROCESS, IDENTIFY
how the information can be used (analyze, interpret, synthesize, prioritize, generate options)

Clinical Reasoning Cycle

• Nursing knowledge
• Roles
• Client
• Environment

Decisions inform actions

• Nursing knowledge
• Roles
• Client
• Environment

Reflect in action
Communicate clearly
Self-regulate performance
Confirm expected outcomes
Demonstrate psychomotor skill
Organize actions in efficient manner
Enact client-centred solutions/goals
Collaborate on delegation, assignment
Coordinate actual care and care delivery
Apply professional and ethical perspectives
Determine appropriate use of technology in care
Monitor external feedback to individualize client care

Set priorities
Make inferences
See patterns over time
Group related cues together
Compare data with normal ranges
Identify inconsistent or missing data
Identify possible bias in interpretation
Match situation with past experiences
Verify and/or validate data/information
Determine sufficiency of data/information
Distinguish between what is and is not relevant
Generate options, solutions, client-centred goals
Communicate and consult with client/other professionals

Fig. 3.1 Unified Process for Thinking and Decision Making: Applying the Clinical Reasoning Cycle.

Other clinical reasoning skills will also be presented in the next three chapters.

## Demonstrate Psychomotor/Technology Skill Associated With Physical and Health Assessment

The physical assessment skills that help with attaining more information about a client issue are key to the first step of nursing care. Nurses must apply the knowledge acquired from courses and other types of education on practical clinical skills and use the technology and equipment needed to conduct a health assessment.

*How Can You Develop This Skill?* Ask to observe and then practise new skills with the supervision of an experienced nurse or instructor. After a skill is learned, continually review it during laboratory practice times, seek opportunities to apply it to client care situations in real clinical settings, and discuss the skill with your peers. Build dexterity by repeating the skill. Learning new skills and technology that are used to improve care can further strengthen your capacity to assess clients and clinical situations.

## FOCUS ON TECHNOLOGY

### *Examples of Tools for Enhancing Assessment*

- Peripheral artery disease can be screened, in part, by assessing the ankle-brachial index (ABI). Systolic pressure is measured and recorded with a handheld noninvasive Doppler probe and a blood pressure cuff, and can be used to calculate the ABI as required.
- Remote presence robotic technology (RPRT) enables health care professionals to provide clinical services at a distance in real time over the Internet. In one pilot project, RPRT increased access to health care services for Indigenous people who live in remote communities in Saskatchewan. A group of community health nurses were supplied with computer tablets so that they could improve care and provide important health care information. The use of this technology was co-developed with Indigenous groups.
- A bladder scanner is a portable ultrasound device used to measure urinary retention (volume of urine remaining in the bladder after voiding). It can identify postvoid residual volume, which can help assess for urinary tract obstructions, the effects of medication, enlarged prostate, and other bladder-related issues.

Khan, I., Ndubuka, N., Stewart, K., et al. (2017). The use of technology to improve health care to Saskatchewan's First Nations communities. *Canada Communicable Disease Report, 43*(6), 120–124; Tyerman, J., & Cobbett, S. L. (2023). *Lewis's medical-surgical nursing in Canada: Assessment and management of clinical problems* (5th. ed.). Elsevier.

## Recognize Relationships Between Concepts and Data

The process of finding information often involves uncovering additional relevant information because evidence, best practice guidelines, or theoretical concepts indicate that more data should be collected. Identifying the relationship between evidence or concepts and more informed approaches to data collection provides a better picture of the client or health care issue at hand and enables better decisions about assessment. For instance, a nurse who collects observed data from a client with a fever, cloudy urine, and frequent voiding will relate that data to a possible urinary tract infection based on evidence and will follow guidelines for continued assessment that include a urine culture and analysis.

*How Can You Develop This Skill?* Study evidence sources, and understand relationships between evidence, concepts and informed data collection in courses and during clinical experiences and interactions with clients, families, and groups. As well, you can understand relationships between concepts and data by creating concept or mind maps that connect key concepts to data or cues, and by engaging in peer consultations.

## Recall Science-Based, Ethics, and Nursing Knowledge

Memorizing frequently encountered facts can facilitate their recall, especially as they relate to normal values and clinical manifestations of physical conditions. Nursing knowledge is science and research based, and grounded in ethical practice. During an assessment, confidentiality, respect for boundaries, and other elements required of an ethical code may be incorporated.

*How Can You Develop This Skill?* Because a large amount of information must be recalled in nursing, use memory tools, such as mnemonics (presented later in this chapter) and pocket notes or cards. Also, consult reference books, including drug manuals, that can assist with accurate recall and application of nursing knowledge. Ethical practice is developed by constant vigilance, review of ethical guidelines, and modelling peers or nurses with experience in various ethical dilemmas.

## Assess Systematically and Comprehensively

This skill is identified in several models of clinical thinking (refer back to Table 2.7) and has long been understood as a foundational skill for nurses. It refers to including everything that is important and relevant to the issue being assessed, and to collecting that information in an organized manner. An assessment plan that follows a systematic approach provides the nurse with a solid foundation for care. As well, a plan that incorporates diverse areas of assessment beyond the physical is more comprehensive. For instance, the assessment of a client's determinants of health can uncover information on their capacity to maintain a state of health beyond a formal health care facility (thinking *BIG* and *small* at the same time). A systematic and comprehensive approach can reduce the chance of missing information.

*How Can You Develop This Skill?* Use the same systematic and comprehensive approach as a baseline assessment tool in your everyday nursing practice. Doing so will improve your assessment performance. For instance, a full head-to-toe assessment or a modified or focused assessment that collects data on a particular body system in a head-to-toe orientation can be practised daily.

## Identify Pre-Existing Bias and Assumptions

This skill is crucial to finding accurate information that reflects the individual, unique client situation. If the nurse does not identify their own biases and assumptions, they risk overlooking important information that is needed to fully assess the client and provide optimal care.

*How Can You Develop This Skill?* Continually reflect on the different perspectives encountered in practice. Exhibit cultural humility by being open to learning about others' beliefs, customs, and practices. Ask yourself questions such as the following: *Am I checking back with the client to confirm what I think I have assessed? Do I really know why the client is responding the way they are? Am I basing my assessment on what I think I already know about this client or on what the client is telling me? Am I seeing this client as an individual who has unique needs?* and *Am I accepting without judgement that this is the client's preference and reality?* Many nursing schools and employers offer additional training that can help you develop this important skill.

## Anticipate Care Needs in Client Context

The ability to engage in anticipatory reflection involves a future-focused consideration of what may occur next, based on past experiences and learning. Predicting or anticipating what a client may need is a skill that seems to overlap with other skills, such as recognizing relationships between concepts and data. It may seem to conflict with identifying (and trying to reduce) pre-existing bias and assumptions. Also, it may seem to jump ahead into processing or analyzing data and other information. However,

when a nurse anticipates the client's care needs, the nurse can help expedite assessments or introduce pre-emptive care that prevents a significant, negative change in health status. It is *very important* to understand that anticipating care may be a starting point when finding information, but it may not be the end point. This is the essence of anticipatory reflection and client-centred care.

*How Can You Develop This Skill?* Develop this skill through experience and involvement in different contexts of care. Review case studies and share experiences with peers as well. When working with a client, you can anticipate what they may need, but always check with the client to see if your prediction was accurate.

## Form Therapeutic Relationship

This skill is essential to establishing trust and confidence in the client, and to practising competent, ethical care. Without this strong professional supportive relationship, finding information on the identified client issue may be a challenge. Barriers in the relationship—that stem from the nurse's or the client's perceptions—may lead to a client withholding information and the nurse missing relevant aspects of the issue, which prevents the collection of accurate, complete data. Professional standards should be adhered to in order to provide effective communication and safe care.

*How Can You Develop This Skill?* Review the processes for establishing safe, ethical, and therapeutic nurse–client relationships introduced in foundational nursing courses. Practise this skill using role play and during real-world clinical experiences. Developing information-finding skills, such as identifying bias and assumptions combined with psychomotor skills, can also help increase the confidence and trust required to build stronger nurse–client relationships.

## Consider Expectations

A subtle skill involved in finding information is the ability to identify expectations of the client (for their own health and health care) and other health care professionals (for the client's health outcomes). If expectations are not determined at an early stage, interpretation of the assessment information and future planning and delivery of care may not lead to the desired result.

*How Can You Develop This Skill?* Develop relationships and use clear communication skills with the client and other health care professionals. Also, understand the roles of others in the care of each client you work with. Initiating conversations with the client on their expectations can facilitate finding information and build bridges that lead to client-centred care.

## THINKING THROUGH THE APPLICATION OF CLINICAL REASONING SKILLS

### Case Scenario on Finding Information

An 80-year-old client is living in a long-term care facility. The client's medical history includes stroke, rheumatoid arthritis, and chronic atrial fibrillation. Their left arm has contractures. This morning, the client states that they have sharp abdominal pain, rated as 8/10 in intensity. The pain is intermittent and does not radiate. The client denies any vomiting, diarrhea, or nausea. A small bowel movement was documented yesterday. The client just voided 650 mL of clear urine. They are able to transfer from bed to wheelchair with assistance. They are able to tolerate medications as prescribed at 0800. The client reports increased abdominal pain after eating breakfast.

Reflect on these questions:
- What information requires immediate attention?
- What findings seem to be related and can be grouped together?
- Is any information missing? What else do you need to know, and how can you find out?
- What clinical reasoning skills would you apply to this scenario when finding information about the client situation?

Knowing the skills that are most useful for the first part of the nurse's thinking process is important. However, it is also important to be aware of obstacles that can arise and adversely affect thinking, and, thus, the process of finding information.

## BARRIERS TO THINKING WHEN FINDING INFORMATION

Inexperience with assessment skills can be a challenge for students and novice nurses. When conducting assessments, there are obvious and less obvious barriers to thinking that affect cue recognition, information gathering, and client observation.

The inability to systematically perceive and process all relevant cues is a key barrier to thinking, clinical judgement and the provision of safe, client-centred care. Inconsistent use of a nursing framework or model may prevent you from incorporating assessments that are directly related to the client's main issues or concerns and from anticipating future nursing care. Missing cues is a concern for nurses and can result if a systematic approach is not applied, especially when caring for clients whose condition and situation may be changing.

Distraction from the focus of a situation or identified client concern is problematic when finding information not just at the outset of the thinking process but at every step. Distraction occurs when one's attention is drawn away from the client or the primary activity. This barrier can include your own unrelated thoughts about other nursing or personal responsibilities, visual or auditory interruptions, your physical discomfort, or uncomfortable environmental conditions. Focusing on irrelevant data and information can be viewed as another type of distraction; it leads the nurse away from the focus of care in that moment.

## THINKING IT THROUGH

### Self-Reflection on Barriers to Finding Information

- What barriers have you noticed when gathering and seeking information?
- Recall instances when you have had trouble getting started with nursing care. Write them down.
- What do you think are the main challenges you have when finding information about a client situation?
- What is the cause (or causes) of the challenges? For example, is it a lack of knowledge about nursing, uncertainty about the tasks within your role, or distraction by too many cues?

Putting the client in the centre of care is what nurses do. However, client-centred care may be jeopardized if the nurse is unaware of their own biases. The terms unconscious bias and *implicit bias* refer to unrecognized stereotypes and ideas that one has about cultures or people that influence one's decision making and behaviours; it occurs outside of conscious awareness (Schultz & Baker, 2017). For instance, a nurse with an unconscious bias *against* a client could unwittingly negatively affect interpersonal interactions and harm the therapeutic nurse–client relationship. Unconscious bias also creates a barrier to cultural safety. In response, the client could view the nurse as unconcerned and, thus, lack trust and confidence in their care. The result may be that the client reduces engagement in their own health care and treatment, which increases health inequities in general. Box 3.1 describes an example of the negative effects of bias in policy and practice on finding information and the safe delivery of health care.

## HELPFUL STRATEGIES FOR FINDING INFORMATION

When conducting assessments and recognizing cues, nurses need to draw on retained knowledge and use it in many different situations. Remember that retained knowledge comes from long-term memory and information that was processed and understood. (Consider

---

**BOX 3.1   Preconceptions and Bias in Policy and Practice: An Example**

*An Indigenous mother recently called 9-1-1 after her 11-year-old daughter experienced a seizure. The daughter has epilepsy and her mother didn't realize that she had stopped taking her medication.*

*Once at the hospital, a nurse asked if the pre-teen had been consuming alcohol or drugs, to which the mother replied no. This question was asked again by at least three additional nurses and a doctor. She felt that this questioning was highly inappropriate given her daughter's age and the fact she is epileptic and was clearly having a seizure. The mother was advised by a nurse that these questions were "protocol."*

*She waited for nearly five hours before a doctor arrived to examine her daughter. Eventually, with no further communication from the staff, they left the hospital. The mother describes the experience for her daughter as "horrible."[a]*

A single negative experience like this one can cause clients to not seek or delay seeking treatment until their condition is serious. Whether a particular practice is part of a workplace's policy, people should be given a clear rationale for assessment and care and reassured that they are not being singled out. Clear, respectful assessment is key to creating safe health care experiences and shared decision making.

[a]British Columbia College of Nurses and Midwives. (2022). *Indigenous cultural safety, cultural humility and antiracism: Practice standard companion guide.* p. 26. https://www.bccnm.ca/Documents/cultural_safety_humility/ps_companion_guide.pdf

---

this when you "cram" for an exam. Doing so puts a strain on your short-term memory, making it hard to fully process and retain knowledge. It is not an effective strategy.) Systematic approaches to thinking, tools to remember the various components to an assessment, and mindful reflection on how one is thinking (recall the concept of metacognition) can help overcome barriers to finding information.

## Using Mnemonics

How can you recall facts and content related to client assessment in a timely manner? Cognitive tools such as mnemonics can help you remember and apply science-based information and nursing knowledge that you need to access frequently.

A **mnemonic** is a device—such as a pattern of letters, ideas, or associations—for remembering facts and information more easily. Health care professionals use mnemonics regularly to recall prior learning during the provision of care (Putnam, 2015; Woodfin et al., 2018). Mnemonics help nurses actively translate concepts into actions and interventions. Moreover, using mnemonics early in a health care professional program can aid diagnostic reasoning (Amey et al., 2017; Senger & Smith, 2020).

Some common mnemonics take the form of alphabetized letters that help jog the memory on what is needed in a complete assessment. When thinking about general approaches to assessments and prioritizing what to assess first (*Where should I start?*), the mnemonic *ABCD* (*a*irway, *b*reathing, *c*irculation, and *d*isability) can help (Tyerman & Cobbett, 2023). In fact, the ABCD survey can be conducted at any point in the care process and is a quick way to prioritize information. It can also help identify important cues that could indicate life-threatening conditions (Table 3.3). Other types of alphabetized mnemonics can help Canadian nursing students recall how to plan care of clients with increased intracranial pressure (Hussein & Jakubec, 2015).

**TABLE 3.3   Cues and Conditions\* Identified in a Primary Survey (ABCD)**

| Airway Cues | Airway Conditions |
|---|---|
| Audible wheezing | Inhalation injury |
| Work of breathing | Obstruction |
| Panic/anxiety | Trauma |
| **Breathing Cues** | **Breathing Conditions** |
| Abnormal respiratory rate | Shock (i.e., anaphylaxis) |
| Chest excursion | Chest injury |
| Pain | |
| **Circulation Cues** | **Circulation Conditions** |
| Heart rate | Direct cardiac injury |
| Blood pressure |   (infarction, trauma) |
| Oxygen saturation | Tamponade |
| Peripheral circulation | Shock (i.e., hypovolemic) |
| | Hemorrhage |
| | Hypothermia |
| **Disability Cues** | **Disability Conditions** |
| Level of consciousness and response | Head injury |
| | Stroke |
| Glasgow Coma Scale score | |

\*Not all inclusive.

Adapted from Tyerman, J., & Cobbett, S. L. (2023). *Lewis's medical-surgical nursing in Canada: Assessment and management of clinical problems* (5th ed.) (p. 1777). Elsevier.

## TABLE 3.4   Assessing Symptoms Using OPQRSTUV

| OPQRSTUV Words | Associated Questions |
|---|---|
| *O*nset | When did it start? How long? How often? |
| *P*rovoking/palliating | What makes it better or worse? |
| *Q*uality | What does it feel like? |
| *R*egion/Radiation | Where is it? Does it spread? |
| *S*everity | Rate on a scale from 0 (no symptom) to 10 (worst possible experience of symptom) |
| *T*reatment | What medications or therapies have been used, and are they effective? |
| *U*nderstanding impact | What do you understand about what is happening? How is this symptom affecting you or your family? |
| *V*alues | What is your goal for managing this symptom? What is most important to you in this situation? |

Adapted from Fraser Health. (2017). *Symptom assessment acronym.* https://www.fraserhealth.ca/-/media/Project/FraserHealth/Fraser-Health/Health-Professionals/Professionals-Resources/Hospice-palliative-care/SymptomAssessmentRevised_Sept09.pdf.

Another alphabetical mnemonic used to assess symptoms such as pain or shortness of breath is *OPQRSTUV* (*o*nset, *p*rovoking/palliating, *q*uality, *r*egion/radiation, *s*everity, *t*reatment, *u*nderstanding impact, and *v*alues). When a client reports a symptom or the nurse observes behaviours that may indicate the client is experiencing a specific symptom, applying OPQRSTUV can be a helpful strategy (Astle & Duggleby, 2024). Using this mnemonic can provide the nurse with more complete information and reduce the risk of missing cues. Table 3.4 presents this mnemonic and assessment questions associated with each component.

An **acronym** is a word, pronounced as such, that is created from the initial letters of other words; it is used to describe something in an abbreviated way. For instance, *SCUBA* diving describes diving while using a *s*elf-*c*ontained *u*nderwater *b*reathing *a*pparatus. A *LASER* beam describes *l*ight *a*mplification by *s*timulated *e*mission of *r*adiation. *LASIK* describes the procedure *l*aser-*a*ssisted in-*s*itu *k*eratomileusis. These acronyms are pronounced "scuba," "laser," and "Lasik," and have become words themselves. They are used so frequently in this form that often the original meaning may not be widely known. In health care, other examples are as follows, which can help you recall the full name of these conditions:

- *AIDS*—*a*cquired *i*mmune *d*eficiency *s*yndrome (pronounced *AIDS*, not spelled out as *A-I-D-S*)
- *SARS*—*s*evere *a*cute *r*espiratory *s*yndrome (pronounced *SARS*, not spelled out as *S-A-R-S*)

*OLD CARTS* (*o*nset, *l*ocation/radiation, *d*uration, *c*haracter, *a*ggravating factors, *r*elieving factors, *t*iming, and *s*everity) is an acronym that can be used to remember questions to ask while assessing the client's history of present illness. This acronym is similar in function to the alphabetic symptom-assessment mnemonic *ABCD*. Use whichever one makes sense to you and your clients, and is most easily remembered. A "sweet" way of remembering the nursing process is thinking of it as easy "as a pie," or *AAPIE* (*a*ssessment, *a*nalysis, *p*lanning, *i*mplementation, and *e*valuation). Acronyms are helpful because they enable easy recall of longer names or descriptions of a process.

An **acrostic** is a saying, phrase, rhyme, or some other composition taken from letters in a group of words in order that is used to improve recall of a number of items or concepts. Acrostics can be useful when conducting a health assessment. For example, to recall and cite the 12 cranial nerves (olfactory, optic, oculomotor, trochlear, trigeminal, abducens, facial, auditory [vestibulocochlear], glossopharyngeal, vagus, spinal accessory, and hypoglossal), the acrostic "On Old Olympus's Towering Tops, a Finn and German Viewed Some Hops" can be used. The resulting composition or poem may not make much sense, but the key is to jog recall and retrieve knowledge quickly so that it can help with seeking and finding information in a health care setting, and when preparing to provide care to a client.

Additional shortened terms are used in health care to facilitate communication. Although they are not necessarily used as memory tools to recall or organize information, *initialisms* are terms pronounced as a series of letters. For example, "shortness of breath" is shortened to the letters *SOB*, "intravenous" is shortened to the letters *IV*, and "body mass index" is shortened to the letters *BMI*. Some sources refer to initialisms as "acronyms" or "abbreviations."

In health care, *abbreviations,* or shortened forms of words or phrases, are used to efficiently communicate information (e.g., "amp" is an abbreviation of *ampoule*). Safety and *accuracy* are so important in the use of abbreviations in health care that the Institute for Safe Medication Practices Canada (ISMP Canada) has generated a list of dangerous abbreviations that should not be used. See the Online Resources at the end of this chapter.

## ❓ THINKING IT THROUGH

### *Self-Reflection on Using Recall Strategies*

- What strategies do you use to help recall what to do when finding information?
- Think about the mnemonics and other memory tools you have come across, and write them down.
- Which do you use more frequently? Why?
- Have you ever created a memory tool of your own? Describe it.
- How can you remember to use recall strategies to augment your thinking, specifically when finding information?

The challenge with these various memory prompts and tools that can be used to learn facts, recall information, or help organize nursing actions is that no single one will work in all areas. For example, other prompts that will be described in later chapters are used to specifically improve the communication of information rather than help to recall facts. Therefore, perhaps ironically, students must think critically about the utility of specific cognitive tools that will enhance their performance as they seek information on a client during assessment. Applying critical thinking traits such as reflection, awareness, and mindfulness can assist with this thinking.

### Practising Mindfulness

Mindfulness is a reflective strategy involving concepts including metacognition, attention, and awareness. To become mindful, a person must pay attention to what is happening in a particular way and with purpose, be present in the moment, and adopt a nonjudgemental stance (Tusaie & Edds, 2009). Mindfulness can be used to address implicit or unconscious bias and reduce the occurrence of inadequate assessments and suboptimal care (Craig, 2022). Ponte and Koppel (2015) developed the *STOP* mindfulness technique for nursing practice to bring awareness to bias and assumptions. Before beginning nursing care, consider practising the following:

- **S**top what you are doing.
- **T**ake slow, deep breaths.
- **O**bserve your thoughts, feelings, and assumptions.
- **P**roceed with client care.

As a form of reflection, the STOP mindfulness technique may also be used during client care, when confirming or needing to redirect care. The act of observing one's thoughts and identifying how they may impact nursing actions in either a positive or negative way is one strategy to become aware of bias. Adhering to standards and competencies, codes of ethics, and client-centred care approaches are others.

When finding information that could inform future thinking and actions, the nurse is mindful of oppression, social justice, and bias. This reflective stance contributes to a safer and more effective care process. When health care practitioners become aware of barriers in their own thinking (and in the health care system), those barriers can be addressed and overcome. In a Canadian study, co-authored by Indigenous Elders and researchers, Two-Eyed Seeing and a sharing circle methodology were used to explore Indigenous clients' experiences of racism and their views on improving cultural safety in health care (Pilarinos et al., 2023). The study proposed that mandatory cultural safety education for health care providers can encourage self-reflection on negative consequences of colonial perspectives, reduce unconscious bias, and improve trust in the health care system and culturally safe client care.

As a nurse, being continually mindful and reflective can improve care, client trust, and the nurse–client relationship. Actions that support self-reflective practice include:

- Be aware of biases that negatively affect practice and make changes to address them.
- Acknowledge others' cultural identities.
- Listen to others' experiences and ask about their concerns and goals.
- Be open to hearing and learning about another's perspective and view of the world.
- Don't make assumptions about another person's feelings or way of thinking.
- Ask for and use feedback on your practice to gain experience and improve (British Columbia College of Nurses and Midwives, 2022, p. 13).

## ✳ TOOLBOX FOR THINKING

Some strategies to use when finding information include:

- Boost your cognitive recall and ability to use stored information by applying mnemonics.
- Practise mindfulness by pausing before a nursing activity and situating yourself in the moment of care.

Finding information can be daunting. Having clinical reasoning skills and various memory tools available to you may help. Another strategy that can be used to find comprehensive information is the NRCE framework (see Chapter 2).

## THINKING THROUGH FINDING INFORMATION: NRCE

Most often, *a primary issue drives the initiation of nursing care.* This issue may be a medical diagnosis, a change in the client's health status, a voiced or perceived client or family concern, a communication from another health care provider, or a result from a laboratory report. In other health care contexts, the primary issue may be a verified change in population health, a reported community need, or an identified gap in policy. How fully the issue is addressed by the nurse depends on the initial information that is assessed, noticed, recognized, and collected.

The NRCE framework used in this textbook can help guide you to recall the wide range of influences on a client care situation when finding information. The NRCE components represent and include primary, secondary, and tertiary sources of information, as well as objective and subjective observations. It is crucial to realize that the four components, which contribute to every step of thinking and decision making (*finding* information, *deciding* how to use the information, *acting* on the decision, and *reviewing* the actions), are interrelated.

*What do I need to assess?* The physical assessment of the client will include objective and subjective observations, and laboratory and diagnostic reports. However, nurses will incorporate more than this information in this first step of the thinking and decision-making process. They will also seek information on the client, the client situation, and the health care environment, which ultimately affect how the client's needs are met and whether outcomes are achieved.

Using the NRCE framework, the nurse can pick up on more than just the physical assessment cues from the client. A good decision that leads to a positive outcome cannot be accomplished if relevant elements of the client situation are missed and if a comprehensive approach is not taken. To illustrate how finding information can be undertaken using the NRCE framework, an example of a client who presents with chest pain will be used. This framework can help you answer the question, *How will I collect relevant information?*

## Nursing Knowledge

The *N* in *NRCE* relates to nursing knowledge. This component highlights the importance of using various sources, critical thinking skills, and reasoning skills in practice. *Nursing knowledge is needed when finding information and at every step of thinking and decision making.*

When seeking information about an issue that is the focus of a nursing care activity, the nurse draws on various sources of knowledge from different disciplines. This knowledge supports the nurse as they conduct physical and other assessments as needed, and recall facts and how concepts relate to one another so that adequate information is gathered. Assessments are relevant to the client issue, admitting diagnosis, and the priority communicated in a hand-off report. Memory strategies can help nurses more easily recall facts and what to assess (e.g., acrostics to remember cranial nerve assessment of clients with neurological conditions, head-to-toe physical assessments).

### Example

A client reports a sudden, crushing pain and pressure in their chest.

The nursing knowledge to consider when finding information includes:

- Anatomy and pathophysiology of the heart
- Mechanisms of pain
- Significance of a family history of cardiac conditions
- Physical assessment (primarily of the cardiovascular and respiratory systems)
- Nurse–client therapeutic relationship theory

If this client was born female and reported atypical discomfort such as neck or jaw pain, the nurse may draw on knowledge about alternate presentations of myocardial infarctions in women to recognize the presenting cue as relevant. Also, while it may seem important to assess the client more comprehensively, it is crucial to focus the initial assessment to help either identify or rule out a significant cardiac event in this case.

## Professional Roles

The *R* in *NRCE* relates to professional roles—the roles and scopes of practice of the nurse and other health care professionals. When finding information, the aim of the nurse is to conduct assessments that are in line with their educational preparation, regulatory requirements, and provincial law. The nurse conducts assessments relevant to their experience and required level of competence and safety. *An awareness of the nursing role in particular is needed when finding information and at every step of thinking and decision making.*

When finding information about an aspect of client care, it is essential for the nurse to understand their scope of practice, required competencies, ethics, and their personal assumptions and biases. Intra- and interprofessional collaboration is a required competency, which means that the nurse must understand the scopes of practice and purpose of other health care professionals' roles (i.e., physician, nurse practitioner, physiotherapist, and dietitian).

A nurse assigned to a client whose assessment requires a blood sample for diagnostic testing must consider several aspects of their professional role before proceeding. Does the nurse's scope of practice include venipuncture? Is the nurse a regulated health care professional who can perform phlebotomy in the jurisdiction in which they practice? Does the nurse have formal education and experience in phlebotomy? Does the nurse have the capacity to manage various outcomes of care? A nurse would not be able to engage in drawing a blood sample as an assessment component if these criteria were not met. On the other hand, a nurse practitioner has a broader scope of practice that includes the authority to order X-rays for diagnostic testing, as well as order and perform ultrasounds (refer to authorization mechanisms for each jurisdiction).

---

### Example

A client reports a sudden, crushing pain and pressure in their chest.

Aspects of professional roles and scopes of practice to consider when finding information include:

- Scope of practice in current nursing position (student nurse, registered nurse, registered practical nurse, nurse practitioner, etc.)
- Ability to order, apply, and interpret electrocardiograms in an acute circumstance
- Roles of other health care professionals who may be present to direct other assessment activities and delegate or assign care
- Professional development and needs of nurse(s)
- Team leadership and role within a team setting
- Communication with other health care providers that is clear, appropriate, and safe

Being clear on your own scope of practice—and its limitations—is necessary for safe assessments and for collaborating on finding information.

---

## Client Context

The *C* in *NRCE* relates to the client context. When finding information that will eventually inform care and decision making, recall that the client is a key source of knowledge. *Attention to the client context is needed when finding information and at every step of thinking and decision making.*

The client's experiences and feelings toward health care and their own health—their values—are respected and incorporated when providing care. An actual assessment may be conducted that is specific to the client's needs, reported concern, situation, or behaviour. This assessment may relate to physical, mental, social, or spiritual aspects of health and well-being. The nurse adapts to the client's communication preferences to obtain assessment data and information in a culturally safe manner; this can include communicating in the client's preferred language or addressing the client in the way they wish to be identified or named. Family and other people in the client's circle may need to be included to gather information, while maintaining client confidentiality. Client dignity is protected, and autonomy is preserved according to the client situation. The context of the client (or the family, defined group, community, or population) is observed fully. The nurse–client relationship is professional, relational, and therapeutic and is based on the nurse's and the client's collaborative understanding of the client's context.

---

### Example

A client reports a sudden, crushing pain and pressure in their chest.

Aspects of the client context to consider when finding information include:

- Family dynamics, health history, and family relationships
- Client internal fears and anxiety about their current experience and external stressors
- Past experiences with similar pain, if relevant, or perceptions of what is happening
- Client understanding of their own health, personal goals, and learning needs
- Cultural, religious, or spiritual backgrounds that have meaning for the client
- Communication preferences or strategies, and possible barriers
- Gender identification

These examples illustrate the depth of understanding that a nurse must have of the client and their unique context to find relevant information and recognize cues. While not all of the aspects listed are specific to chest pain, you can see how this information is needed to establish a trusting nurse–client relationship that is foundational for initiating the care process and finding accurate, truthful clinical data and other information.

---

## Health Care Environment

The *E* in *NRCE* relates to the health care environment. The setting that the client is in—acute care, long-term care, palliation, at home, or (more broadly) in a provincial or national context—must be considered when finding information. *Understanding the health care environment is needed when finding information and at every step of thinking and decision making.*

Noticing the client's surroundings, recognizing what is happening around the client, assessing the environment, and gathering information from sources external to the client increase the nurse's situation awareness. Elements of the health care environment that the nurse would take note of when finding information include the following: the amount, nature, and condition (ECG) of equipment needed to conduct required assessments; the nurse-to-client ratio on a unit; policies and procedures; the organizational culture; and professional and occupational supports for the safe collection of information. It is also important to consider how these elements may influence assessments.

**Example**

A client reports a sudden, crushing pain and pressure in their chest.

Elements of the health care environment to consider when finding information include:

- Availability and working condition of ECG and other equipment needed to conduct assessment
- Presence of qualified care providers to contribute to assessment activities
- Use of policies and procedures for initiating emergency care (i.e., code)
- Distractions in the immediate setting that occur while finding information (e.g., other conversations, interruptions)
- Existence of perceived or actual safety supports
- Institution-approved processes or guidelines as criteria for initiating care

Table 3.5 presents a summary of the NRCE components applied to finding information in a nursing scenario on chest pain. You may notice that the NRCE topics and areas can overlap and are interconnected. For example, an immunosuppressed client reporting chest pain in a particular acute care environment may have limited family visits because of infection control policies or a COVID-19 pandemic. The client's nurse may be challenged to communicate with and gather relevant information on a client whose condition is changing because they are a new graduate and have not encountered the presenting clinical situation before. This example highlights how nursing knowledge of relevant physical and other assessments, professional roles, client needs and preferences, and institutional policy are interconnected and affect one another. It also demonstrates the complexity of nursing care and the need to think thoughtfully and systematically.

It is important to understand that because each clinical situation and client circumstance is different, not all components of the NRCE framework will apply with equal weight each time. At some points, only one, two, or three components—either $N$ or $R$ or $C$ or $E$—will be most important. That is fine. Recall that this framework is meant to help guide thinking and to ensure that as holistic a picture as possible of the client is captured. It is important to note

| TABLE 3.5 | Using NRCE When Finding Information on a Client Reporting Chest Pain |
| --- | --- |
| **NRCE** | **What to Consider** |
| **Nursing** Knowledge | <ul><li>Anatomy and pathophysiology of the heart</li><li>Mechanisms of pain</li><li>Family history of cardiac conditions</li><li>Physical assessment of cardiovascular and respiratory systems (e.g., *ABCD* as a mnemonic)</li><li>Nurse–client therapeutic relationship</li></ul> |
| Professional **Roles** | <ul><li>Scope of practice in current nursing position</li><li>Use of ECGs in an acute circumstance</li><li>Roles of other health care professionals for directing, delegating, or assigning care</li><li>Reflection on professional development and needs of nurse(s)</li><li>Leadership of team and role within a team setting</li><li>Communication with other health care providers</li></ul> |
| **Client** Context | <ul><li>Family dynamics and relationships</li><li>Client internal fears and anxiety, and external stressors</li><li>Past experiences or perceptions of what is happening</li><li>Client's personal health goals and learning needs</li><li>Cultural, religious, or spiritual background</li><li>Communication preferences or strategies, and possible barriers</li><li>Gender identification</li></ul> |
| Health Care **Environment** | <ul><li>Equipment needed to conduct assessment</li><li>Presence of qualified care providers</li><li>Use of policies and procedures for initiating emergency care (i.e., code)</li><li>Distractions in the immediate setting</li><li>Existence of perceived or actual safety supports</li><li>Institution-approved processes or guidelines as criteria for initiating care</li></ul> |

that nurses must continually look beyond the obvious and critically think at every step of thinking, no matter the nursing framework or model they use for thinking and decision making.

Finding information is the first step in *thinking it through*. However, significant overlap exists with a couple of skills involved in deciding what to do: analyzing and interpreting (Chapter 4). For example, when *analyzing* findings, the

nurse may *interpret* that something is missing or not making sense, or that more questions need to be answered to make a reasonable plan or goal. Finding important information is foundational to care. Therefore, the nurse will return to this first step of the thinking and decision-making process when information gaps need to be filled or when it becomes apparent that an aspect of noticing was missed. Going back to find more information is sometimes necessary.

**TABLE 3.6   Case Study: Application of the Clinical Reasoning Cycle to Finding Information**

| Client Situation | Nursing Model and Application of Thinking | | |
| --- | --- | --- | --- |
| | Clinical Reasoning Cycle[a] | Clinical Reasoning Skills Used | Possible Nursing Responses (Barriers, Strategies) |
| 64-year-old male, recent widower, arrives at hospital at 0715 with reported chest pain; history of dyslipidemia, obese | | | |
| **Handover report at 0720:** Client arrived with chest pain that woke him up this morning. Pain at 7/10. IV started normal saline to keep vein open. ECG administered; physician called. Oxygen at 6 L/min, saturation 97%. | ***Consider the client situation:*** Describe facts, contexts, situations, and people. | Identify pre-existing bias and assumptions. Anticipate care needs in client context. Form therapeutic relationship. Consider Expectations. | Check biases and assumptions. Ensure knowledge of anatomy, clinical manifestations. Provide supportive care environment. Confirm goals of care with client. |
| **Assessments at 0725:** Temperature—37°C (98.6°F) Pulse rate—112 bpm Respiratory rate—22 bpm Blood pressure—145/90 mm Hg Restless, reports anxiety, diaphoretic | ***Collect cues/information:*** • Review available information from handover reports, history and charts, previous medical and nursing assessments. • Gather new information. • Recall knowledge from the sciences, pharmacology, nursing therapeutics and scope of practice, client learning, and the health care environment. | Demonstrate psycho-motor/ technology skill associated with physical and health assessment. Recognize relationships between concepts and data. Recall science-based, ethics, and nursing knowledge. Assess systematically and comprehensively. | Measure current vital signs. What will they tell you? Can you anticipate what they may be? Consider the link between vital signs and client presentation. Recall strategies for assessing pain. |
| | Process information (interpret, discriminate, relate, infer, match, predict) | *Consider next steps. What will you do with what you have found out?* | |
| | *Identify problems/issues . . .* | | |
| | *Establish goal(s) . . .* | | |
| | *Take action . . .* | | |
| | *Evaluate outcomes . . .* | | |
| | *Reflect on process and learning . . .* | | |

Note: Only the steps relating to finding information are covered in the descriptions in this table.
[a]Levett-Jones, T., Hoffman, K., Dempsey, J., et al. (2010). The "five rights" of clinical reasoning: An educational model to enhance nursing students' ability to identify and manage clinically "at risk" clients. *Nurse Education Today, 30*(6), 515–520.

# FINDING INFORMATION: A CLINICAL REASONING CYCLE CASE STUDY

This chapter demonstrated how various skills and strategies can be used when finding information in nursing practice. The NRCE framework can be applied as a guide to help you fully assess, notice, recognize, and collect information from all relevant areas. Now, we will consider how finding information can be applied in practice, using the clinical reasoning cycle (CRC) (Levett-Jones et al., 2010) as an example nursing model. The CRC will be applied to a simple case study, using the example of a client who presents with chest pain. As you may recall, the CRC (described in Chapter 2) includes "consider the client situation" and "collect cues/information," two steps that are particularly salient to

finding information. Refer back to Table 2.4 for details on the steps in this nursing model.

The case study in Table 3.6 incorporates key ideas covered in this chapter, including the clinical reasoning skills described earlier. As well, it addresses possible responses to barriers to thinking and strategies to overcome those barriers.

In each of the next three chapters, a different nursing model will be applied to a case study. Using a different nursing model each time will illustrate that any model can be applied to any case or client situation, and that any step of the thinking process (*finding* information, *deciding* what to do, *acting* on the decision, and *reviewing* the action) can be thought through using specific skills and a common framework.

## SUMMARY

This chapter built on the basic concepts in the first two chapters and presents the first step of the thinking process: finding information. Without adequate information, the nurse will not be informed in any future thinking and will be unable to provide safe, competent, and ethical client-centred care. The approaches and skills used for finding information in this chapter were illustrated in a case study using the clinical reasoning cycle (Levett-Jones et al., 2010). However, they can be applied to any model.

## KEY POINTS TO REMEMBER

These are the key points to remember from this chapter.

### About the Importance of Finding Information as a First Step

- Having the most appropriate information, which includes data, evidence, and resources, on which to base thinking is essential for optimal care and nursing practice.
- Research evidence is a basis for professional and efficient decision making in practice.
- Check assumptions about whether evidence—science and research based—is valid, relevant, and appropriate to the context of client care.
- Nursing theories help provide a systematic view of nursing phenomena so that the phenomena can be explained or predicted.
- Nursing, health, client or person, and environment are overarching and consistent concepts that are embedded in nursing theories and shape nurses' thinking and professional work.
- Having discipline-specific knowledge and a theoretical base is part of what defines nursing as a profession and guides nurses' thinking processes, including how they seek information.
- Nursing theories often help nurses to place clients at the centre of care.

- Client-centred care reflects the importance of the nurse coming to know the whole client when assessing the client condition, or when seeking and gathering information.
- *Situation awareness* is being cognizant of what is happening around you and understanding what that information means, now and in the future.
- Situation awareness comprises three levels: perception of elements in the environment, comprehension of the current situation, and projection of future status.
- Perception of elements in the environment, the first level in situation awareness, involves assessment in a holistic manner to produce optimal results in future decision making.

### About Skills Used When Finding Information

- The unified process for thinking and decision making (see Figure 3.1) includes a number of skills that can be useful when finding information:
  - Demonstrate psychomotor/technology skill associated with physical and health assessment.
  - Recognize relationships between concepts and data.
  - Recall science-based, ethics, and nursing knowledge.
  - Assess systematically and comprehensively.
  - Identify pre-existing bias and assumptions.

- Anticipate care needs in client context.
- Form therapeutic relationships.
- Consider expectations.

### About Barriers to Thinking When Finding Information

- Barriers to thinking when finding information may lead to missing cues or focusing on irrelevant information at the start of the thinking process.
- Unconscious or implicit bias is a barrier to finding accurate and relevant information.

### About Helpful Strategies for Finding Information

- Strategies that can be used to overcome barriers to finding information include systematic approaches to thinking, mnemonics, and mindfulness techniques.

### About Thinking Through Finding Information: NRCE

- This textbook's NRCE framework provides a holistic view of assessing, noticing, recognizing, and gathering information in the first step of the thinking process.

### About a Case Study on Finding Information

- A case study showed how the key ideas in this chapter can be brought together in the first step of the nurse's thinking and decision-making process toward optimal client care.

## CONCLUSION AND THINKING IT THROUGH

The skills identified in this chapter are needed for clearer thinking when finding information about a client situation, and for assessing, noticing, recognizing, and collecting data.

Remember that critical thinking is a general term that describes the purposeful, informed, and self-regulated ability to connect ideas aimed at increasing the likelihood of a desired outcome. It is *a full set of adaptable skills, attitudes, and knowledge* that is needed in nursing practice.

In the next few chapters, more skills that support other steps of the thinking process will be explored. You will note that they will also be useful elsewhere in your daily life.

## CLASS ACTIVITIES TO CHECK THINKING

### Think-Aloud Pair Problem Solve (TAPPS)

Form pairs. Decide who will be a problem solver and listener for Problem A. The problem solver reads the problem aloud and talks through a response to the problem, while the listener reminds the problem solver to think aloud, asks clarification questions, offers encouragement to keep thinking, but refrains from providing possible answers. Switch roles for Problem B.

For each of these problems, apply a thinking strategy for finding information.

- **Problem A:** A 75-year-old client admitted to hospital for undiagnosed delirium is not eating. They pick at the cereal, sandwiches, and stew and potatoes provided on the meal trays. The client's family states that they always cooked their own food at home. The nurse is concerned about adequate nutritional intake.
- **Problem B:** A nursing student is suddenly tearful during a clinical shift and withdrawn during post-conference discussions. The student is usually shy and lacks confidence. The student's peer wonder how they should respond.

When finished, discuss with each other any differences and similarities in finding information about client issues and professional issues.

### Activities and Discussion Questions

1. Identify a nursing assessment (or clinical manifestations related to a clinical situation) that you find difficult to remember. Create an acronym, acrostic, or some other memory tool that will help you to recall that knowledge more easily. Share it with your peers.

2. Reflect on a recent assessment activity that you performed in a clinical or laboratory setting. Group your assessment actions into the NRCE framework components (N, R, C, and E). Consider what may have been missed or overlooked.

3. Visit the website of the Implicit Association Test at https://implicit.harvard.edu/implicit/takeatest.html. Choose a category to explore any hidden biases you may have. From the results, individually reflect on what this may mean to the assessments and observations you make during your interactions with clients. Would you miss, or overlook, collecting data because of any biases you identify? Make a plan to address any results you discover.

## CASE STUDY REVIEW

In small groups, discuss the case study that was described in Table 3.6. How will the clinical scenario continue, and how could it conclude? Base your thinking on the clinical reasoning cycle and the information that was discovered. Consider your current nursing knowledge.

## EVIDENCE-INFORMED THINKING ACTIVITY

Review information in Table 3.1. Select a type of physical assessment (pain, blood pressure, pressure injury, or another of your choosing) and find at least two resources that can help you complete a detailed assessment. The resources may be a measurement tool or scale, best practice guideline, survey, etc., and may be associated with other related assessments such as psychological, cultural or social aspects of health. Answer the following questions.

1. What evidence is there to support the resources that you found (how do you know that they are valid and reliable)?
2. How will information gained from using more than one resource provide a better assessment (or not)?

## QUESTIONS TO ASSESS LEARNING

### Review Questions

1. Which phrase best reflects the meaning of unconscious bias in nursing?
   a. Deliberate and intentional discriminatory behaviour toward clients
   b. Conscious and evidence-informed decision based on objective evidence
   c. Automatic and unintentional prejudice or stereotype that influences judgements and actions
   d. Random and unpredictable pattern of favouritism toward certain client groups
2. Which statement best describes the importance of situation awareness (SA) in nursing care?
   a. SA enables the nurse to effectively multitask.
   b. The ability to assess cues in a holistic way is increased by SA.
   c. Only nurses in critical care settings use SA.
   d. SA is used to administer medications accurately.
3. What is the benefit of using mnemonics when finding information in nursing practice?
   a. Allows for the nurse to quickly retrieve learned information
   b. Provides a fun way to describe illnesses to clients
   c. Always presents information alphabetically
   d. Clarifies the rationale for seeking information

## ONE LAST THOUGHT

How will you know that you have found sufficient, relevant information about an issue before moving to the next steps in the thinking process?

## ONLINE RESOURCES

*Acceptable abbreviations for prescription health product labels in Canada* (2017). Canada: ISMP. https://www.ismp-canada.org/download/Acceptable-Abbreviations-Canada.pdf.
*Common nursing mnemonics* (2021). Western Governors University. https://www.wgu.edu/blog/common-nursing-mnemonics2110.html#close.
*Do not use: Dangerous abbreviations, symbols and dose designations* (2006). Canada: Institute for Safe Medication Practices. https://ismpcanada.ca/wp-content/uploads/2022/02/ISMP-CanadaListOfDangerousAbbreviations.pdf.

Example of the use of a client education mnemonic in Canada—Page, C. (2019). Evaluating the effectiveness of a mnemonic to guide staff when providing patient education to autologous hematopoietic stem cell transplant patients. *Canadian Oncology Nursing Journal, 29*(2), 123–131. https://www.ncbi.nlm.nih.gov/pmc/articles/PMC6516336/.

## REFERENCES

Amey, L., Donald, K. J., & Teodorczuk, A. (2017). Teaching clinical reasoning to medical students. *British Journal of Hospital Medicine, 78*(7), 399–401. doi:10.12968/hmed.2017.78.7.399.

Astle, B., & Duggleby, W. (2024). *Potter and Perry's Canadian fundamentals of nursing* (7th ed.). Elsevier Inc.

British Columbia College of Nurse and Midwives. (2022). *Indigenous cultural safety, cultural humility and anti-racism: Practice standard companion guide.* https://www.bccnm.ca/Documents/cultural_safety_humility/ps_companion_guide.pdf.

Canadian Cardiovascular Society. (2020). Hypertension Canada's 2020 comprehensive guidelines for the prevention, diagnosis, risk assessment, and treatment of hypertension in adults and children. https://doi.org/10.1016/j.cjca.2020.02.086

Carper, B. A. (1978). Fundamental patterns of knowing in nursing. *Advances in Nursing Science, 1*(1), 13–23.

Chinn, P. L., Kramer, M. K., & Sitzman, K. (2022). *Knowledge development in nursing: Theory and process.* Elsevier.

Craig, D. J. (2022). Strategies to recognize and address implicit bias in healthcare. *Nursing News, 46*(4), 14–15.

Ellis, J. A., Ootoova, A., Blouin, R., et al. (2011). Establishing the psychometric properties and preferences for the Northern Pain Scale. *International Journal of Circumpolar Health, 70*(3), 274–285.

Endsley, M. R., & Jones, D. G. (2012). *Designing for situation awareness: An approach to user-centred design* (2nd ed.). CRC Press.

Fawcett, J. (1995). *Analysis and evaluation of conceptual models of nursing* (3rd ed.). F. A. Davis.

Fraser Health. (2017). *Symptom assessment acronym.* https://www.fraserhealth.ca/-/media/Project/FraserHealth/FraserHealth/Health-Professionals/Professionals-Resources/Hospice-palliative-care/SymptomAssessmentRevised_Sept09.pdf.

Hockenberry, M. J., & Wilson, D. (2006). *Wong's nursing care of infants and children* (8th ed.). Elsevier Mosby.

Hussein, M. T. E., & Jakubec, S. L. (2015). An alphabetical mnemonic teaching strategy for constructing nursing care plans. *Journal of Nursing Education, 54*(1), 57–59. https://doi.org/10.3928/01484834-20141224-03.

Khan, I., Ndubuka, N., Stewart, K., et al. (2017). The use of technology to improve health care to Saskatchewan's First Nations communities. *Canada Communicable Disease Report, 43*(6), 120–124.

Levett-Jones, T., Hoffman, K., Dempsey, J., et al. (2010). The "five rights" of clinical reasoning: An educational model to enhance nursing students' ability to identify and manage clinically "at risk" patients. *Nurse Education Today, 30*(6), 515–520.

Melnyk, B. M., & Fineout-Overholt, E. (2015). *Evidence-based practice in nursing and healthcare: A guide to best practice* (3rd ed.). Lippincott Williams & Wilkins.

Orsted, H., Keast, D., Foret-Lalande, L., et al. (2018). *Best practice recommendations for the prevention and management of wounds.* Canada: Wounds. https://www.woundscanada.ca/docman/public/health-care-professional/165-wc-bpr-prevention-and-management-of-wounds/file.

Pandey, M., Kamrul, R., Michaels, C. R., et al. (2022). Identifying barriers to healthcare access for new immigrants: A qualitative study in Regina, Saskatchewan, Canada. *Journal of Immigration and Minority Health, 24*(1), 188–198. doi:10.1007/s10903-021-01262-z.

Pilarinos, A., Field, S., Vasarhelyi, K., et al. (2023). A qualitative exploration of Indigenous clients' experiences of racism and perspectives on improving cultural safety within health care. *Canadian Medical Association Journal Open, 11*(3), E404–E410. doi:10.9778/cmajo.20220135.

Ponte, P. R., & Koppel, P. (2015). Cultivating mindfulness to enhance nursing practice. *American Journal of Nursing, 115*(6), 48. https://doi.org/10.1097/01.NAJ.0000466321.46439.17.

Putnam, A. L. (2015). Mnemonics in education: Current research and application. *American Psychological Association, 1*(2), 130–139. https://doi.org/10.1037/tps0000023.

Registered Nurses' Association of Ontario. (2013). *Assessment and management of pain.* https://rnao.ca/sites/rnao-ca/files/AssesssAndManagementOfPain_15_WEB-_FINAL_DEC_2.pdf.

Registered Nurses' Association of Ontario. (2015). *Person and family-centred care.* https://rnao.ca/sites/rnao-ca/files/FINAL_Web_Version_0.pdf.

Registered Nurses' Association of Ontario. (2016). *Assessment and management of pressure injuries for the interprofessional team.* https://rnao.ca/sites/rnao-ca/files/Pressure_Injuries_BPG.pdf.

Schultz, P. L., & Baker, J. (2017). Teaching strategies to increase nursing student acceptance and management of unconscious bias. *Journal of Nursing Education, 56*(11), 692–696. https://doi.org/10.3928/01484834-20171020-11.

Senger, B. A., & Smith, D. W. (2020). Augmenting a focused bedside history for prelicensure nursing students. *Journal of Nursing Education, 59*(3), 178. https://doi.org/10.3928/01484834-20200220-14.

Stubbings, L., Chaboyer, W., & McMurray, A. (2012). Nurses' use of situation awareness in decision-making: An integrative review. *Journal of Advanced Nursing, 68*(7), 1443–1453.

Tower, M., Watson, B., Bourke, A., et al. (2019). Situation awareness and the decision-making processes of final-year nursing students. *Journal of Clinical Nursing, 28*(21–22), 3923–3934. https://doi.org/10.1111/jocn.14988.

Tusaie, & Edds, K. (2009). Understanding and integrating mindfulness into psychiatric mental health nursing practice. *Archives of Psychiatric Nursing*(5), 23. https://doi.org/10.1016/j.apnu.2008.10.006.

Tyerman, J., & Cobbett, S. L. (2023). *Lewis's medical-surgical nursing in Canada: Assessment and management of clinical problems* (5th ed.). Elsevier.

White, J. (1995). Patterns of knowing: Review, critique and update. *Advances in Nursing Science, 17*(4), 73–86. https://doi.org/10.1097/00012272-199506000-00007.

Woodfin, K. O., Johnson, C., Parker, R., et al. (2018). Use of a novel memory aid to educate perioperative team members on proper patient positioning technique. *AORN Journal, 107*(3), 325–332. https://doi.org/10.1002/aorn.12075.

# Deciding What to Do

4

## LEARNING OUTCOMES

*After reading this chapter, you will be able to:*

- Identify the importance of provincial or territorial standards and entry-to-practice competencies when possible making decisions in nursing practice.
- Explain how evidence and theory contribute to decisions in health care settings.
- Describe the relationships between the concepts of analysis, interpretation, synthesis, prioritization, and decision making.
- Summarize how nursing regulations, workplace laws, and practical experience contribute to the decision-making process.
- Apply the ethical decision-making model to nursing decisions.

## GLOSSARY

**Analysis:** the process of uncovering patterns and trends in information; the second phase of the decision-making or judgement process, where data is used to determine key issues and relationships about a client's status, situation, and environment

**Decision making:** selecting the best option from the alternatives that are available; in nursing, it requires the use of critical thinking and clinical reasoning

**Generating options (or solutions):** identifying expected outcomes and using hypotheses to define future interventions; highlighting desired outcomes and what should be avoided

**Interpretation:** the process of assigning meaning to information; it relies on analysis of the data

**Prioritization:** the ranking of client or nursing-related issues using criteria for urgency or importance, so that a sequence of nursing actions can be determined

**Risk:** the probability or likelihood that something may occur; in nursing, it is associated with the severity of any anticipated consequence of that risk; it is represented by a situation where there is a possibility of loss or injury, or a situation that may create a hazard

**Synthesis:** the combining or mixing of everything that is known to form a whole idea or a new perspective; interpretation and synthesis are closely related

This chapter explores decision making and decision-making drivers in nursing practice. The decision-making process requires an understanding of how the information gathered in step one of the thinking and decision-making process can be used. The step of *deciding what to do* can be described as *analyzing, interpreting, synthesizing,* and *prioritizing.* When analyzing and interpreting information about the client or the environment, nurses rely on evidence and theory as well as the parameters of their nursing role and scope of practice.

When synthesizing and prioritizing information, nurses combine what is known to identify connections and then rank issues in order of importance. A number of clinical reasoning skills can support nurses as they decide what to do. The NRCE framework is applied to the step of deciding what to do to highlight the wide range of influences on decision making, and it is illustrated using a client scenario. Also, later in the chapter, an ethical decision-making model is applied to a case study to demonstrate how decisions can be made in practice.

4

71

## WHAT IS DECISION MAKING?

A decision occurs when the best option from the available alternatives is selected. Decision making is the process of choosing between various courses of action or competing goals, with a certain outcome in mind. This second step in *thinking it through*—deciding how to use the information found in step one—is key to determining a future course of action and its outcomes.

What do we know about decision making? According to the evidence, a number of factors affect decision making. For instance, a person's experience—whether they are a novice or an expert—determines thinking patterns and knowledge organization during the decision-making process (Muntean, 2012). Also, discipline-specific knowledge influences the scope of decision making. As well, one's creativity and critical thinking skills affect how decisions are made. The thinking strategies a person uses affect the success of decision-making outcomes, which means that monitoring the quality of the thinking process is important (Gambrill, 2012). It is exciting to know that nursing practice that incorporates constructive feedback can foster good decision making. Better decision making can be learned.

Think back to System 1 and System 2 thinking (see Chapter 1). Recall that System 1 thinking is intuitive, reflexive, and seemingly effortless; and when it is associated with good outcomes, it is often attributed to expertise (Halpern, 2014; Kahneman, 2011). Slow thinking, or System 2 thinking, is deliberate, effortful, and provides the foundation for the ability to think fast (Halpern, 2014; Kahneman, 2011). Both of these ways of thinking are important and useful. To provide a foundation for more expert thinking, slow and deliberate System 2 thinking must be cultivated.

The information collected during the initial step of nursing care (which involves assessing, noticing, recognizing, and collecting) is used to make a decision about what to do to address the identified issue or problem. Thinking to arrive at a decision involves a number of steps: the information gathered needs to be sorted and sifted through, organized, and ordered in terms of relevance; also, it must be questioned as part of the decision-making process. Sometimes, not all of the information gathered is needed, and not all of the information is of equal importance. Therefore, information and complex data need to be managed—analyzed, interpreted, synthesized, and prioritized—to *generate options* on which a final decision is made (Blondy et al., 2016). In nursing, clinical reasoning skills are required to understand how information can be used.

### Making a Good Decision

A *good decision* is one that addresses the identified issue or problem effectively, given the information that was available *at the time*. Whether a decision is good or not depends on the context. If the context changes after a decision is made, the interpretation of the outcome of the decision may also change. Additionally, there are no agreed-upon standards for what constitutes an *accurate decision*.

A good decision tends to have the following characteristics:
- the correct application of relevant, available information;
- a systematic and repeatable approach to thinking;
- a realistic perspective, in that it anticipates the way in which the actions may be carried out;
- a positive impact on others, with a focus on supporting human potential;
- and a decision-maker who is accountable (whether the decision-maker is an individual or a group).

A good decision also includes a collaborative approach to gathering information and shared decision making.

One way of evaluating decisions is to consider how they are made. Was the manner in which the decision was made satisfactory? This question focuses on the decision-making *process*. The process used to select the best option from the available alternatives can be considered as appropriate, or "good" if it considers the relevant information and various options systematically. An error in decision making, or a bad decision, can occur if there is a deviation from a systematic decision-making process that increases the likelihood of an undesired outcome (Gambrill, 2012). Interestingly, if the decision-maker focuses strictly on the process of making a decision (rather than on what or who the process is about), less-than-optimal outcomes may also occur.

Determining whether a decision is good can also be *outcome focused*. Was the end result satisfactory? Did the decision have the desired effect? Outcomes, as measurable results, are essential in health care settings, and thus the term *effective decision making* is often used instead of *good decision making*.

A number of resources can support nurses as they decide what to do. The section that follows provides examples of such resources, which can serve as foundations, or rationales, for deciding what to do.

## FOUNDATIONS FOR DECIDING WHAT TO DO

While many resources can inform a decision, certain resources are often consulted by nurses when deciding what to do. Evidence and theory, and the nursing role and scope of practice are examples of resources that nurses consider when analyzing and interpreting information and client care situations. Also, models such as Maslow's hierarchy of needs (1943) and acronyms such as *ABCD* and *CURE* are used to synthesize information and prioritize options and client-centred care.

### Analyzing and Interpreting

Analysis is the process of uncovering patterns and trends in information, and of establishing relationships among data. When analyzing information, consider the available presenting clinical data and compare them against your knowledge of areas such as normal laboratory result ranges, clinical manifestations of related conditions, typical and atypical physical or psychological responses to a particular situation, and any past experiences with similar situations. As well, use best practice guidelines and medically based algorithms to gain insight into ways of thinking about the presenting clinical data and to inform decisions. Also ask yourself whether it is within a nurse's role to address the particular client care situation. Analysis can also involve information on professional practice issues. Interpretation, or the process of assigning meaning to information, entails clearly identifying what is occurring in relation to the concern or issue.

## Evidence and Theory

The ability to recall and analyze science- and nursing-based knowledge and theory will help you apply this information to the issue at hand in the decision-making process. What does it mean to analyze information? Once you have facts that were collected from assessing a client and noticing the client situation, asking yourself several questions will help you analyze whether the information is appropriate, relevant, and useful to addressing the identified issue:

- Is the information reliable and valid in relation to what is known?

- Does this information represent a change in status or condition?
- Has this situation happened before, and is there a pattern or trend (i.e., whether it repeats, and if it does, when)?
- Does the information have a science- or theory-based connection to the identified issue (i.e., whether relationships exist among the collected data)?

Interpretation of what is occurring will be based on the results of the analysis of patterns and trends. Use science-based and evidence-informed thinking to interpret or find the meaning of what has been observed or noticed. For instance, you may ask yourself:

- What does this mean for the client's identified issue?
- How could this affect the client and their overall situation?
- Could what has been observed or noticed represent a significant change to the client and their situation?
- Does something else need to be done to confirm my interpretation (i.e., find more information or involve others)?

Thoughtful analysis of the available information and interpretation of what it means will guide you toward synthesis and prioritization. From there, generating options will lead to a decision.

Box 4.1 considers the scenario of a client who states that they feel hot 3 days after a surgical procedure. This simple

---

**BOX 4.1    Analyzing and Interpreting Information: An Example**

The client states, "I feel hot." Based on this client-identified concern and other information available to the nurse, analysis and interpretation are necessary.

| Information Available | Analyses | Interpretations |
|---|---|---|
| Body temperature: 38.3°C Pulse: 110 beats per minute | Vital sign data may be related; higher than the day before. | Nurses have knowledge and responsibility to address the client's statement. |
| Many blankets are on bed; client is visibly shivering. | Trends are evident since surgery occurred. | It represents a significant change in condition. |
| Room temperature is warm. | Environment may be contributing to elevated temperature. | Risk of not addressing this change now may mean further complications and delayed return to desired state of health. |
| Emergency bowel resection for obstruction, post-operative day 3. | Other clinical manifestations may be associated with elevated temperature. | |

example shows what analysis and interpretation of information can look like in the clinical setting.

## Nursing Role and Scope of Practice

Knowing the responsibilities of your nursing role—whether as a registered nurse, practical nurse, or student—is very important when deciding what to do in a client care situation and in a health care environment. Your professional designation and role as a registered professional are defined by several factors:

- Provincial or territorial legislation that describes actions that may be undertaken in the nursing role (nursing practice and regulated health professions acts)
- Laws that may pertain to where you work (public hospital, long-term care facility, federal government agency)
- Provincial or territorial regulatory body's practice standards for direct care, administration, education, and research practice areas
- Entry-level competency requirements
- Codes of ethics and ethical standards of practice
- Specialty standards of care (i.e., critical or perioperative care)
- Employer's policies and procedures, including the description of responsibilities for the nursing position held

*Scope of practice* is defined as the range of roles, functions, responsibilities, and activities for which nurses are educated, authorized, and competent to perform (College of Registered Nurses of Newfoundland and Labrador, 2022). A nurse's scope of practice, which is guided by the above factors relating to their role, is also influenced by the following:

- Individual competency and acquired practical experiences
- Educational level and continued formal learning opportunities (certification)
- Employer's authorization to perform particular nursing actions
- Client needs and health goals

Scopes of practice in nursing are always evolving and expanding. As a result, nurses must continuously reflect on their own abilities and competence, and ensure that their actions and decisions are based on current evidence and nursing activities they are legislated to perform in the health care setting (Lankshear & Martin, 2019).

Nurses are required to respond to client needs. At the same time, they must reflect on their own knowledge, skills, and abilities to determine whether they are the right professional to provide care to a particular client. Think about a nurse on a postoperative unit who is caring for a client when the client's condition deteriorates to the point where critical care is required. In this instance, the client must be transferred to a Critical Care Unit and be cared for by a nurse with additional specialized skills who is able to provide the necessary level of care. A clear understanding of your responsibilities and scope of practice in your particular role is crucial to deciding what to do.

Deciding what to do is based on the analysis of patterns, trends, and relationships among data, and an interpretation of the meaning of this information. These thinking activities support the next parts of decision making: making connections to identify a potential new problem and choosing which issues and actions are most important.

## Synthesizing and Prioritizing

Once available information is analyzed and interpreted, what is understood needs to be synthesized. Synthesis refers to the combining or mixing of everything that is known to form a whole idea or *a new perspective*. It follows the analysis and interpretation of information and describes a mental activity that "depends on cognitive skills and competencies, situational and contextual factors, preparation and knowledge acquisition skills, interpersonal and interaction skills, and personal qualities" (Blondy et al., 2016, p. 668).

Synthesis takes place during client care when the nurse identifies that there is in fact a new, acknowledged problem or a change in condition. For example, combining data about elevated body temperature in a postoperative client and changes observed over 3 days since surgery, and an understanding of risk of infection with surgery will lead the nurse to the new idea of a possible postoperative infection. Then, the importance of this new idea must be prioritized in relation to other issues in the current care of the client.

Prioritization involves ranking client- or nursing-related issues using criteria in order of urgency or importance, so that a sequence of nursing actions can be determined. It addresses the question, "What should I do first?" Client situations are always changing, which means that priorities are always changing. Because a client's identified issue is often associated with other aspects of their condition or situation, all salient issues need to be considered in context to determine the priority of each.

Generating options (or solutions) is an activity that relates closely to prioritization. Generating options or solutions involves identifying expected and preferred outcomes, and what should be avoided. *Goal setting* is a similar activity which incorporates options or proposed solutions. Goals and anticipated outcomes for clients are ideally collaboratively determined with the client and reflect clear decisions that are made about the care that will be provided (Astle & Duggleby, 2024). Goals are prioritized so that those that are urgent or short term are met before those that are less urgent or longer term.

Risk is another significant component of determining priorities for care. **Risk** is the probability or likelihood that something may occur. In nursing, it is associated with the severity of any anticipated consequence of that risk. Risk is represented by a situation where there is a possibility of loss or injury, or a situation that may create a hazard. Making decisions about risk in a clinical or nursing situation is very challenging, and, by its nature, is a source of uncertainty and anxiety for nurses.

If, based on analysis and interpretation of the available evidence, the potential risk of a severe consequence or complication is synthesized and identified, then an appropriate response would be to prioritize care to ensure that the risk is reduced. The saying, "better safe than sorry" may come to mind. However, this decision would not be based on an adage like this one. Instead, it would be grounded in evidence that demonstrates that the benefits of addressing the issue outweigh the costs of not addressing the issue. In other words, identifying a significant issue early on so that it can be prevented from worsening, based on rationale, is preferrable to a threat to health.

In the scenario described in Box 4.1, it would be reasonable, given the information, to interpret the situation as a possible postoperative infection, rather than any other alternative, and that it is an identified change in condition that a nurse must help address. Now refer to Box 4.2 for the continuation of this scenario. Interpretation of the client situation evolves to synthesis and prioritization. If a possible infection is not acted on, the client's condition may deteriorate to septic shock or some other complication, and the client's hospital stay could be lengthened.

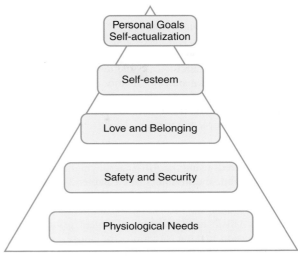

Fig. 4.1 Maslow's Hierarchy of Needs.

When deciding what to do, it is important for nurses to thoughtfully consider the available information and bear in mind that a risk factor for most clients may not be a risk factor for an individual client.

### Maslow's Hierarchy of Needs

Nurses can prioritize client needs using a model such as Maslow's hierarchy of needs (Figure 4.1). This model is well known and simple to understand when setting priorities.

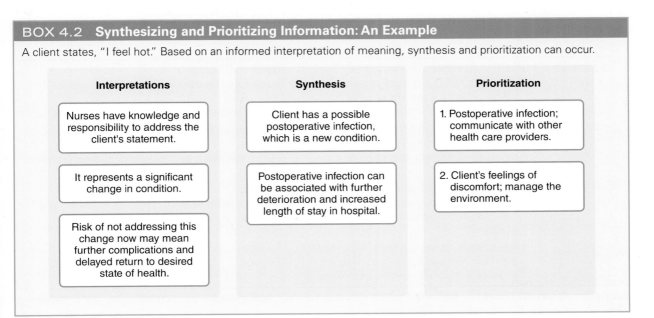

**BOX 4.2   Synthesizing and Prioritizing Information: An Example**

A client states, "I feel hot." Based on an informed interpretation of meaning, synthesis and prioritization can occur.

| Interpretations | Synthesis | Prioritization |
| --- | --- | --- |
| Nurses have knowledge and responsibility to address the client's statement. | Client has a possible postoperative infection, which is a new condition. | 1. Postoperative infection; communicate with other health care providers. |
| It represents a significant change in condition. | Postoperative infection can be associated with further deterioration and increased length of stay in hospital. | 2. Client's feelings of discomfort; manage the environment. |
| Risk of not addressing this change now may mean further complications and delayed return to desired state of health. | | |

The needs lower in the hierarchy must be satisfied before those higher up can be attended to. This model reminds nurses that physiological needs and safety and security—especially in situations that are life threatening or present a risk to basic physiological functioning—must be met before higher-level needs. In this model, needs relating to a client's self-esteem and self-actualization are ranked as higher-level needs, at the top of the pyramid.

## ABCD

Similarly, nurses can prioritize the client's physiological and safety needs using the *ABCD* acronym *a*irway, *b*reathing, *c*irculation, and *d*isability (see Chapter 3). This handy acronym can be used to find information and structure a client assessment.

Using ABCD to identify initial urgent priorities in a quick decision-making situation, the nurse would first ensure that there are no obstructions or threats to the client's airway. If synthesis indicates that the airway is obstructed, care of the airway is the priority, and the decision-making process is shortened. If the airway is patent and not compromised, breathing (ventilation, respiration) is the next priority, followed by circulation (cardiac, vascular, hemorrhage). Assessment of disability (level of consciousness and response) or a brief neurological examination completes this survey (Tyerman & Cobbett, 2023). ABCD is useful to rank synthesized information and can also be applied to prioritize care among multiple clients.

## CURE

The CURE hierarchy helps nurses better understand how to manage the competing physiological needs of several clients. *CURE* stands for *c*ritical needs, *u*rgent needs, *r*outine needs, and *e*xtras (Kohtz et al., 2017). Specifically, it helps nurses categorize different clients' needs so that they can prioritize what actions to take and when. Table 4.1 presents CURE client needs with examples.

## Client Preferences

A nurse's ability to determine client needs also depends on their knowledge of and collaboration with the client. The client's perceptions of what is important to them are also a factor in priority setting. It may be challenging for the nurse and client if their views on what is important differ and if the client's preferences for care do not align with Maslow's hierarchy or physical safety. By engaging in client education or clearer communication with the client on their health situation, the nurse may help the client understand why one activity needs to be performed before another. When differing views cannot be easily resolved, an ethical dilemma may result.

When assessing client needs, it is important for experienced nurses to listen to their instincts, as they are informed by nursing knowledge and past situations. Intuition (see Chapter 7) is more than a "gut feeling" and is part of clinical judgement (Tanner, 2006; Nielsen et al., 2007). Skills such as intuition that develop over time may help the nurse when advocating for a client and deciding what to do.

| TABLE 4.1 | **CURE: A Tool for Prioritizing Client Needs** | |
|---|---|---|
| **CURE Client Needs** | **Description** | **Examples** |
| Critical needs | Needs that require immediate action; they align with ABCD and Maslow's physiological needs (critical aspects of care) | Airway compromise<br>Respiratory distress<br>Chest pain<br>Signs of stroke |
| Urgent needs | Needs that require prompt attention; needs addressed after critical ones met; they cause client discomfort or represent a safety risk | Postoperative pain<br>Fall alarm<br>Clarification of a prescription prior to administration |
| Routine needs | Scheduled care in a typical day; the majority of care is standard and planned; these needs do not supersede critical or urgent needs | Prescribed medication administration<br>Physical assessment<br>Care of a chronic stable condition |
| Extras | Non-essential needs, but ones that promote client comfort and satisfaction; they are provided if other needs have been met | Hair care<br>Massage |

Adapted from Kohtz, C., Gowda, C., & Guede, P. (2017). Cognitive stacking: Strategies for the busy RN. *Nursing, 47*(1), 18–20. https://doi.org/10.1097/01.nurse.0000510758.31326.92.

Making a decision about what to do is the last thought activity in this step of the thinking and decision-making process. After deciding what to do (identifying appropriate solutions based on client-centred goals, etc.), the nurse develops a plan and acts on the plan (see Chapter 5).

---

**KNOWLEDGE CHECK-IN**
- What is meant by a *good decision*?
- Describe the terms *analysis* and *interpretation* in your own words and provide examples.
- How are evidence and scope of practice used when analyzing and interpreting information?
- Give examples of synthesis and prioritization of information when thinking in nursing practice.

---

## SKILLS USED WHEN DECIDING WHAT TO DO

In nursing, thinking is a purposeful, controlled action that is rational and logical. To that end, nurses make decisions based on the data collected, and other information they are aware of. Certain skills help with deciding what to do. Figure 4.2 presents the unified process for thinking and decision making that incorporates the ethical decision-making model discussed in Chapter 2. As an example of a nursing model that can be applied to the unified process, the ethical decision-making model (in the blue centre) includes the following steps: assessing; reflecting on and reviewing potential actions; selecting and engaging in an ethical action; and reflecting on and reviewing the action. As is the case with other models, each of these steps is associated with specific clinical reasoning skills. This chapter will explore the skills needed when analyzing, interpreting, synthesizing, and prioritizing information, and generating options for action. These skills are listed in the grey-shaded area of the figure. The ethical decision-making model will be applied to a case study on decision making, later in this chapter.

### Clinical Reasoning and Other Skills Used When Deciding What to Do

The following clinical reasoning and other skills support the process of decision making. These skills are applied after the preceding step of finding information.

### Set Priorities

As discussed earlier, prioritization is key when deciding what to do. The inability to identify what to do first could result in the delay of essential treatment. Interestingly, setting priorities is an important skill to use *throughout the entire thinking process*. Asking yourself what to do first is essential during assessment, goal setting, implementing care, and evaluating care. The nurse cannot do everything at once, so they must decide what is most important to do now and what can reasonably wait. Setting priorities also promotes efficient and effective care.

*How Can You Develop This Skill?* Be aware of client needs and consult with other health care professionals to better understand care priorities. Master time management (discussed in Chapter 8) to facilitate your ability to set priorities and arrange tasks to deliver optimal care. Priority setting often receives the most attention from nursing students and educators when learning in clinical practice situations. Case studies and practice applying various nursing models will help you develop the habit of thinking in terms of priorities.

### Make Inferences

An *inference* is made when a conclusion is reached, based on evidence and reasoning. It can be simple (deducing that a postoperative client who grimaces when moving may be in pain), or it can involve more complex analyses and interpretations. Drawing the correct conclusion is important to making the correct decisions about client care. Compare this skill with making an *assumption*, which is not based on evidence.

*How Can You Develop This Skill?* Confer with the client on what you are thinking and verify the information. Ensure that you are drawing on current science- and nursing-based knowledge and theory, and validating data that has been gathered without jumping to conclusions or making assumptions. This skill is tied to other skills such as identifying bias in interpretation.

### See Patterns Over Time

Identifying *patterns,* which are sets of data that follow a recognizable form or that occur in a familiar and predictable arrangement, help the nurse see the big picture and contribute to decision making. When a pattern is identified as representing a certain problem or condition, it may also direct the nurse to employ other skills, such as identifying missing information and grouping other cues. Patterns may also represent normal conditions or behaviours. When patterns occur and recur (establishing a trend), they usually do so for a reason. Trends are changes in a particular direction over time.

*How Can You Develop This Skill?* Recall your learning about which arrangement of cues, or clinical manifestations, are associated with which condition or problem. Also, if you identify but are not certain about a particular pattern, ask the client to fill in any information gaps to validate (or invalidate) the pattern or confer with an experienced nurse who can help confirm an emerging pattern.

### Group Related Cues Together

Grouping related information enables the nurse to analyze a client situation. It requires the nurse to have extensive

Identify quality improvement approaches and
  evidence gaps
Evaluate effectiveness of actions and outcomes
Debrief with peers/self, other professionals
Incorporate new knowledge and evidence
Review personal learning plan
Predict future client needs
Reflect on actions

Demonstrate psychomotor/technology skill associated
with physical and health assessment
Recognize relationships between concepts and data
Recall science-based, ethics, and nursing knowledge
Assess systematically and comprehensively
Identify pre-existing bias and assumptions
Anticipate care needs in client context
Form therapeutic relationship
Consider expectations

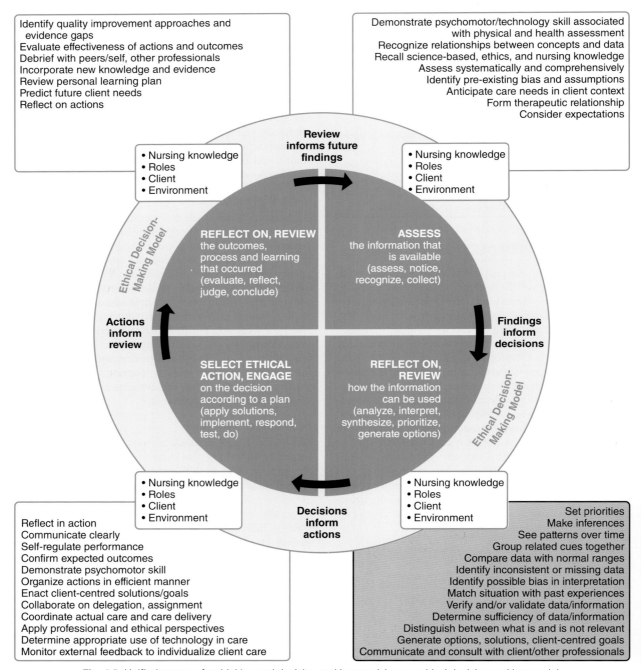

Reflect in action
Communicate clearly
Self-regulate performance
Confirm expected outcomes
Demonstrate psychomotor skill
Organize actions in efficient manner
Enact client-centred solutions/goals
Collaborate on delegation, assignment
Coordinate actual care and care delivery
Apply professional and ethical perspectives
Determine appropriate use of technology in care
Monitor external feedback to individualize client care

Set priorities
Make inferences
See patterns over time
Group related cues together
Compare data with normal ranges
Identify inconsistent or missing data
Identify possible bias in interpretation
Match situation with past experiences
Verify and/or validate data/information
Determine sufficiency of data/information
Distinguish between what is and is not relevant
Generate options, solutions, client-centred goals
Communicate and consult with client/other professionals

Fig. 4.2  Unified process for thinking and decision making: applying an ethical decision-making model.

knowledge of evidence and theory in order to identify and group related cues together in a coherent and logical manner. For example, a nurse is caring for a client with an elevated heart rate, reported postsurgical incisional discomfort, and no recent documented analgesia administration. The client is restless and cannot focus on postoperative discharge instructions. After gathering these cues and reflecting on them, the nurse may conclude that the client is in pain instead of disinterested in learning self-care after surgery.

*How Can You Develop This Skill?* Use a body systems approach to thinking if the main client issue is physiological; recall how body systems affect one another. Refer to your psychological knowledge if the client is experiencing personal or social issues. Recall that mental health and psychological well-being may be associated with physical well-being. Pay attention to the timing of clinical manifestations in the client and think about cause and effect. Also, create flow charts, concept maps, or mind maps to help you learn relationships between client cues.

## Compare Data With Normal Ranges

This skill is learned early in a nurse's educational program and requires knowledge of normal ranges for laboratory tests. Laboratory values provide critical insight into a client's situation, and missing or not understanding these data could allow a condition to go untreated. The ability to distinguish between what is normal and what is abnormal does not only apply to laboratory values. It also applies to anticipated or expected client behaviours, group characteristics, and population changes. For example, an older client may be less likely to exhibit an increase in temperature in the initial stages of infection.

*How Can You Develop This Skill?* Remember normal ranges by using pocket notes for common values encountered in your area of practice or by referring to a normal values resource on the unit. If you are unsure about what a laboratory value indicates, ask a mentor or colleague. Consider that when developing this skill, you need to use other skills, such as "identify possible bias in interpretation." Ask yourself, *Is a value or behaviour outside the normal range really abnormal for a particular client (i.e., the client may be on medication that affects a laboratory result)?* Analytical skills are needed when comparing data with normal ranges.

## Identify Inconsistent or Missing Data

Recognizing problems with data, such as two items of information or cues that contradict each other, or gaps in data, is essential to correct analysis and interpretation, and for ensuring accuracy. This skill complements other skills, such as "verify and/or validate data/information." Inconsistent data may indicate that an assessment needs to be

confirmed or that further information needs to be gathered. This skill is a reminder of the iterative nature of thinking, and that sometimes going back to the preceding step of finding information and assessing the client is necessary.

*How Can You Develop This Skill?* Develop a solid understanding of science- and nursing-based knowledge to be able to recognize data that are incoherent or absent. Confirm or re-check assessment data with the client. Refer to available nursing resources or best practice guidelines to ensure that your assessment is accurate. Referring to guidelines may remind you about what was missed. At times, it may be necessary to ask another nurse with more experience for their advice: it can be hard to identify what is missing if you do not know what is missing. Reading case studies in journals is another way to learn about clinical manifestations of various conditions not often seen in your daily practice.

## Identify Possible Bias in Interpretation

While interpreting information, avoid making assumptions about its meaning. The professional, cultural, and spiritual perspectives of the nurse, and their personal assumptions about the information and what it means for the client may not be accurate and represent bias. An error associated with bias in interpreting a client situation could lead to incorrect synthesis, a detrimental decision, and mistrust in the nurse–client relationship. This is an example of an error that can be avoided.

*How Can You Develop This Skill?* Adopt a stance of inquiry. Form a habit of asking yourself, *Am I assuming my interpretation is right because that is what I know most about?* Be aware that bias may be unconscious. Be open to other possibilities and viewpoints. Even if you have encountered a similar client situation in the past, check with the client to establish more accurate interpretations of what is occurring.

## Match Situation With Past Experiences

Matching past experiences with the present situation enables the nurse to recognize the nature of the current issue more quickly and to think efficiently and with more confidence. This skill aligns with the skill "see patterns over time" in this step of the thinking and decision-making process. It draws on the lived experience of the nurse and the client, which can be shared and contribute to deciding what to do, especially if solutions to past issues have resulted in positive outcomes.

*How Can You Develop This Skill?* Ask yourself, *Have I seen this before?* and ask the client, "Has this happened to you in the past?" to provide information that helps establish patterns or trends. Understand that matching a current situation to a similar past experience does not necessarily mean that any actions that follow will also be the same. For novice nurses, case studies or hearing other nurses' stories can help build a repertoire of clinical scenarios. Gain as much practical experience as you can.

### Verify and/or Validate Data/Information

To validate data is to confirm that it is accurate. Without ensuring that a piece of information is true or valid, any decisions that are based on it may be problematic. Confirming the accuracy of information is particularly important for critical data on which any other decision may be dependent. For instance, for a client whose blood pressure is suddenly and unusually low, repeating the measurement in the other arm or having a colleague double-check would validate the information before making a decision about hypotension or possible hypovolemic shock.

*How Can You Develop This Skill?* Adopt a stance of inquiry. To create a habit of thinking in this way, always question whether the available information is the best and the most accurate. Cultivating mentorships with your peers that support checking data is another way to develop this skill.

### Determine Sufficiency of Data/Information

The ability to determine whether enough data or information exists to make a decision is another skill that many novice nurses seek to acquire. This skill is similar to "identify inconsistent or missing data," but it focuses more so on whether the information on hand has adequate depth. For instance, is it enough to know that a client is in severe pain or is more information using the OPQRSTUV tool required?

*How Can You Develop This Skill?* Ask yourself, *Will it make a difference to gather more information?* If no, and there is enough information to make a rational decision and a competent action plan, then moving on with what you have may be most efficient. Take cues from the client to explore any information gaps and determine what they think is sufficient, particularly in relation to the client's various personal or cultural needs.

### Distinguish Between What Is and Is Not Relevant

*Relevance* refers to how closely or appropriately a cue, piece of information, or data is connected to the main, identified issue. Establishing the relevance of information is important so that unnecessary or less important information does not influence decision making in a negative way and does not prolong the nurse's ability to make a decision. Consider a client who reports that they have not had a bowel movement in 2 days. In the immediate, this information may not be as relevant as the client's observed shortness of breath, coughing, and hyperthermia and so it may be considered accordingly. The skill "group related cues together" can help you distinguish between what is relevant and what is not as well.

*How Can You Develop This Skill?* Cultivate a habit of asking yourself, *How does this information fit with the big picture?* and *Does this information make sense in relation to what is known so far?* as you think about the available information. Continue to gain experience and exposure to new client situations to further develop this skill.

### Generate Options, Solutions, Client-Centred Goals

This skill is usually applied toward the end of the process of deciding what to do, after analysis, interpretation of the client situation, synthesis of the whole situation, and prioritization have occurred. As part of making a decision, the nurse generates options or solutions to address the main identified issue, based on the available evidence. At this point, specific, measurable, attainable, relevant, and realistic alternatives are proposed. Ideally, they include input from the client in a specified time frame. If an option is selected, a plan of care is created that becomes the basis for the next step in the thinking and decision-making process: acting on the decision (see Chapter 5).

*How Can You Develop This Skill?* Draw on past experiences or brainstorm with colleagues about options to consider. Involve the client. Use the *SMART* goal acronym (*s*pecific, *m*easurable, *a*ttainable, *r*elevant, and *t*imed) to recall the essential components of setting a goal. Practise creating or writing goals, as doing so is more challenging than it may seem. For Indigenous clients, consider the Truth and Reconciliation Commission of Canada's call to action 22, which is "to recognize the value of Aboriginal healing practices and use them in the treatment of Aboriginal patients in collaboration with Aboriginal healers and Elders where requested" (Government of Canada, 2015, p. 3). For all clients, check that the goals make sense for them and are a fit with their goals for optimal health.

### Communicate and Consult With Client/Other Professionals

Involving the client in deciding what to do is essential. This approach is not only a professional standard but also a component of ethical practice. Other health care professionals who are working with the client or with a group or population must also be involved.

*How Can You Develop This Skill?* Communicate clearly and as often as needed, using professional language and accepted health care terminology, to ensure transparency and accuracy of decision making. Additionally, understand the roles and scopes of practice of other health care professionals. Knowing what others do can facilitate communication and enable efficient information sharing and decision making.

## THINKING THROUGH THE APPLICATION OF CLINICAL REASONING SKILLS

### Case Scenario on Decision Making

A 29-year-old, pregnant with their first child, presents to the health clinic to establish prenatal care. The client is unsure of the date of their last menstrual period and notes that prepregnancy weight was 49.9 kg. Nausea has been reported for the last few weeks, and they have not had much to eat or drink. Current weight is 44.5 kg. The following findings are documented: pulse 88 beats per minute; blood pressure 106/70 mm Hg; urinalysis positive for ketones; history of intimate partner violence and chlamydia. The client currently lives with a parent and attends college part-time.

Reflect on these questions:

- Given the available information, what cues are missing? Which are more important than others?
- Of these more important cues, which may be related to one another?
- What do you make of this information? What is its meaning?
- What are priorities in this scenario?
- Who can you communicate with to help the client?
- Which clinical reasoning skills would you apply to this scenario when making a decision?

## Deciding Not to Act

Sometimes, the best and most appropriate decision is to not respond or perform an intervention, and instead to observe or monitor the client situation (Shellian & Levinson, 2016). This choice to "do nothing" is based on the same process of evidence and data analysis. In a way, it is actually "doing something." Maintaining the current state or situation and being ready when needed are actions that can result from a nursing decision.

A nurse may question whether a test or treatment is needed. For a client who has type 2 diabetes, and who is not taking insulin or other medication that could increase their risk of hypoglycemia, the nurse would not act to advise routine self-monitoring of blood glucose levels (Canadian Nurses Association, 2020). The nurse may decide to act if the client's condition changed such as in acute illness or pregnancy and would work with other health care professionals to determine a course of care.

These clinical reasoning skills enable the nurse to anticipate and predict care, and decide what to do. You will note that many of the ways to develop these skills include a foundation in science, evidence, and nursing knowledge. A nurse cannot make decisions and provide care without this basic understanding.

## BARRIERS TO THINKING WHEN DECIDING WHAT TO DO

Logic and sound rationale are key to making good decisions. However, errors in logical thinking may affect decision making (Gambrill, 2012). Barriers that can impede appropriate decision making often relate to personal, relational, and organizational issues (Robijn et al., 2020). These barriers include slow or poor interpretation of physiological changes, an inability to clearly articulate client changes, apprehension about communicating with other health care professionals, and challenging organizational culture (Clayton, 2019).

### Personal Barriers

When deciding what to do, personal barriers can influence the decision-making process. Factors such as maturity, past experiences, and concerns about one's own health affect a nurse's confidence in making decisions, but other challenges that are less obvious require reflection.

Logical fallacies, which are common errors in thinking, are arguments that are found to be false when examined using logical reasoning (Walton & Waddell, 2025). There are many types, and a few examples are listed in Table 4.2. Taking logical fallacies as facts can result in poor decisions because they are based on unsound thinking. Note that logical fallacies are not the same as biases (see Chapter 3), which are caused by our own values, experiences, and preferences.

Feelings of stress or pressure, a lack of nursing knowledge, and a high cognitive load are other personal and individual barriers that can arise when analyzing, interpreting, synthesizing and prioritizing information. *Cognitive load* refers to the relative demand on thinking required for a particular task or tasks. The amount of information and facts that working memory can process at once varies depending on competing mental tasks, one's psychological or physical state (i.e., fatigue, burnout), and the complexity and demands of the task at hand (Burgess, 2010). A high cognitive load may negatively affect decision-making ability.

### Relational Barriers

Communication with clients and health care professionals can be challenging. Novice nurses may be hesitant to communicate and consult with clients, clients' families, and colleagues because they are unsure of what to ask or cannot clearly identify their concerns. A lack of understanding of others' views can result from ineffective or absent communication. Nurses may not appreciate or understand the roles of other health care workers and so may not factor them into a collaborative decision-making process. Also, they may be fearful of disappointing someone such as a mentor, feeling embarrassed, or of making an erroneous decision and harming a client.

Ethical situations often arise in the context of human interactions, communications, and relationships. Your personal

**TABLE 4.2    Examples of Logical Fallacies**

| Fallacy | Problem | Example |
|---|---|---|
| **Ad populum:** A proposition is claimed to be accurate solely because a majority or many people believe it to be so. | The majority may be wrong or may not have enough knowledge. | "Many people believe that free access to health care is important. Therefore, it is worth saving at all costs." |
| **Appeal to authority:** An assertion is said to be true because of the position or authority of the person making the statement. | The authority's statement may be inaccurate, not relevant to the argument, or may be out of context. | "Nurses should focus on cleaning tasks because Florence Nightingale said it was important to do so." |
| **Hasty generalization:** Too small of a sample size was used to support a sweeping generalization. | It involves jumping to a conclusion without adequate evidence. | "That nurse couldn't access a vein in this client, so no one will be able to start an IV line in this client." |
| **False dichotomy:** An assumption is made that only two possible solutions exist, so disproving one solution means that the other solution should be used. | It ignores other alternative solutions or rationales. | "If COVID-19 vaccinations work, then why are some vaccinated people getting sick?" |

values and preferences may differ from those of others. Also, the situation you are faced with may not present a clear answer (no right or wrong response), making it more difficult to make a decision. The following types of ethical issues may occur when communication, value differences, expected or intended actions, and situations are challenging (Burkhardt et al., 2018):

- *Ethical dilemma:* a situation in which there are conflicting moral claims or values; no matter the choice, there will be consequences
- *Ethical uncertainty:* a state that occurs when the correct action to take on a problem, or what moral principles apply, is unclear
- *Ethical distress:* a reaction to a situation or interaction where there are problems that seem to have clear solutions, yet one is unable to follow their beliefs because of external or institutional constraints (Note: This last point of distress relates to workplace practices and culture, and can result in anger, frustration, poor performance, and overall poor decision making for the nurse.)

Racism profoundly impacts a nurse's ability to make clinical decisions in nursing practice, often manifesting as implicit biases from colleagues or clients. These biases which negatively affect relationships can undermine the nurse's confidence, leading to second-guessing of their clinical judgments and decisions. Research (Beagan, et al., 2022) indicates how racial discrimination in healthcare settings can create a hostile work environment, contributing to stress and burnout among affected healthcare professionals. The effects of such barriers influence the  environment as well as the nurse's mental well-being and pose a risk to client care by limiting nurses' abilities to relate to others, advocate effectively or make decisions.

**💡 THINKING IT THROUGH**

***Self-Reflection on Barriers to Deciding What to Do***

- What decision-making barriers have you encountered in your practice setting?
- Recall instances when you have had trouble interpreting the meaning of information. Do these instances have anything in common?
- What do you think are the main challenges you have when trying to decide what to do? What is the cause(s) of the challenges? Why are they happening?

## Organizational Barriers

Organizations have their own value systems: a vision, a mission or purpose, and principles that they uphold when operating. They may also have less obvious or hidden cultural systems that act as barriers to decision making. For example, an organizational culture may devalue creative thinking, make teamwork difficult, or not acknowledge nurses' voices when client or occupational safety concerns arise. As with a client's beliefs, organizational cultural beliefs can affect how clinical and ethical situations are perceived and how subsequent decisions are made in practice environments.

Other organizational barriers include physical distractions in the environment (e.g., noise, announcements, movement, visual disturbances, and interruptions) and mental distractions to analyzing, interpreting, synthesizing, and prioritizing (e.g., stress, too many competing problems, interruptions). Distractions and interruptions can be particularly problematic during high-stakes activities such as medication administration (McGillis Hall et al., 2010).

## HELPFUL STRATEGIES FOR DECIDING WHAT TO DO

It takes time to develop decision-making skills and overcome barriers that arise when trying to make a decision.

### Personal Strategies

To help address personal barriers that arise when deciding what to do, mindfulness, reflection, and metacognition are key stances to adopt (see Chapters 2 and 3). Thinking positively about your knowledge, applying what you know, and finding answers to what you do not know is a motivating approach to professional development. These self-regulated types of activities apply to analysis, interpretation, synthesis, and prioritization, and indeed, to every step of the thinking and decision-making process in nursing practice.

Exposure to decision-making opportunities through nursing practice experiences is an active and effective strategy to develop related skills and overcome personal barriers (Nibblelink & Brewer, 2018). Thinking about what to do is often influenced by previous experiences rather than by the actual clinical situation in which decisions are made (Cappelletti et al., 2014). For instance, if you received negative feedback on a decision you made in the past, you may be hesitant to make other decisions in the same environment or with a similar client. However, with collaboration and mentorship, the more practice you gain, the better you can become with making confident decisions.

### Relational Strategies

Relational barriers can be reduced by engaging in a therapeutic relationship with the client. Cultivating respect and trust with the client can enable good communication and assessments and allow you to check back and confirm observations and your thinking with the client's views.

Shared decision making (SDM) is a process whereby decisions are made by the client and the health care provider(s) using client preferences and the best available evidence (Coulter & Collins, 2011). SDM supports the provision of therapeutic care. As one example, research by Inuit-led organizations that span Nunavut and the Ontario cancer health systems described the use of SDM by Indigenous populations and health partners to make decisions about health. The SDM approach upheld "Inuit Quajimajatuqangit principles in health care systems and, in particular, Aajiiqatigiinniq: Decision making through discussion and consensus" (Jull et al., 2021, p. 8). Such client-centred approaches are used when caring for clients from all backgrounds.

Activating team supports that are available will facilitate collaboration. No one can know everything, so be aware of any resources that may be accessible to you. Consulting with others who have more experience is a way of analyzing and interpreting information, which is also part of the decision-making process. When novice nurses are pressured for time, applying thinking and decision-making models may feel less efficient than asking for information and advice directly from other more experienced nursing team members. However, with practice, using models will strengthen your ability to provide comprehensive, efficient care based on sound evidence. Ultimately, you must decide what needs to be done in collaboration with the client who is assigned to your care.

In addition to regular reflective practice (Danda, et al., 2022), mechanisms for addressing relational effects of racism need to be implemented at an organizational level to support nurses experiencing unsafe environments. Anti-racism and cultural safety courses and training can help expose existing racist thinking or microaggressions and prompt awareness, personal reflection and collegial advocacy. These and other approaches that examine institutional policies and practices are considered alongside organizational strategies.

### ❓ THINKING IT THROUGH

#### Self-Reflection on Using Strategies When Deciding What to Do

- What strategies do you use when trying to make a decision?
- Do you have your own team supports or mentors in nursing practice?
- When consulting with others, do you share your own thoughts as well as seek alternative views? Consider how you can develop your knowledge instead of just asking someone else what you should do next.

### Organizational Strategies

Becoming familiar with an institution's procedures can assist you with making decisions. When you share ideas and observations about the health care environment, doing so in a way that seeks improvement and positive change is more constructive. Include possible solutions if you can, rather than focusing on the negative or being resistant to change.

In terms of organizational culture, nurses at all levels (staff, administrators, educators) have a responsibility to develop and support a safe environment where everyone can speak up and share ideas. For instance, an approach to performance evaluation or hiring that is equity-focused,

**TABLE 4.3    Summary of Decision-Making Barriers and Strategies to Address Them**

| Barriers | Strategies |
| --- | --- |
| Lack of confidence | Gain exposure to new situations. Recall successes and learn from errors to move forward. |
| Logical fallacies | Reflect on your thinking. Be aware of logical thought and metacognition. Check with others. |
| High cognitive load | Focus on the main concern and relevant outcomes. Use a systematic approach, such as a model for thinking and decision making. |
| Communication hesitancy | Collaborate with colleagues. Develop clear communication patterns. Adopt a respectful and professional stance. |
| Lack of understanding of others' values and views | Inquire about client and peer opinions by asking yourself, *Am I making decisions with everyone's input in mind?* Adopt an ethical stance to thinking. |
| Racism in practice settings | advocacy for self and others; courses and training in anti-racism behaviours and system approaches to change |
| Nurses' voices not acknowledged | Advocate for yourself and others. Communicate professionally about client and workplace issues as they arise. Maintain communication with colleagues and administrators. |
| Distractions (physical, mental) | Remove yourself from a busy area, or ask for a minute to think so you are not interrupted. Maintain a tidy work environment. Practice mindfulness and focus on one issue at a time, if possible. Take a short break. |

and professional development that does not blame and shame nurses who make errors can encourage and support appropriate decision making in practice. Advocating for safe behaviours and attitudes, and for client safety, is important for confidence and clinical decision-making.

Different strategies can be used to address distractions to thinking. Mindfulness practices can help reduce mental distractions. Some institutions have a no-interruption zone where health care providers can prepare medications without the distraction of conversation (Doyle & McCutcheon, 2015). Finding a small, quiet space or sitting down in a chair to think can remove you from distractions in a physically busy setting. Other institutions have mentoring programs that help new graduates develop confidence in making decisions.

### Summary of Strategies for Decision Making

Table 4.3 presents a summary of barriers to decision making and some strategies to overcome them. As you review these strategies, think about others you can use that are most relevant to you in your practice. Deciding what to do is a crucial point in the thinking and decision-making process, so it is important to be fully aware of how you can develop the skills that will lead to optimal health outcomes for clients.

The benefits of support and experience and the use of strategies in decision making are clear (Nibblelink & Brewer, 2018). Until a novice nurse acquires sufficient experience to be confident and competent, they can employ a more analytical approach when decision making (Price et al., 2017) and engage with models or frameworks.

### ✳ TOOLBOX FOR THINKING

Some strategies to use when making decisions include:
- Apply mindfulness, reflection, and metacognition to help you focus on what is relevant and will support you in seeking answers to any questions you may have.
- Use shared decision making when collaborating with clients and other professionals or personal mentors on best options for care.
- Learn about institutional policies or procedures that protect time for making decisions and support equity and professional development through mentorship to strengthen nursing practice.

### THINKING THROUGH DECIDING WHAT TO DO: NRCE

The NRCE framework used in this textbook can help guide you to recall the wide range of influences on a client care situation during decision making. In the client scenario described in this section, the focus is on the second step of the thinking and decision-making process. Enough information has been found to proceed with deciding what to do. The client scenario in this section relates to medical assistance in dying (MAID) in Canada (Government of Canada, 2024). This NRCE framework can help you answer the question, *What must I consider when deciding what to do?*

## Nursing Knowledge

The *N* in *NRCE* relates to nursing knowledge. When deciding what to do, the nurse considers whether they have the requisite knowledge, skills, and abilities to think and perform in a particular client- or health-related situation. Interpretation of the information that has been gathered on the client's health is based on nursing knowledge and critical thinking skills. For instance, when abnormal values or cues are identified, the nurse needs enough knowledge of pathophysiology to group this information together with other clinical manifestations. "Cue recognition is the foundation of all decision making and is built through knowledge that is gained in nursing school" (Muntean, 2012, p. 20).

Consider what you know about nursing theory, standards and guidelines, the skills and procedures that you can perform, and how these are all applied and communicated in practice. Sasso et al. (2016) found that nursing students perceived differences between what they learned during their academic education and what they observed during their subsequent clinical practicum experiences. Differences in what was learned and what was observed further affect nursing students and newly graduated nurses, who attempt to reconcile these differences. They report feelings of insecurity in their health care activities and in decision making in relation to ethical situations, which may negatively affect the care provided to clients. In your work, think about how the knowledge you have acquired translates into evidence-informed, safe, and ethical care through decision-making processes.

### Example

A client who is terminally ill indicates to the nurse that they would like to access MAID. The nurse has a conscientious objection (CO) to MAID that has been reported and documented to their employer.

The nursing knowledge to consider when deciding what to do includes (but may not be limited to):

- Process and legal knowledge of mechanisms and procedures for MAID
- Therapeutic communication theory and approaches with client and other potential collaborators and health care providers (i.e., family, other health care professionals)
- Nursing best practices and guidelines that apply to the holistic care of a client with a terminal illness who is requesting MAID
- Availability and application of ethical decision-making models that support perspectives, biases, or alternative values of those engaged in decision making and decision support

## Professional Roles

The *R* in *NRCE* relates to professional roles—the roles and scopes of practice of nurses and other health care professionals. Recall that the nursing role and scope of practice include specific responsibilities and standards of care. When making decisions, nurses know that a medical diagnosis is a decision that is beyond the scope of the nursing profession (with some exceptions for nurse practitioners). Nurses must have a clear understanding of their distinct role. For example, in Ontario, registered nurses (RNs) and registered practical nurses (RPNs) can participate in providing nursing care and collaborating with a nurse practitioner (NP) or physician who is able to legally provide MAID to a client (College of Nurses of Ontario, 2021).

Additionally, interpretation may require consultation with others to obtain more information and validate care processes. Consultation is especially important in complex and ethical decisions and for synthesizing information. Detailed documentation of interprofessional roles and health care providers' contributions may be needed if a nursing plan is to be implemented over time and shared with others through delegation or collaboration on certain aspects of a client's care.

### Example

A client who is terminally ill indicates to the nurse that they would like to access MAID. The nurse has a CO to MAID that has been reported and documented to their employer.

The professional roles and scopes of practice to consider when deciding what to do include:

- Provincial or territorial practice standards for nurses in providing care; and the responsibility and duty to uphold care (i.e., cannot allow CO to obstruct access to care)
- Scopes of practice of other involved health care professionals
- Delegation, supervision, and leadership role capacity

## Client Context

The *C* in *NRCE* relates to the client context. The interpretation of client-generated information and of observed data, including the client's perspectives and experiences, requires verification and validation. It may also require requests for additional information. Analysis and interpretation of a client experience over time, compared with previously obtained or reported data, may be needed. The process of interpreting and analyzing information helps ensure that client views are clearly understood and not judged.

Increased nurse–client interaction could lead to the discovery of more information or specific needs that support synthesis of ideas for approaches to care and the overall decision-making process. The challenge for novice nurses is that clients may have other questions or preferences that could result in an analysis of information unrelated to the original issue at hand, increasing the cognitive load of the nurse and distracting them from priorities in client care (Muntean, 2012).

### Example

A client who is terminally ill indicates to the nurse that they would like to access MAID. The nurse has a CO to MAID that has been reported and documented to their employer.

Aspects of the client context to consider when deciding what to do may include (but are not limited to):

- Past experiences in health care situations
- Personal goals and perceptions of health and well-being
- Cultural and spiritual perspectives and preferences
- Client educational needs about MAID

## Health Care Environment

The *E* in *NRCE* relates to the health care environment, which is also an important influence on how decisions are made. In an institution, a number of resources support deciding what to do. They include standard operating procedures; staffing set-ups; clear organizational structures; available communication technologies; conference rooms or places to have discussions with clients or families that maintain privacy and confidentiality; and occupational health supports for practising professionals. In an interprofessional environment, these resources are available to nurses and other health care providers who participate in decision making. The provincial or territorial setting in which health care is delivered also influences how decisions are made. This setting includes external factors such as law, financial supports for the delivery of care to the population, and the pool of available health care providers.

### Example

A client who is terminally ill indicates to the nurse that they would like to access MAID. The nurse has a CO to MAID that has been reported and documented to their employer.

Elements of the health care environment to consider when deciding what to do include:

- Laws that relate to the institutional environment
- Complexity of care that is typically managed in the setting
- Staffing and health care delivery structures
- Distractions and conflicts that arise in the environment during the delivery of care
- Policies and procedures that support safe care (and accessibility and training related to MAID)
- Mental health and self-care practice supports
- Safe (i.e., no-blame or blame-free) organizational or unit culture

Table 4.4 presents a summary of the NRCE components as applied to decision-making activities (analyze, interpret, synthesize, and prioritize information, and generate

| TABLE 4.4 | Using NRCE When Making Decisions With a Client Who Requests MAID |
|---|---|
| **NRCE** | **What to Consider** |
| **Nursing** Knowledge | • Process and legal knowledge of mechanisms and procedures for MAID<br>• Therapeutic communication theory<br>• Perspectives, biases, and alternative values of those engaged in decision making and decision support<br>• Availability and application of ethical decision-making models that pertain to nursing |
| Professional **Roles** | • Provincial or territorial practice standards for nurses; and the responsibility and duty to provide care<br>• Scopes of practice of other involved health care providers<br>• Delegation, supervision, and leadership role capacity |
| **Client** Context | • Past experiences in health care situations<br>• Personal goals and perceptions of health and well-being<br>• Cultural and spiritual perspectives and preferences<br>• Client educational needs |
| Health Care **Environment** | • Laws that relate to the institutional environment<br>• Complexity of care that is typically managed in the setting<br>• Staffing and health care delivery structures<br>• Distractions and conflicts in the environment<br>• Policies and procedures that support safe care<br>• Mental health and self-care practice supports<br>• Safe organizational or unit culture |

## TABLE 4.5   Case Study: Application of the Ethical Decision-Making Model to Deciding What to Do

| Ethical Situation* | Nursing Model and Application of Thinking | | |
|---|---|---|---|
| | Ethical Decision-Making Model[a] | Clinical Reasoning Skills Used | Possible Nursing Responses (Barriers, Strategies) |
| The resident of a small rural long-term care facility has requested and been approved for MAID using intravenous-administered drugs. The family is supportive. The client has selected the day as the anniversary of their spouse's death and wants to die at "home" (the facility). The nurse scheduled to be on duty for that day has a conscientious objection (CO) to MAID, which has been reported to their employer.<br>The main issue is a conflict of personal versus professional values (client's right to autonomy and choice versus the nurse's responsibility to enable access to MAID, and the nurse's moral convictions and CO to actively or passively participating).<br>All available options for addressing the ethical issue must be identified. So too how any choices may be perceived, valued, and implemented. | Assessing<br><br>**Reflecting on and reviewing potential actions** | As described in the ethical situation.<br><br>Make inferences.<br>Identify possible bias in interpretation.<br>Match situation with past experiences.<br>Verify and/or validate data/information.<br>Determine sufficiency of data/information.<br>Distinguish between what is and is not relevant. | Check biases and assumptions: the nurse identified a CO to MAID.<br>Check knowledge: the nurse has no previous experiences of MAID at this facility. |
| Professional obligations must be acknowledged when deciding on an action.<br>The rural facility does not have a large nursing staff. Most are personal support workers. A nurse is needed to assist in this case.<br>Moving the client to another facility would enable the nurse to work, but the client's desire to die at "home" would not be met.<br>The ideal outcome is for the client and nurse to be equally supported in their desires and needs. | **Selecting an ethical action (maximizing good)** | Set priorities.<br>Generate options, solutions, and client-centred goals.<br>Communicate and consult with client/other professionals. | Consult with the supervisor and medical health care professional to ensure an ideal outcome.<br>Consider whether MAID can be scheduled when the nurse is not on shift. Coordinate with the medical health care professional.<br>Consider switching nurses' schedules for that day. |
| | Engaging in ethical action<br><br>Reflecting on and reviewing the ethical action | *Consider the next steps. What actions will occur with what has been decided?* | |

*Modified from an ethical situation in Panchuk, J., & Thirsk, L. M. (2021). Conscientious objection to medical assistance in dying in rural/remote nursing. *Nursing Ethics, 28*(5), 766–775 (pp. 769–772). doi:10.1177/0969733020976185.
[a]Canadian Nurses Association. (2017). *Code of ethics for registered nurses.* https://www.cna-aiic.ca/en/nursing/regulated-nursing-in-canada/nursing-ethics.

options). As with the first step of the thinking and decision-making process (finding information), some areas overlap. For instance, the nurse's knowledge of the process, policy, and regulation of MAID and their competency in being able to apply it in the health care setting is strongly supported by institutional or employer policy and procedures.

## DECIDING WHAT TO DO: AN ETHICAL DECISION-MAKING MODEL CASE STUDY

In this section, the ethical decision-making model (see Chapter 2) will be applied to a simple case study, using the example of a client who would like to access MAID. The case study provides an example of how to approach the second step of the thinking and decision-making process: deciding what to do. Refer back to Table 2.6 for details on the steps involved in this model.

The case study in Table 4.5 incorporates key ideas covered in this chapter, including the clinical reasoning skills described earlier. As well, it addresses possible responses to barriers to thinking and strategies to overcome those barriers.

## SUMMARY

This chapter outlined concepts, skills, strategies, and models that support the nurse during decision making. Analysis, interpretation, synthesis, and prioritization are all needed to successfully generate reasonable options for care of the client. Decisions on the appropriate care for a client will incorporate as much input as possible from the client and others in the circle of care. A client scenario was presented to illustrate how the ethical decision-making model can be applied as an example for guiding decision making in nursing practice. However, other models can assist with this step of the thinking and decision-making process as well.

## KEY POINTS TO REMEMBER

These are the key points to remember from this chapter.

### About Decision Making

- A decision occurs when the best option from the available alternatives is selected.
- Decision-making literature shows that expertise with decision-making varies, novices and experts use different thinking processes, discipline-specific knowledge is important, creativity and critical thinking are needed, the thinking strategies used affect success, and monitoring the quality of the thinking process is important.
- Information and complex data need to be analyzed, interpreted, synthesized, and prioritized to generate options on which a final decision is made.
- A *good decision* is one that addresses the identified issue or problem effectively, given the information that was available *at the time*.
- Decision making is both outcome focused and process focused; what is decided and how it was decided are both important when making good decisions.

### About Foundations for Deciding What to Do

- Nurses must use analyzing, interpreting, synthesizing, and prioritizing skills before a choice is made on what to do.
- Analysis is the process of uncovering patterns and trends in information, and of establishing relationships among data.

- Interpretation is the process of assigning meaning to information and entails clearly identifying what is occurring in relation to the concern or issue.
- Nursing knowledge, evidence-informed approaches, and science can help analyze and interpret information.
- Understanding the responsibilities in your nursing role and your scope of practice can guide you in analysis and interpretation of a client situation.
- Synthesis occurs when everything that is known is brought together to form a whole idea or a new perspective about a client situation, such as when the nurse identifies a significant change in the client's condition.
- Prioritization involves ranking client or nursing-related issues using criteria for urgency or importance, so that a sequence of nursing actions may be planned or established in the path ahead.
- Risk is another significant component when determining priorities for care and can be described as the probability or likelihood that something may occur. It is associated with the degree of severity of any anticipated consequence of that risk. It is an important consideration when identifying priorities.
- Maslow's hierarchy of needs, the *ABCD* acronym, and the related *CURE* hierarchy can be used by the nurse as tools to establish priorities based on client needs.

## About Skills Used When Deciding What to Do

- The unified process for thinking and decision making (see Figure 4.2) includes a number of skills that can be useful when deciding what to do:
  - Set priorities.
  - Make inferences.
  - See patterns over time.
  - Group related cues together.
  - Compare data with normal ranges.
  - Identify inconsistent or missing data.
  - Identify possible bias in interpretation.
  - Match situation with past experiences.
  - Verify and/or validate data/information.
  - Determine sufficiency of data/information.
  - Distinguish between what is and is not relevant.
  - Generate options, solutions, client-centred goals.
  - Communicate and consult with client/other professionals.

## About Barriers to Thinking When Deciding What to Do

- Barriers to using these skills when decision making in nursing include personal errors or challenges to thinking, relational or communication difficulties, and organizational impediments.

- Relational racism and other institutional structures that overlap with organizational barriers can negatively affect a nurse's decision making.

## About Helpful Strategies for Overcoming Barriers to Deciding What to Do

- Strategies that can help the nurse overcome barriers include thinking about one's thinking, gaining experience, engaging with others in clear and respectful communication, and advocating for supportive and safe health care environments.
- Courses and training that increase awareness of racism can assist with personal reflection and institutional policy improvements.

## About Thinking Through Deciding What to Do: NRCE

- This textbook's NRCE framework provides a holistic view of analyzing, interpreting, and synthesizing information to prioritize and decide what to do.

## About a Case Study on Deciding What to Do

- A case study on an ethics-related client scenario showed how key ideas in this chapter, with the use of the ethical decision-making model as a guide, can be applied to the decision-making process and client care.

## CONCLUSION AND THINKING IT THROUGH

Understanding the components of decision making helps the nurse form a foundation for reasoning processes and logic thought. Decision-making is analytical and requires the decision-maker to combine client cues, interpret and synthesize, and to form a logical determination of an eventual intervention that will address a particular client need (Corcoran-Perry & Bungert, 1992). While identified as the second step in thinking it through in nursing practice, decision making is a recurring mental activity that takes place at many points and in different ways. For instance, when finding information during the first step of the process, you need to decide what to assess first and make choices about what is relevant and what is not.

A decision occurs when the best option from the available alternatives is selected. Once this happens, a path forward is established. Next, a plan of care is created and implemented to support the identified solutions and nursing actions. This topic will be presented in Chapter 5.

## CLASS ACTIVITIES TO CHECK THINKING

### Think-Aloud Pair Problem Solving (TAPPS)

Form pairs. Decide who will be a problem solver and listener for Problem A. The problem solver reads the problem aloud and talks through a response to the problem, while the listener reminds the problem solver to think aloud, asks clarification questions, offers encouragement to keep thinking, but refrains from providing possible answers. Switch roles for Problem B.

For each of these problems, analyze, interpret, synthesize and prioritize options for care.
- **Problem A:** A 35-year-old client on a labour and delivery unit states, "My water just broke." Membranes noted to rupture clear fluid, and bloody show is apparent. Client reports pain at 9/10 with contractions. A pulsating umbilical cord was palpated during the vaginal exam; fetus at 0 station, 8 cm dilated, and 80% effaced. Vital signs: Temperature 37.2°C (99°F); pulse 110 beats per

minute (bpm); respiratory rate 20 breaths/minute; blood pressure 90/62 mm Hg. Fetal heart rate: 90 bpm with minimal variability and prolonged decelerations.

- **Problem B:** A client on a surgical unit who has had recent abdominal surgery coughs forcefully and then states, "I feel like something gave way under my bandages." The nurse removes the dressing and observes a loop of bowel protruding through the incision.

Which of these two problems was more challenging to work through? Why?

### Activities and Discussion Questions

1. Identify a simple clinical situation that requires a decision. This may include whether to administer a prn (as needed) medication to a client, or whether to notify a physician of a change in client condition either immediately or later on. You may think of another situation that you may have recently experienced. Then, *draw a map* of the decision-making process that starts after you have completed the required assessment. Share your map with a classmate and have them explain to you your own decision making based on the map. Is it accurate?

2. Review the clinical reasoning and other skills that may be used when making decisions. Select two and write a short description of how you think you will use them in your own thinking.

3. Choose one barrier and strategy from Table 4.3. Describe to a classmate what your own challenges are with the identified barrier and what you will personally do to overcome it.

## CASE STUDY REVIEW

Review the case study in Table 4.5.

### Questions

1. On your own, consider your personal views on MAID and how they would influence your thinking in such a situation. Consult your jurisdiction's information and guidance on MAID if you are unfamiliar with this process.
   a. Think about the challenge of providing care in a situation that you disagree with. What would you do?
   b. Make a list or write a short reflection to help clarify your thoughts.
   c. How do your personal views and reflections fit with your obligations as a professional nurse?
   d. How could this affect your decision making in a similar situation?

2. With a classmate, review how the case study can be completed. What are the steps to take and why?

## EVIDENCE-INFORMED THINKING ACTIVITY

Consider the following scenario in which a nurse's decision differs. A nurse has been caring for a client who requires intensive wound care after a third degree burn injury to both legs. The client is so grateful for the nurse's expertise and caring approach that they offer the nurse $200.00 in cash as an expression of thanks.

- *Decision A:* The nurse decides to graciously accept the money and vows to continue to care for the client in a professional and caring manner.
- *Decision B:* The nurse decides to refuse the money, thanks the client for the generous offer, and proceeds with providing care.

## QUESTIONS TO ASSESS LEARNING

### Review Questions

1. A nurse has discovered a pattern in a client's blood pressure that increases just before or during a medical appointment. The nurse also confirms that doctors make the client "nervous." What processes are used by the nurse when connecting these points of information?
   a. Prioritizing and judging
   b. Analyzing and interpreting
   c. Synthesizing and deciding
   d. Recognizing and identifying

2. A client living with type 2 diabetes mellitus currently has a very high blood glucose level and is increasingly confused. The client, who is at home and very lonely, is asking that the nurse help them place a video call to their daughter who lives in another province because "I can't understand the computer or see the screen very well." What should the nurse use to *prioritize* care in this situation?
   a. Maslow's hierarchy of needs
   b. Client preference
   c. Reference to policies about confidentiality
   d. Personal values about family

3. Which strategy *does not* demonstrate mindfulness when administering medications?
   a. Directing a colleague to ask their question after the task is completed
   b. Focusing on every step of the task
   c. Answering questions from clients about the medications
   d. Finding a quiet place to perform dosage calculations

4. A nurse says, "The most experienced nurse on the unit said this was the correct way to perform this procedure, so it must be right." This rationale is based on which logical fallacy?
   a. False dichotomy
   b. Ad populum
   c. Hasty generalization
   d. Appeal to authority

## ONE LAST THOUGHT

How will you define a good decision in your own nursing practice? Make a list of how you currently identify decisions that you identify as optimal. Reflect on your confidence with proceeding to act on the last clinical decision that you made. Explain your level of confidence in relation to your decision.

## ONLINE RESOURCES

*Logical fallacies* (2024). Purdue University. https://owl.purdue.edu/owl/general_writing/academic_writing/logic_in_argumentative_writing/fallacies.html.

*Medical assistance in dying: Overview* (2024). Government of Canada. https://www.canada.ca/en/health-canada/services/health-services-benefits/medical-assistance-dying.html.

*Mind maps in education expand learning potential* (2024). Mindmaps.com. https://www.mindmaps.com/mind-maps-for-education/.

*Nursing management and professional concepts eBook: Chapter 2.3 tools for prioritizing*—WisTech Open (n.d.): https://wtcs.pressbooks.pub/nursingmpc/chapter/2-3-tools-for-prioritizing/#:~:text=The%20CURE%20hierarchy%20uses%20the,patient%20needs%20require%20immediate%20action

*Short film and anti-racist resource.* Danda, M., Pitcher, C., & Key, J. (2022). Hearing our voices: Nurses speaking out about decentering whiteness in health care. https://www.youtube.com/watch?v=C66xZSLMdCk

## REFERENCES

Astle, B., & Duggleby, W. (2024). *Potter and Perry's Canadian fundamentals of nursing* (7th ed.). Elsevier.

Beagan, B. L., Bizzeth, S. R., Sibbald, K. R., & Etowa, J. B. (2022). Epistemic racism in the health professions: A qualitative study with Black women in Canada. *Health. 28*(2), 203–215. https://journals.sagepub.com/doi/pdf/10.1177/13634593221141605.

Blondy, L. C., Blakeslee, A. M., Scheffer, B. K., et al. (2016). Understanding synthesis across disciplines to improve nursing education. *Western Journal of Nursing Research, 38*(6), 668–685. https://doi.org/10.1177/0193945915621720.

Burgess, D. J. (2010). Are providers more likely to contribute to healthcare disparities under high levels of cognitive load? How features of the healthcare setting may lead to biases in medical decision making. *Medical Decision Making: An International Journal of the Society for Medical Decision Making, 30*(2), 246–257. https://doi.org/10.1177/0272989X09341751.

Burkhardt, M. A., Nathaniel, A. K., & Walton, N. (2018). *Ethics and issues in contemporary nursing* (3rd Cdn ed.). Nelson.

Canadian Nurses Association. (2017). *Code of ethics for registered nurses.* https://www.cna-aiic.ca/en/nursing/regulated-nursing-in-canada/nursing-ethics.

Canadian Nurses Association. (2020). *Nine tests and treatments to question in nursing.* https://choosingwiselycanada.org/recommendation/nursing/.

Cappelletti, A., Engel, J. K., & Prentice, D. (2014). Systematic review of clinical judgment and reasoning in nursing. *Journal of Nursing Education, 53*(8), 453–458. doi:10.3928/01484834-20140724-01.

Clayton, W. R. (2019). Overcoming barriers impeding nurse activation of rapid response teams. *Online Journal of Issues in Nursing, 24*(3), 1–10. https://doi.org/10.3912/OJIN.Vol24No03PPT22.

College of Nurses of Ontario. (2021). *Guidance on nurses' roles in medical assistance in dying.* https://www.cno.org/globalassets/docs/prac/41056-guidance-on-nurses-roles-in-maid.pdf.

College of Registered Nurses of Newfoundland and Labrador. (2022). *Scope of practice framework.* https://www.crnnl.ca/site/uploads/2022/06/scope-of-practice-framework.pdf.

Corcoran-Perry, S. A., & Bungert, B. (1992). Enhancing orthopaedic nurses' clinical decision making. *Orthopedic Nursing, 11*(3), 64–70.

Coulter, A., & Collins, A. (2011). *Making shared decision-making a reality: No decision about me, without me.* The King's Fund.

Danda, M., Pitcher, C., & Key, J. (2022). Hearing our voices (part 2): Empowering nurses to take anti-racist action in health care. *Canadian Nurse.* https://www.canadian-nurse.com/blogs/cn-content/2022/05/24/hearing-our-voices-part-2-empowering-nurses-to-tak.

Doyle, G. R., & McCutcheon, J. A. (2015). *Clinical procedures for safer patient care.* BCcampus. https://opentextbc.ca/clinicalskills/.

Gambrill, E. (2012). *Critical thinking in clinical practice: Improving the quality of judgments and decisions* (3rd ed.). Wiley.

Government of Canada. (2015). *Truth and Reconciliation Commission of Canada: Calls to action.* https://publications.gc.ca/site/eng/9.801236/publication.html.

Government of Canada. (2024). *Medical assistance in dying.* https://www.canada.ca/en/health-canada/services/medical-assistance-dying.html.

Halpern, D. (2014). *Thought and knowledge: An introduction to critical thinking* (5th ed.). Psychology Press.

Jull, J., Sheppard, A. J., Hizaka, A., et al. (2021). Experiences of Inuit in Canada who travel from remote settings for cancer care and impacts on decision making. *BMC Health Services Research, 21,* 328. https://doi.org/10.1186/s12913-021-06303-9.

Kahneman, D. (2011). *Thinking fast and slow.* Canada: Anchor.

Kohtz, C., Gowda, C., & Guede, P. (2017). Cognitive stacking: Strategies for the busy RN. *Nursing, 47*(1), 18–20. https://doi.org/10.1097/01.nurse.0000510758.31326.92.

Lankshear, S., & Martin, D. (2019). Getting comfortable with "it depends": Embracing the impermanence of scope of practice. *Nursing Leadership, 32*(1), 30–41. doi:10.12927/cjnl.2019.25850.

Maslow, A. H. (1943). A theory of human motivation. *Psychological Review, 50*(4), 370–396.

McGillis Hall, L. M., Ferguson-Paré, M., Peter, E., et al. (2010). Going blank: Factors contributing to interruptions to nurses' work and related outcomes. *Journal of Nursing Management, 18*(8), 1040–1047. https://doi-org.ezproxy.library.yorku.ca/10.1111/j.1365-2834.2010.01166.x.

Muntean, W. (2012). *Nursing clinical decision-making: A literature review.* https://www.ncsbn.org/research-item/nursing-clinical-decisionmaking-a-literature-review.

Nibbelink, C. W., & Brewer, B. B. (2018). Decision-making in nursing practice: An integrative literature review. *Journal of Clinical Nursing, 27*(5–6), 917–928. https://doi.org/10.1111/jocn.14151.

Nielsen, A., Stragnell, S., & Jester, P. (2007). Guide for reflection using the clinical judgement model. *Journal of Nursing Education, 46*(11), 513–516.

Panchuk, J., & Thirsk, L. M. (2021). Conscientious objection to medical assistance in dying in rural/remote nursing. *Nursing Ethics, 28*(5), 766–775. doi:10.1177/0969733020976185.

Price, A., Zulkosky, K., White, K., et al. (2017). Accuracy of intuition in clinical decision-making among novice clinicians. *Journal of Advanced Nursing, 73*(5), 1147–1157. doi:10.1111/jan.13202.

Robijn, L., Deliens, L., Rietjens, J., et al. (2020). Barriers in the decision making about and performance of continuous sedation until death in nursing homes. *The Gerontologist, 60*(5), 916–925. https://doi.org/10.1093/geront/gnz165.

Sasso, L., Bagnasco, A., Bianchi, M., et al. (2016). Moral distress in undergraduate nursing students: A systematic review. *Nursing Ethics, 23*(5), 523–534. https://doi.org/10.1177/0969733015574926.

Shellian, B., & Levinson, W. (2016). When more is not always better: Choosing nursing interventions wisely. *Nursing Leadership (Toronto, Ont.), 29*(4), 8–9. doi:10.12927/cjnl.2016.24989.

Tanner, C. (2006). Thinking like a nurse: A research-based model of clinical judgment in nursing. *Journal of Nursing Education, 45*(6), 204–211.

Tyerman, J., & Cobbett, S. (2023). *Medical-surgical nursing in Canada: Assessment and management of clinical problems* (5th ed.). Elsevier.

Walton, N. A., & Waddell, J. I. (2025). *Yoder-Wise's leading and managing in Canadian nursing* (3rd ed.). Elsevier.

# Acting on Decisions

## LEARNING OUTCOMES

*After reading this chapter, you will be able to:*

- Incorporate the concepts of inclusivity and diversity, and the unique needs of clients in collaborative planning.
- Explain the importance of communication during care planning and implementation.
- Compare and contrast various health care professionals' contributions to team-based care.

- Describe how self-regulation can affect the delivery of care.
- Identify the clinical reasoning skills used when taking action in an individual client situation and a larger community context.

## GLOSSARY

**Collaboration:** the process whereby a client or family member participates in the development and delivery of a plan of care, or when professionals interacting in real time discuss a client's presenting symptoms, describe their views on treatment, and jointly develop a plan of care

**Consultation:** the process of confirming or checking information with a client or family, or seeking advice, validating plans of care, or corroborating perceptions of a client's needs with another professional

**Coordination:** working together with a client or client family for a common goal; at least two professionals communicating and working in parallel or in a back-and-forth fashion to achieve a common client-centred goal, while delivering care separately

**Implementation:** initiation and completion of planned actions or nursing interventions; it includes documenting or recording the care provided

**Interprofessional collaboration:** "a partnership between a team of health providers and a client in a participatory, collaborative and coordinated approach to shared decision-making around health and social issues" (Canadian Interprofessional Health Collaborative, 2010, p. 24)

**Planning:** a description of how client-centred outcomes will be achieved, which is developed once priorities

and outcomes for addressing a problem are identified; planning involves collaborating, consulting, and communicating, and can address several client issues at once

**Professional communication:** communication that conveys a role of responsibility and accountability for one's actions and is clear, courteous, individual, trustworthy, and assertive; with other health care professionals, follows evidence-informed frameworks

**Reflection-in-action:** the ability of a nurse to observe ("read" or notice) the client and their response to a nursing intervention, and to adjust the interventions as needed based on that observation (Tanner, 2006)

**Self-regulation:** the ability to reflect on thinking and identify one's learning needs, set goals, select useful resources, and self-evaluate accomplishments and subsequent development that is required to improve

**Taking action:** carrying out the solutions that address the highest priorities; similar to intervention, it includes the most appropriate activities and the tasks/skills required to perform the intervention (administering, communicating, teaching, documenting, coordinating, etc.)

The quality of a nurse's decision making becomes evident when planning for and acting on a decision. Once a decision is made, planning begins on how that decision will be implemented. An understanding of nursing theory, nursing practice, effective client and interprofessional collaboration, and the health care context can help guide the delivery of planned care. Later in this chapter, the nursing process is used as an example to demonstrate how decisions can be acted on in a local community setting.

## MOVING FORWARD ON A DECISION: MAKING A PLAN OF CARE

Once a decision is made, it is time to act. Action, or response, is focused on carrying out the decision that was made to address a particular client issue or health care–related problem. Action involves applying a solution, planning how the identified goals will be met, and choosing which activities should be performed in response.

Recall that in the second step of the thinking and decision-making process, options for care were generated and compared, and several possible solutions were considered. Then, client-centred goals were chosen and prioritized. These goals were selected for their appropriateness for the client situation. When deciding what to do, it is important to consider the value and relevance of the various options and possible solutions, and then collaboratively identify goals or desired outcomes *before* a plan is created. Otherwise, the plan of care and subsequent nursing actions may be unclear, directionless, inefficient, and ineffective.

A plan of care maps out nursing activities and demonstrates the nurse's accountability in partnering with the client to deliver care. Planning requires that the nurse apply critical thinking skills and enact priorities and outcomes that have been identified. The way to meet these priorities and outcomes is described in the plan of care. Implementation of the plan involves initiating and completing the planned actions or nursing interventions, and documenting or recording the care provided (Astle & Duggleby, 2024).

### Confirming the Plan's Goals

Client-centred goals are used as a basis for developing a meaningful plan of action. Therefore, check with the client and their family or significant others as needed to ascertain whether anything has changed and whether the goals are still relevant and agreeable to the client. Doing so is especially important if time has passed since the goals were selected and the client's situation or condition has changed.

Confirm that the goals are *SMART* (*s*pecific, *m*easurable, *a*ttainable, *r*elevant, *t*imed) and client centred. If goals were created to address a professional nursing issue that is not directly client related, the goals should be SMART and issue centred as well. Following confirmation of the goals, the plan is communicated and shared.

### Engaging in Professional Communication

Professional communication conveys a role of responsibility and accountability for one's actions and is clear, courteous, individual, trustworthy, and assertive. The process of planning involves certain aspects of communication. Specifically, consultation, collaboration, and coordination (3Cs) help create a plan that is actionable and clear to those involved in the care process (Table 5.1). While these communication activities can occur in other phases of the care process and contribute to thinking as a nurse, they are essential to formulating a plan to meet a client's goals. Consultation occurs when seeking verification and confirmation of plans of care. Collaboration depends on the scope of practice of the professional (in terms of how their knowledge and skill set can contribute to care) and on the client's abilities, and it often occurs in complex situations (Cohen et al., 2015). Generally, coordination involves planning and resource management to ensure that activities are complementary and promote optimal health.

### Developing a Client-Centred Plan

The individual needs of the client are incorporated into planning care. Recall that when finding information on a client's situation, identified concern, or health issue (see Chapter 3), the individuality of the client is recognized and respected. This includes but is not limited to observations of their values, beliefs, and preferences for culture, spirituality, gender identity or sexual orientation, and lived experiences with their health and health care settings. If a client chooses to have limited or no involvement in their own care, nurses are responsible for communicating and documenting this choice and to continue to revisit it during care. In some circumstances, however, care actions must occur quickly, and clients may not be fully involved in decision making. This topic is discussed further in Chapter 7.

The nurse must engage in clinical reasoning when thinking and communicating about how to best adapt a plan for a client so that an optimal outcome can be achieved. Box 5.1 presents a comparison of two approaches to developing a plan of care for a client.

| TABLE 5.1 | Communication: 3Cs Used in Planning and Implementing Care | |
| --- | --- | --- |
| **Activity** | **Description** | **Examples** |
| Consultation | Confirming or checking information with a client or family to ensure development of a relevant plan. Seeking advice from other health care professionals, validating plans of care, or corroborating perceptions of a client's needs with other professionals | A client on several medications for a long-term mental health condition is experiencing uncontrolled nausea during pregnancy. The nurse contacts the obstetrician for a prescription, but they are not sure of an appropriate medication. The obstetrician calls to leave a message for the pharmacist. The pharmacist returns the call after conferring with their colleague and recommends promethazine (Phenergan). The obstetrician communicates back to the nurse with a plan for medication. |
| Collaboration | Working together with a client or client's family for a common goal; promotes responsibility and self-expression, and strengthens client problem solving and understanding of their health situation. Two or more health care providers interacting in real time to discuss the order of care, a client's presenting symptoms, or their views on treatment to jointly develop a plan to deliver care | After conducting an assessment, the nurse identifies that a client who has been diagnosed with type 2 diabetes mellitus has not been managing the disease well. The nurse tells the client that a dietitian and the diabetes nurse educator may be able to help, and the client agrees. The nurse arranges for the professionals to meet together and with the client. The dietitian teaches about diet options that fit with the client's culture and preferences, and the diabetes educator reviews the client's ability to self-monitor. |
| Coordination | A process that may occur with the client's or family member's participation in delivery of care. Two or more health care professionals working in parallel or in a back-and-forth fashion to achieve a common client-centred goal, while delivering care separately | A nurse is just about to enter a client's room with a nursing student to conduct an assessment. The nurse is called by a health care aide who explains that a different client who speaks Urdu and is about to be discharged requires teaching. The nurse agrees, confirms the client's room number, and tells the aide that they will speak with the client after the assessment and to call the translator. In the meantime, the aide gathers discharge materials in Urdu and provides it to the client. The nurse proceeds to assess the client as scheduled. Once that care is completed, the nurse meets with the translator and proceeds to teach the client, who has been reviewing the discharge materials. |

Adapted from Cohen, D. J., Davis, M., Balasubramanian, B. A., et al. (2015). Integrating behavioral health and primary care: Consulting, coordinating and collaborating among professionals. *Journal of the American Board of Family Medicine, 28* (Suppl 1), S21–S31. https://doi.org/10.3122/jabfm.2015.S1.150042.

Generally, if adapting common procedures or standard plans of care to meet a client's needs, consider the following factors:

- Necessity: Ask yourself, *Is a change to the standard approach to care required to meet the client's needs? AND*

- Safety: Ask yourself, *Is the change going to introduce a new risk or threat to the safe care of the client, or to nurses or the environment?*

Identifying the way to efficiently organize, share, and execute even a simple plan or task will help you choose what to do first (Box 5.2). This activity helps avoid wasting

---

**BOX 5.1    Comparing Approaches to Developing a Client-Centred Plan**

**Scenario:** A client of Indigenous heritage enters the palliative care unit while awaiting arrangements for palliative home care. The client has advanced cancer and wishes to forgo further treatments. They have been living independently in their own home in an Indigenous community. However, their condition has deteriorated in the last few weeks. Their partner is at the bedside. The client and partner are requesting a smudging ceremony.

| Less Optimal Case Planning | More Optimal Case Planning |
|---|---|
| **Nurse:** I see that you are experiencing some pain; your pulse is weak and irregular, and you appear restless. | **Nurse:** I see that you are experiencing some pain; your pulse is weak and irregular, and you appear restless. |
| **Client:** Yes, I would like to ask for a smudging ceremony. It would bring me peace and comfort. | **Client:** Yes, I would like to ask for a smudging ceremony. It would bring me peace and comfort. |
| **Nurse:** It is important for you that we control your pain first, and unfortunately because of the fire codes, such a ceremony is not possible. Is there anything else you need? | **Nurse:** I see that this is important to you. I am going to ask what can be done and plan for you and your partner to hold this ceremony. What do you think? |
| **Client:** No, that was it . . . | **Client:** Okay. |
| | **Nurse:** Do you have the name of someone you would like us to contact? |
| | **Partner:** I can provide the name of a Knowledge Keeper. |
| | **Nurse:** Thank you. I'm going to get your pain medication and find out how you can conduct a smudging ceremony here. I will do this as soon as I can and update you on what I find out. |

Kristoff, T. (2022). Co-constructing a diverse hybrid simulation-based experience on First Nations culture. *Clinical Simulation in Nursing, 67*, 33–38. https://doi.org/10.1016/j.ecns.2022.02.012; Mullin, J., Lee, L., Hertwig, S., et al. (2001). A native smudging ceremony: A young native patient in palliative care teaches his caregivers a lesson in spirituality and cultural diversity. *The Canadian Nurse, 97*(9), 20–22.

---

**BOX 5.2    Tips for Planning to Act**

- Take time to strategize when and how the task will be completed; test it out if possible.
- Take and keep notes. Create a checklist of next steps.
- Ensure familiarity with relevant policies and procedures.
- Gather information and/or supplies, and bring extra items as needed.
- Maintain a tidy and organized environment: "a place for everything, and everything in its place."
- Keep supplies clean, and return unused items.
- Know when to communicate with others and organize reporting.

supplies and time, engaging in repeated communication, and possibly confusing the client about the care they will receive. It also helps increase your confidence in and control of your practice.

## Formalizing a Plan

A plan of care can take different forms, depending on institution or agency resources. It can be paper based or computerized (electronic), or a standardized critical pathway of care for groups of clients experiencing a particular situation. These plans can be customized and shared among nurses and other health care professionals. Plans are formalized to ensure consistent delivery of care and future actions.

The *computerized plans* included in the electronic health care record (EHR) are primarily used by nurses and serve as a foundation for formally documenting client care. EHR systems support clinical decision making, client risk assessment, and barcode medication administration. Computerized plans also allow client care to be customized, and for information to be added or deleted from general menus. While nurses may find it time consuming to create and maintain records and associated plans of care (Strudwick et al., 2022), these records and plans are essential for professional communication. They also provide a means for sharing information among relevant health care professionals in a confidential and clear manner that supports the legal requirements of care.

Community-based settings also require formal plans for client care. These plans are created and shared in clinics, health offices, or between care providers working with clients in their own homes. These plans may be computerized or paper based, depending on the employer resources and the process for comprehensive documentation and provision of rationale for care. They may include a broader assessment of the client situation and a home and family assessment. Aspects of the plan of care involve the client and self-care activities that support the identified health goals.

*Critical pathways* serve as multidisciplinary resources for the standard or routine care of clients with similar clinical needs (D'Entremont, 2009). They apply to about 80% of clients in a particular cohort or group (such as clients undergoing a hip arthroplasty). While they often require some individual adjustment and cannot replace a nurse's clinical reasoning and decision making, they facilitate information sharing and coordination of the delivery of care. Critical pathways are based on evidence-informed knowledge and support best care practices at the institution that creates them. At certain decision points in the client's course of care (daily or hourly), they recommend activities and therapies, and describe interventions. For certain conditions, critical pathways can replace the need to fully develop a client plan (Astle & Duggleby, 2024).

Plans may also be worked through, tested, or discussed verbally or (more formally) on paper or electronically. The 3Cs (collaboration, consultation, coordination) are often engaged in during face-to-face or virtual discussions with other health care professionals. Short, single-action plans may be communicated verbally and then formally documented. Increasingly, simple plans or changes to plans are shared via text or email using the institutional messaging or chat features of EHR and documentation platforms. Clients who are involved in planning their care also use more accessible technologies (such as email or telehealth) to seamlessly communicate with health care providers as needed. Recall that confidentiality standards and institutional policy should be followed in all communications.

Formalizing and sharing a plan of care is also guided by the perspectives of the client (i.e., the individual, family, group, community, or population). Clients may have preferences for sharing their plan with a friend or family member who they would like to be involved. Client consent and permission is needed to share plans of care. An understanding of the client's culture, personal experiences, diverse background, and Indigenous views and knowledge plays a large role in supporting client preferences in a formalized plan of care. Not including the input of a client who is able to participate in their care jeopardizes their dignity and autonomy.

## IMPLEMENTING THE PLAN OF CARE

Once a plan of care has been established with relevant input from other health care providers involved in the client's care and the client, acting on that plan occurs next. The totality of what has been considered culminates in the implementation of care to maintain or improve health. How care is implemented varies widely, depending on the nursing care setting, the client's environment, and the resources available, all of which would have been factored into the planning step.

Once the decision is made that care will proceed, scheduling and coordinating care are crucial next steps. However, these activities are often overlooked in planning. If an intervention is required immediately, the policies and procedures that the nurse and other health care providers need to employ to safely guide the response must be taken into account. If an intervention is required at a specific time or by a particular deadline, the nurse must arrange for it to happen. Coordination with other health care providers in the care setting is crucial to ensure that care takes place when it should and as it should.

The nurse who acts on a decision and implements care relies on nursing knowledge and an understanding of activities that will help deliver care. Implementation involves the use of technology, teaching, teamwork processes (assigning, delegating, and supervising), and self-regulation (discussed in Chapter 1). These activities are important because they inform how implementation occurs and can be applied to many client situations and health care circumstances. *All involve clinical reasoning skills* to ensure the delivery of safe, competent, and ethical nursing care.

### Using Technology

Technology is commonly used when delivering care to measure and monitor trends, administer therapy, and support health. However, as technology is always changing, it is being used increasingly in the processes of decision making and implementing care.

Hospitals are beginning to incorporate technological innovations on a larger scale. As one example, Ontario's Mackenzie Health's Cortellucci Vaughan Hospital was the first smart hospital in Canada. It features fully integrated technology systems and medical devices that communicate digitally to maximize information exchange and facilitate improved client care (Mackenzie Health, 2023). Nurses can use this technology to access information and communicate plans more easily. Become familiar with the technological tools available to you and develop your competence with digital health technology. Bear in mind that any new technology has advantages and disadvantages.

## FOCUS ON TECHNOLOGY

### *Balancing Care in a Digital World*

A number of digital health technologies have become integrated in health care and nursing practice:

- *Artificial intelligence/big data:* It can be used when planning and responding to outbreaks or pandemics with contact tracing and population health response to care. Transparency and privacy are concerns for nurses and clients.
- *Social media and online information:* Diverse sources of health information can assist with implementing care and client education. Quality and reliability are necessary. It is important to use proper "netiquette" when engaging in online activities and advocating for clients.
- *Virtual and augmented reality:* It is used to assess and deliver treatments or clinical interventions to remote communities. It enhances teaching and coaching, and supports communication. It should use low-cost devices and software or integrate easily with existing technology resources. It can enhance clinical learning in education settings.
- *Telehealth:* As a virtual model of care delivery and communication, it can include coaching and triaging clients, and it can help reduce isolation and improve safety during outbreaks in long-term care settings.
- *Mobile devices:* The use of smartphones and health care applications enables real-time conversations, supports remote advice, and can be used to supplement client teaching.
- *Precision health care:* The delivery of care tailored to the individual client using genomic health data. Only certain clients may have access to this innovation, which leads to possible inequities.

Booth, R. G., Strudwick, G., McBride, S., et al. (2021). How the nursing profession should adapt for a digital future. *BMJ, 373*(1190). http://dx.doi.org/10.1136/bmj.n1190.

### Engaging in Client Teaching

As a core nursing competency, teaching is implemented to respond to the needs and goals of the client. It includes therapeutic communication and collaboration with the client and can incorporate the use of technology. A primary purpose of client teaching is to empower clients to control, maintain, or improve their own health more independently.

Often, client education is formalized to ensure the delivery of safe care. Instructing clients about discharge information and postoperative care at home, self-monitoring for complications or new symptoms, self-administration of new medications, and dietary changes (e.g., for diabetes) are examples of important teaching actions to prevent untoward health events. Teaching actions are documented and typically recorded in the client's health record. Supplemental teaching occurs often and is more informal but is no less important.

Clients have access to online information and may question the actions of health care providers, especially once clients start experiencing the delivery of a particular treatment or therapy. Teaching may be needed in such cases to provide clients with further information about the care they are receiving and what constitutes reliable, valid online resources. Client education is therefore a continual and ever-present nursing action.

### Working in Teams

In nursing, teamwork is usually part of care implementation. Leadership theories in nursing influence how nurses perform in teams, in the context of their various roles and within small and larger organizations. Nursing programs provide information on teamwork, leadership, and followership, and the various ways in which planning and implementation are organized based on nursing roles. *Followership* refers to the act of engaging with other leaders and managers by contributing to the work that must be done (Walton & Waddell, 2025); it is an important component of teamwork.

Professional practice standards across provinces and territories include nursing competencies related to teams, teamwork, and communication and reporting among team members. In particular, interprofessional collaboration is emphasized for its role in client safety. **Interprofessional collaboration** is "a partnership between a team of health providers and a client in a participatory, collaborative and coordinated approach to shared decision-making around health and social issues" (Canadian Interprofessional Health Collaborative, 2010, p. 24). How relationships among professionals develop and are maintained facilitates the implementation of care to achieve optimal health outcomes (Canadian Interprofessional Health Collaborative, 2010).

When acting on decisions, nurses often engage in delegation, assignment, and supervision. The concepts of delegation, assignment, and supervision are often confused, but they are distinct (Table 5.2). When planning and implementing care, you need to understand the differences between these mechanisms for performing nursing actions in a team environment. All three require critical thinking and clinical reasoning skills, an understanding of regulated and unregulated nursing roles, and knowledge of provincial or territorial practice standards.

**TABLE 5.2   Comparing Delegation, Assignment, and Supervision**

| Activity | Description | Examples |
|---|---|---|
| Delegation (oral or written) | The formal, complex process of granting authority to act to another who would not normally have the legal authority to do so; the delegator must have the authority and competence in a controlled act to be able to delegate it and is responsible for the decision to delegate, within specific parameters | The nurse *delegates* the controlled act of heparin administration by injection to an unregulated care provider. |
| Assignment (oral or written) | Allocating responsibility of care or aspects of care to another health care provider who has competence to address any challenges of the assignment in the health care environment | The nurse manager in a long-term care facility *assigns* care of clients to the registered practical nurse. |
| Supervision (direct, indirect, or remote) | Monitoring and directing specific activities of others for a defined period; based on complexity of care, nature of task, available resources, and level of competence of the supervisee; may relate to an assignment; not the same as managerial activities | The nurse directly *supervises* the nursing student's care of a client who requires insertion of a Foley catheter. |

Note: Refer to provincial or territorial regulatory body practice documents and standards.
Canadian Nurses Protective Society. (2021). *INFOLaw: Delegation to other health care workers.* https://cnps.ca/article/delegation-to-other-health-care-workers/; College of Nurses of Ontario. (2023). *Scope of practice* (p. 10).https://www.cno.org/globalassets/docs/prac/49041-scope-of-practice.pdf.

## Practising Self-Regulation

**Self-regulation** is the ability to reflect on thinking and diagnose one's learning needs, set goals, select useful resources, and self-evaluate accomplishments and subsequent development that is required to improve. It involves self-correction—with or without limited feedback from others—so that errors can be anticipated, reduced, or rectified. Consider the example of a nurse who is implementing care for a client who had a recent open reduction and internal fixation for a fractured ankle and who is helping move and ambulate the client. The nurse will anticipate a typical response by the client to pain, even if the client has taken an analgesic. This anticipation would be based on knowledge of the client, experience, and textbook learning of psychological and physiological pain. The nurse's ability to identify changes in the client's pattern of pain response or an unusual response to moving or ambulating requires in-the-moment reflection. Based on a client's actual pain response, the nurse may adapt their actions, select another approach to ambulation, or consult with another health care provider about more appropriate approaches for pain control and ambulating the client. Later, the nurse will think back on this experience with the client and identify changes for implementing similar care of clients in the future.

Why is self-regulation important when responding to clients' needs and implementing care? It will guide your actions and fine-tune your performance as a nurse. Additionally, it will support the overall development of your professional skills.

> **KNOWLEDGE CHECK-IN**
> - How do the 3Cs support planning in nursing care?
> - Identify ways to clearly share a plan with a client or other health care providers.
> - Provide a few examples of how technology, client teaching, and teamwork are used when implementing a plan.
> - Why is self-regulation important when responding to a client's needs and performing care?

## SKILLS USED WHEN ACTING ON DECISIONS

In this chapter, the nursing process is used to describe the third step of the thinking and decision-making process: acting on decisions. This step includes planning and implementing. Refer to Figure 5.1 for an overview of this familiar process, which has been embedded in the unified process for thinking and decision making. The nursing process activities of assess, analyze, implement, and evaluate are included in the blue centre areas. Notice how planning is considered as an *action* on a decision, as much as implementation is. Many skills are common to both planning and implementing care for a client. These skills are highlighted in the grey-shaded area. The nursing process will be applied to a case study on acting on a decision, later in this chapter.

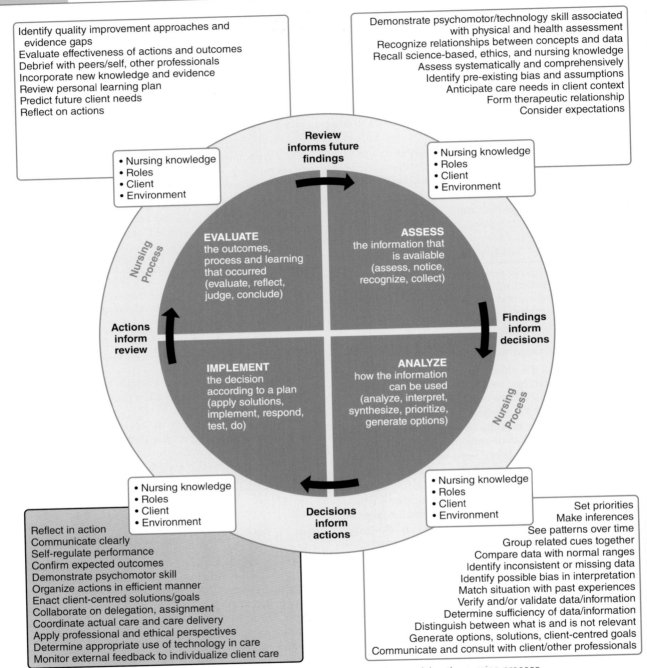

Identify quality improvement approaches and
  evidence gaps
Evaluate effectiveness of actions and outcomes
Debrief with peers/self, other professionals
Incorporate new knowledge and evidence
Review personal learning plan
Predict future client needs
Reflect on actions

Demonstrate psychomotor/technology skill associated
  with physical and health assessment
Recognize relationships between concepts and data
Recall science-based, ethics, and nursing knowledge
Assess systematically and comprehensively
Identify pre-existing bias and assumptions
Anticipate care needs in client context
Form therapeutic relationship
Consider expectations

- Nursing knowledge
- Roles
- Client
- Environment

- Nursing knowledge
- Roles
- Client
- Environment

Review
informs future
findings

Nursing Process

EVALUATE
the outcomes,
process and learning
that occurred
(evaluate, reflect,
judge, conclude)

ASSESS
the information that
is available
(assess, notice,
recognize, collect)

Actions
inform
review

Findings
inform
decisions

IMPLEMENT
the decision
according to a plan
(apply solutions,
implement, respond,
test, do)

ANALYZE
how the information
can be used
(analyze, interpret,
synthesize, prioritize,
generate options)

Nursing Process

- Nursing knowledge
- Roles
- Client
- Environment

Decisions
inform
actions

- Nursing knowledge
- Roles
- Client
- Environment

Reflect in action
Communicate clearly
Self-regulate performance
Confirm expected outcomes
Demonstrate psychomotor skill
Organize actions in efficient manner
Enact client-centred solutions/goals
Collaborate on delegation, assignment
Coordinate actual care and care delivery
Apply professional and ethical perspectives
Determine appropriate use of technology in care
Monitor external feedback to individualize client care

Set priorities
Make inferences
See patterns over time
Group related cues together
Compare data with normal ranges
Identify inconsistent or missing data
Identify possible bias in interpretation
Match situation with past experiences
Verify and/or validate data/information
Determine sufficiency of data/information
Distinguish between what is and is not relevant
Generate options, solutions, client-centred goals
Communicate and consult with client/other professionals

**Fig. 5.1** Unified process for thinking and decision making: applying the nursing process.

## Clinical Reasoning and Other Skills Used When Acting on Decisions

The following skills are key when planning and taking action in nursing practice. They are reasoning skills that follow a decision about a direction for care of a client (once options for care are generated or client goals are identified).

### Reflect in Action

Reflection is a skill that is often associated with an end point. It is used to determine how well a process or an activity was implemented and whether improvements should be made in the future. Recall that reflection is a cyclical process (see Chapter 2), which means that it does not only occur at the end point of a nursing action, or once all care has been completed. When acting on, responding to, or implementing a decision that has been made, you have the opportunity to reflect in action, or "in the moment." Consider reflection as a continual check-in with yourself and your client, and the start of the evaluation process.

*How Can You Develop This Skill?* Practise reflection skills during nursing laboratory or virtual simulation experiences by conducting self-check-ins using questions such as, *Are my plans and actions based on sound knowledge and decision making?* While performing a task or implementing care with a client, ask yourself, *Is what I am doing appropriate at this time?* and *How is the client reacting to the care that is currently being implemented?* Use built-in institutional procedures as tools to assist you with this inquiry, such as checklists for blood product administration, surgical preparation, or discharge from care.

### Communicate Clearly

Clear communication skills and processes are essential to developing a meaningful plan for and with a client, involving all relevant health care professionals, and implementing care. Communication is one of the most common challenges in health care.

*How Can You Develop This Skill?* Refer to information that you learned about communication in courses and health care settings. Become familiar with common communication strategies and practise using them. Observe nursing mentors: notice how they choose language, use body posturing to engage, and employ other verbal and nonverbal ways to ensure that clients and colleagues understand their meaning. Take ownership of your part in a conversation. You are responsible for any issues that may arise from another person's interpretation of what you say.

### Self-Regulate Performance

An important component of acting on decisions, self-regulation of one's nursing performance and activities is necessary for competent care delivery. Recall that self-regulation involves reflection and self-correction, which includes anticipating and rectifying mistakes.

*How Can You Develop This Skill?* Engage in thinking about your own learning needs, setting goals for your learning, choosing resources, and reflecting on your own accomplishments in both your personal and professional life. Ask yourself, *Is what I am doing/thinking correct? How do I know?* Developing self-regulation skills is an ongoing activity. It may be helpful to check in with others on your performance to confirm your interpretation of how you can improve.

### Confirm Expected Outcomes

When planning and implementing care, continually confirming expected outcomes with the client is important. Confirmation takes place formally during planning and in the moment while implementing care or performing tasks that help the client address immediate health issues. This skill is valuable in the informed consent process and fulfills the ethical obligation of the nurse to deliver client-centred care.

*How Can You Develop This Skill?* Make a habit of confirming with clients their care goals or desired outcomes. The following are sample questions for checking in with the client: "Are you still in agreement with this approach to your care?" and "Are there any changes we can make with you?"

### Demonstrate Psychomotor Skill

Particularly when acting on plans, the ability to physically carry out a nursing task is crucial to efficient, effective, safe, and competent care. While not a cognitive skill, successfully performing direct nursing care requires the application of significant knowledge, reflection, and an understanding of the client context. Actions physically demonstrate a nurse's ability to think through information.

*How Can You Develop This Skill?* Build your physical skills and the ability to manipulate and manage equipment, perform therapeutic techniques, and assist with the movement of clients or use of supplies through practice. Go to simulation laboratories and practice settings to receive guidance and feedback on your performance in a nursing skill, and take the time to repeat what you have learned with any available practice kits or supplies on your own. Also watch videos of various skills to help you remember what to do.

### Organize Actions in Efficient Manner

Recall the ways in which you can prioritize information (see Chapter 4), and incorporate them into planning and implementing care.

*How Can You Develop This Skill?* Know that once the decision is made about how care will be delivered, planning (organizing this care) and then implementing (following the plan) become the focus. Use a systems approach to carrying out actions. Think about what must be done first in terms of priority, and then consider how to act efficiently (e.g., not wasting supplies, reducing backtracking or repeating actions, establishing a clear space where care will be delivered). Visualizing your actions and how you will move from one activity to the next may help. Refer to Box 5.2 for more tips.

### Enact Client-Centred Solutions/Goals

After an assessment of the client's needs, goals were identified in collaboration *with* the client. Enacting these goals requires knowledge of how to plan for and implement them—for instance, who to contact, what processes or systems to activate, and where to refer clients.

*How Can You Develop This Skill?* Develop your knowledge of options and a wider range of resources through practice and communication, and your confidence in acting on decisions will grow. Do not be afraid to ask experienced colleagues questions such as, "Who should I contact about this referral for the client?" or "Where can the client access this culturally specific resource?" Include the client in this process of planning and implementing goals to understand their preferred supports so that you can advocate for resources for the client as necessary. Doing so will ensure that client needs are met and that they receive optimal care.

### Collaborate on Delegation, Assignment

Approaches to teamwork, such as delegating or assigning tasks, can facilitate the delivery of collaborative, efficient, and effective care. The success and safety of such approaches depend on a clear understanding of the scopes of practice (roles and responsibilities) of the different health care providers involved in care. Ensure that you understand the provincial and territorial requirements for formal delegation and any restrictions on delegating or receiving a delegation.

*How Can You Develop This Skill?* Observe others who perform delegation or assignment, and make a note of who is involved, and how it is communicated and documented. When an aspect of care is assigned to you, be sure that you can deliver that care, know who to contact if there are concerns, and report clearly when the task is completed. Refer to the decision tree in Figure 5.2.

### Coordinate Actual Care and Care Delivery

The ability to coordinate activities and the implementation of care can be complex. Several health care providers may be involved, or other departments or agencies may need to be included in providing a client's care. Often, this complexity is overlooked and can delay the start or completion of planned care.

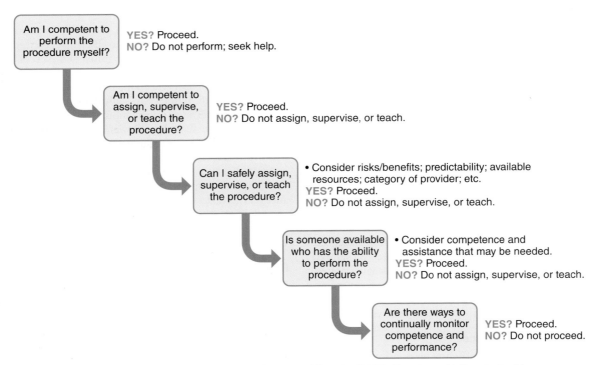

**Fig. 5.2** Decision Tree. (Adapted from College of Nurses of Ontario. (2022). *Practice guideline: Authorizing mechanisms* [p. 13]. [Retired])

*How Can You Develop This Skill?* Identify the participants in the care of the client. Participants can include not only the client but also the client's significant other/family members as well as health care professionals involved in the care of the client. Determine who may be involved in the resourcing of supplies or systems and who may affect the environment (or community) in which care is delivered. Communicating clearly is an important skill that is also used in coordinating care.

## Apply Professional and Ethical Perspectives

When acting on decisions (as in all other steps of the thinking and decision-making process), professional standards and codes of ethics must be followed. These principles influence assessment, analysis, and decision making with or about clients, and it is when you take action on a decision that your professionalism and ethics become very apparent. Your behaviour and performance (e.g., confidentiality, privacy, respect, trust) display the thinking processes that have led to the nursing action.

*How Can You Develop This Skill?* Know the Canadian Nurses Association (2017) Code of Ethics for Registered Nurses and your provincial or territorial ethical practice standards. Successful completion of the jurisprudence exam, required for registration in nursing in most areas in Canada, will demonstrate your knowledge of this content.

## Determine Appropriate Use of Technology in Care

Digital health technologies are now embedded in client and health care settings, from handheld devices for accessing information and data to system-wide electronic records for sharing diagnoses and plans of care. The skill of understanding which technology is appropriate to use in practice relates to professional and ethical knowledge, and to the evidence on the use of particular technologies in client care. Technology can sometimes fail. For example, automatic blood pressure monitors may be inaccurate. Therefore, it is the responsibility of the nurse to use clinical reasoning skills and to question the appropriate use of equipment, systems, and results that may be generated through electronic systems and technology overall.

*How Can You Develop This Skill?* Continually review new nursing knowledge and evidence on technology to inform your practice. Review available updates on how health information can be shared using the latest technology. Also, pay attention to how technology can be incorporated in the care of clients with specific health needs. Although it is important to become familiar with technology that is intended to contribute to client health, do not rely on it completely. As one example, consider the use of the Internet by clients as a medical resource. If a client shows you a social media site promising a quick cure for their type 1 diabetes mellitus, talk with the client about the appropriate use of online medical information. Nursing knowledge is essential to understanding how to use technology in client care.

## Monitor External Feedback to Individualize Client Care

Noticing and responding to how a client reacts to an intervention in the moment is necessary to maintain safety and trust, and to deliver appropriate physical and mental health care that meets client needs. This reflective activity puts you "in tune" with the client in a direct care situation. It requires emotional intelligence that can identify subtle changes in the client response and can begin to inform your evaluation of how successful an intervention will be.

*How Can You Develop This Skill?* Practise situation awareness (see Chapter 3), and actively observe the client's facial expressions, body movements, and verbal reactions. This way of being with the client requires your full attention. Consider ways to reduce the effects of any distractions when you are performing an intervention. Be aware that distractions include the psychomotor task itself. Also, being new to performing a skill can take away attention from the client. Develop your skills and take your time with client care.

 **THINKING THROUGH THE APPLICATION OF CLINICAL REASONING SKILLS**

### Case Scenario on Acting on Decisions

A 34-year-old client living as human immunodeficiency virus (HIV) positive for the last 3 years has experienced frequent watery diarrhea for the past 4 days and is reporting abdominal cramping. The pain level is rated at 8/10. Lung sounds are clear bilaterally, pulse is regular, and capillary refill is >2 sec. The client is alert and oriented, and exhibits visible jaundice; the white blood count is high. Culture and sensitivity results are pending. Infection control precautions and treatment of an underlying infection with antibiotics are selected as an initial approach to care. The client's partner is present and wishes to stay with them.

Reflect on these questions:
- How will a complete plan of care be established for this client? What needs to be set up, and who needs to be included, etc.?
- What actions will be implemented? What will you do first, next, etc., and why?
- Which clinical reasoning skills will you use to respond to the decision in this scenario?

# BARRIERS TO THINKING WHEN ACTING ON DECISIONS

Certain barriers to thinking can prevent nurses from clearly understanding the implementation of care and how to meet the client's health care goals. Sometimes, nurses are confused about the distinction between an assessment and an action intended to change or improve the client's health. A lack of clarity about these activities can have implications when communicating to other health care providers and for thinking about what to do next. To clarify the difference in their minds, nurses can ask, *Is this activity meant to measure aspects of or changes in the client's condition or situation?* and *Is this activity meant to help change or improve the condition or situation?* For instance, applying an electrocardiogram (ECG) monitor may seem like a response or an action (and it may be part of a plan of care), but the purpose of this activity is to find out more information about a client's health rather than change or improve their health. An ECG is considered an assessment activity, not an intervention, and consequently ECG results require analysis, interpretation, synthesis, and prioritization as to whether action is needed. Part of the plan of care may be to provide ongoing assessment or monitoring, which demonstrates the iterative nature of the entire thinking process in nursing practice.

Other barriers to thinking that can affect acting on a decision include:

- *Low self-confidence:*
  The nurse's level of confidence in their own abilities to perform nursing activities will depend on their understanding of how to apply nursing knowledge, past experiences, the complexity of the client's needs, and the resources available to them. Confidence in communicating plans and putting those plans into action will develop over time and with practice.
- *Concerns about occupational and physical safety:*
  They may prevent timely action on a plan and, thus, may delay client care. Concerns may include a lack of knowledge about equipment use, personal safety resources, a task-related procedure, or an agency policy.
- *An inability to reflect in the moment:*
  This barrier can arise due to distractions in the environment and can affect the delivery of care. Distractions can be external (e.g., noises, the client being treated, other assigned or nearby clients, other demands) and internal (e.g., high cognitive load from a lack of familiarity with the client or task at hand).

## ? THINKING IT THROUGH

### Self-Reflection on Barriers to Acting on Decisions

Recall instances where you were hesitant or not able to respond in a timely manner to a decision.
- What do you think were your main challenges when acting on or responding to a client goal or applying identified solutions in a client care situation?
- What caused these challenges? Why did they happen (e.g., lack of knowledge about a skill, not sure if it was within your role, low confidence level)?

# HELPFUL STRATEGIES FOR ACTING ON DECISIONS

A number of strategies can help nurses overcome barriers in developing and sharing plans and implementing client care. Based on your self-assessment and an understanding of your thinking in practice situations, consider ways to group, organize, and prioritize actions to ensure a decision about care is followed through. You may also have other approaches that work for you.

Decisions made in health care often need to be directly communicated to another health care professional or worker, or shared with the client, family, group, community, or population. Clearly and consistently communicating decisions in the health care setting, and how and why the decisions were made, supports safe practices (Boersma & Freeman, 2022). Therefore, adopting a structured approach to communication in the health care setting can enable efficient and effective action on a collaborative decision.

Using well-known communication structures that are applied by other health care providers helps ensure that information is:

- *anticipated/expected* in the same way;
- *conveyed* using the same approach; and
- *received* more readily because it was presented using that structure.

Table 5.3 presents key communication tools used in health care. Recall that such simple, short mnemonics can be used consistently in practice and across disciplines to reduce medical errors (Starmer et al., 2014). Other tools may be used by your health care employer that form an expectation for how communication occurs with professionals and groups. Communication may appear to be a linear (or step by step) process.

## TABLE 5.3  Communication Tools in Health Care

| Structured Tool | Description |
|---|---|
| ISBAR-R<br>(used for communication and client hand-off) | **I**ntroduction/identify: identify yourself and your role<br>**S**ituation: identify the purpose of the communication<br>**B**ackground: provide a summary of the client's background<br>**A**ssessment: share recent, relevant client assessments<br>**R**ecommendation: state any recommendation for the client's care<br>**R**epeat back/receive: repeat back any important information; receive questions |
| N-PAS<br>(used for client hand-off) | **N**urse: tool specific to nursing and used for client hand-off<br>**P**atient summary: demographics; admitting diagnosis; mental status; physical assessment; ambulatory and code status; allergies; pertinent medical history; vital signs; lab reports; relevant assessment including necessary precautions, medications, family situation; etc.<br>**A**ction plan: nursing interventions planned, scheduled procedures, ongoing monitoring, discharge and education teaching<br>**S**ynthesis: step where sender and receiver ask questions and clarify information |
| I-PASS<br>(used for client hand-off) | **I**llness severity: stable, "watcher," unstable<br>**P**atient summary: summary statement, relevant events leading up to current situation or admission, health progress, ongoing monitoring, plan<br>**A**ction list: scheduled care, timelines, and most responsible people<br>**S**ituation awareness and contingency planning: what is currently happening; planning for what may change<br>**S**ynthesis by receiver: step where receiver summarizes what was heard, asks questions, clarifies and restates key actions |

Boersma, K., & Freeman, M. (2022). Effective nurse handoffs. *Nursing, 52*(4), 51–54. doi: 10.1097/01.NURSE.0000823256.78368.d7; Kostiuk, S. (2015). Can learning the ISBARR framework help to address nursing students' perceived anxiety and confidence levels associated with handover reports? *Journal of Nursing Education, 54*(10), 583–587. https://doi.org/10.3928/01484834-20150916-07.

However, it often requires that you return to previous steps in thinking to ensure that the information communication is based on is appropriate and grounded in solid evidence. Clinical reasoning is needed to convey information, decisions, and plans of care accurately. When you communicate a plan using communication tools and deliver a course of action, continually reflect back on whether client needs are being met.

At times, nurses may also use texts or emails on secure networks to contact physicians or other health care professionals when communicating client plans. Communication tools can used to organize and share information consistently in this format as well.

Anticipating client treatments can assist with the creation of a plan and how it can be delivered. In this regard, mnemonics are useful tools for identifying which therapies are expected during care planning. For instance, the *ABCD* mnemonic, which takes on a new meaning in the context of a medical diagnosis of stroke, describes *a*ntiplatelets/anticoagulants, *b*lood pressure, *c*lot extraction, and *d*iagnostics as important foci of intervention activities (El-Hussein & Green, 2021). Any strategy that helps nurses understand medical plans and actions can facilitate nursing planning and interventions.

Strategies related to mindfulness can reduce errors during the implementation of care and administration of medication (Ekkens & Gordon, 2021). The skill of **reflection-in-action**, or reflecting in the moment (Schön, 1983), may be useful, particularly if auditory or visual distractions are present. Being mindful of your actions will enable you to question and double-check the accuracy and relevance of your activities in providing optimal care.

## THINKING THROUGH ACTING ON DECISIONS: NRCE

The NRCE framework used in this textbook can help guide you to recall the wide range of influences on a client care situation when acting on decisions. Nursing knowledge, professional roles, client context, and the health care environment all affect planning and implementation. In this section, the scenario of a community influenza outbreak is used to illustrate how planning and implementation can occur after an outbreak is declared. This framework can help you answer the question, *What appropriate response should be provided?*

### Nursing Knowledge

The *N* in *NRCE* relates to nursing knowledge. When considering a plan of action, the nurse may function as a leader or facilitator of care. The nurse works with other associated health care professionals and carefully reviews and incorporates the following:

- Science and evidence to address the client goals that were identified
- Theory that relates to therapeutic skills, leadership, communication, and ethics
- Knowledge of improving or maintaining health (physical care and interventions, teaching and counselling)
- Psychomotor skill and actions related to the implementation (doing) of direct client care

#### Example

An influenza outbreak is declared in a community. The public health nurses implement specific plans and actions to contain the outbreak and prevent spread.

 The nursing knowledge to consider when planning and acting in practice includes (but may not be limited to):
- Process of transmission of influenza
- Clinical manifestations of influenza and associated complications
- How illness may affect diverse client groups differently
- Relevance and frequency of diagnostic testing methods to be employed
- Vaccination schedules and procedures, prophylaxis

### Professional Roles

The *R* in *NRCE* relates to professional roles—the roles and scopes of practice of nurses and other health care professionals. While leadership skills are required at many points in the thinking and decision-making process, they are most necessary when acting on decisions. Being familiar with the staffing complement and other health care professionals available to deliver care is important for understanding how care can be planned and enacted. The nursing role involves adopting a professional demeanour, performing competently within one's scope of practice, and supporting other health care providers in their roles in client care. It also involves actions such as assignment, supervision, check back, follow-up, and continual reflection. Confidence in action comes from familiarity with the nurse's role and clear communication with others.

#### Example

An influenza outbreak is declared in a community. The public health nurses implement specific plans and actions to contain the outbreak and prevent spread.

 The professional roles and scopes of practice to consider when planning and acting in practice include (but are not limited to):
- Notification of municipal, provincial, or territorial authorities and stakeholders
- Assembly of teams to provide multiple levels of care (administrative, clinical, housekeeping, pharmacy, etc.)
- Mechanisms of authority and delegation that can facilitate efficient and effective care
- Scheduling relevant professionals and staff based on need

### Client Context

The *C* in *NRCE* relates to the client context. During planning and action, the client context focuses on the client's involvement in care and the client as a recipient of care. Communication is client specific and mindful of neurodiversity, learning preferences, language, and inclusion of client perceptions, needs, personal values, and care partners. For instance, language interpreters or modifications to teaching materials based on client need may be offered to ensure that identified goals are met. Advocacy entails an active response to client needs and the context of their health situation.

 General observation of a client's reactions to a plan of care and associated nursing actions requires that the nurse make in-the-moment adaptations based on these reactions. This type of reflection is integral to ongoing assessment and marks the beginning of an evaluation of nursing and/or medical care. If others are delivering care, nurses still monitor client response and outcomes as part of their ongoing actions toward optimizing client health.

## Example

An influenza outbreak is declared in a community. The public health nurses implement specific plans and actions to contain the outbreak and prevent spread.

Aspects of the client context to consider may include (but are not limited to):

- Provision of direct care to those who contract the illness
- Initiation of case management processes
- Communication to client and family about possible visitor restrictions
- Support of client's mental health
- Maintenance of cultural and spiritual preferences

## Health Care Environment

The *E* in *NRCE* relates to the health care environment. In the health care environment, space, resources, and policies significantly influence how care is planned and delivered. Physical privacy, areas to conduct care delivery, room temperature, and supply availability are all important environmental factors the nurse must consider when planning to provide optimal care. Planning also involves the health care setting's policies on inclusivity and respect for client preferences, which help guide interactions with the client and client's family, as well as standards to adhere to when delivering care in less-than-optimal environmental conditions (e.g., outbreaks, technology or power outages, staffing shortages, occupational injury).

Nurses need to be aware of other institutional procedures that communicate the need for action. Many agencies include codes—with standard colours—that are associated with emergencies or specific situations that require health care professionals to respond in specific ways. Review examples of codes at an agency where you are placed.

## Example

An influenza outbreak is declared in a community. The public health nurses implement specific plans and actions to contain the outbreak and prevent spread.

Elements of the health care environment to consider when deciding what to do may include:

- Provincial or territorial public health regulations
- Cohorting of clients affected by influenza (isolating)
- Supplies available for precautions
- Environmental cleaning
- Application of institutional policies and procedures

Table 5.4 presents a summary of the NRCE components as applied to planning and implementation activities. As in

| TABLE 5.4   Using NRCE When Planning and Implementing Care in an Influenza Outbreak | |
|---|---|
| **NRCE** | **What to Consider** |
| **Nursing** Knowledge | • Process of transmission of influenza<br>• Clinical manifestations of influenza and associated complications<br>• How illness may affect diverse client groups differently<br>• Relevance and frequency of diagnostic testing methods to be employed<br>• Vaccination schedules and procedures, prophylaxis |
| Professional **Roles** | • Notification of municipal, provincial, or territorial authorities and stakeholders<br>• Assembly of teams to provide multiple levels of care (administrative, clinical, housekeeping, pharmacy, etc.)<br>• Mechanisms of authority and delegation that can facilitate efficient and effective care<br>• Scheduling relevant staffing based on need |
| **Client** Context | • Provision of direct care to those who contract the illness<br>• Initiation of case management processes<br>• Communication to client and family about possible visitor restrictions<br>• Support of client's mental health<br>• Maintenance of cultural and spiritual preferences |
| Health Care **Environment** | • Provincial or territorial public health regulations<br>• Cohorting of clients affected by influenza (isolating)<br>• Supplies available for precautions<br>• Environmental cleaning<br>• Application of institutional policies and procedures |

previous steps of the thinking and decision-making process, there may be some overlap among finding information, decision making, and even the next step of reviewing actions.

Consider the NRCE components as you review the following case study.

## ACTING ON DECISIONS: A NURSING PROCESS CASE STUDY

In this section, the nursing process (see Chapter 2) will be applied to the public health situation of an influenza outbreak in a small community. This case study illustrates how to approach the third step of the thinking process: acting on decisions. Interestingly, this third step does not initially appear to be a "thinking" step because it is action oriented toward a plan and the implementation of care goals. However, it should be evident by now that a lot of clinical reasoning is needed to ensure that the correct plan and actions occur. Therefore, thinking and action go hand in hand, and in fact represent reflection-in-action.

The case study in Table 5.5 incorporates key ideas covered in this chapter, including the clinical reasoning skills

| TABLE 5.5    Case Study: Application of the Nursing Process to Acting on Decisions | | | |
|---|---|---|---|
| **Client Situation** | **Nursing Model and Application of Thinking** | | |
| The local public health authority has identified that the *area population, as a client,* is experiencing an influenza outbreak. | **Nursing Process** | **Clinical Reasoning Skills Used** | **Possible Nursing Responses (Barriers, Strategies)** |
| A local retirement community had been monitoring a resident who had respiratory symptoms. Assessment was conducted for both COVID-19 and influenza. Influenza A was detected. Now, another separate retirement community and two units in the local hospital have reported the same influenza. An influenza outbreak was identified. | Assessment and Analysis | As described in client situation. | |
| | **Planning** | Confirm expected outcomes. Collaborate on delegation, assignment. Coordinate actual care and care delivery. Determine appropriate use of technology in care. Organize actions in efficient manner. Reflect in action. Communicate clearly. | Reduce spread and treat clients who are symptomatic. Implement antivirals; know that timing is important for initiating treatment and prophylaxis; identify who to administer to. Discuss the plan with interprofessional community leads and plan staff education. Use technology to review dashboards and other statistics for reported cases. |
| Two nurses work part-time at each of the agencies where outbreaks occurred. A recent survey of handwashing practices conducted at the hospital indicated 66% adherence to the policy. A goal to eliminate the outbreak was set. | **Implementation** | Self-regulate performance. Demonstrate psychomotor skill. Enact client-centred solutions/goals. Apply professional and ethical perspectives. Monitor external feedback to individualize client care. | Administer antiviral therapy until the outbreak is over. Ensure client familiarity with the medication (client education, communication, risks and reactions, etc.) Address any issues related to informed consent for antivirals. Communicate to all staff and encourage self-assessment of symptoms. Provide staff education. Undertake ongoing monitoring of residents/clients and new cases. Complete provincial reporting as required. |
| | Evaluation | *Consider next steps. How will you evaluate these actions?* | |

described earlier. As well, it addresses possible responses to barriers to thinking and strategies to overcome those barriers. Note that the nursing process was chosen as the model for this case study because of its steps of planning and implementation.

## SUMMARY

This chapter explored planning—how client-centred goals will be met—and implementation—how nursing care to meet those goals will be delivered. Planning involves professional communication, taking into account the client's needs, and plan sharing. Implementation involves the use of technology, client teaching, teamwork processes (assigning, delegating, supervising), and self-regulation. Barriers to thinking when acting on a decision—such as low self-confidence, concerns about occupational and physical safety, and an inability to reflect in the moment—can be overcome by using communication tools, building anticipatory skills, and practising mindfulness. A case study using the nursing process illustrated how nurses act on decisions by planning and implementing care.

## KEY POINTS TO REMEMBER

These are the key points to remember from this chapter.

### About Moving Forward on a Decision: Making a Plan of Care

- Planning requires the nurse to apply critical thinking skills and to enact priorities that have been identified.
- If the client's situation or condition has changed, confirm that the goals remain client centred and are *SMART* (*s*pecific, *m*easurable, *a*ttainable, *r*elevant, *t*imed).
- Professional communication conveys a role of responsibility and accountability for one's actions and is clear, courteous, individual, trustworthy, and assertive.
- Consultation occurs when seeking verification and confirmation of plans of care.
- Collaboration depends on the scope of practice of the professional (how their knowledge and abilities can contribute to care) and on the client's abilities.
- Coordination often involves planning and resource management to ensure that activities are complementary and promote optimal health.
- The nurse must engage in clinical reasoning when thinking about how to best adapt a plan for a client so that an optimal outcome can be achieved.
- If adapting a plan, ask yourself, *Why am I adapting the plan?* (necessity) and *Is this necessary and safe to do?* (safety).
- Ensure your plan is efficient and effective to the best of your ability and knowledge. Doing so will help you decide what to do first. This type of prioritization helps avoid wasting supplies and time, repeated communication, and possibly confusing the client about the care they will receive.
- A plan of care can be paper based or computerized (electronic), or a standardized critical pathway of care for groups of clients experiencing a particular situation.
- Planning is a dynamic process that continues to change once the client's needs are met and as new information is obtained.

### About Implementing the Plan of Care

- How care is implemented varies widely, depending on the nursing care setting, the client's environment, and the resources that are available.
- Scheduling and coordination of care are often overlooked; communication and coordination with others must occur to deliver care in a timely way.
- Technology enables access to information and the communication of plans. Become familiar with the technological tools available to you and develop your competence with digital health technology.
- Client teaching is a nursing action that responds to the needs and goals of the client and includes therapeutic communication and collaboration with the client. It can include the use of technology.
- Client education empowers clients to control, maintain, or improve their own health more independently.
- The actions of delegation, assignment, and supervision are distinct from one another and require an understanding of scopes of practice and provincial or territorial regulation.
- Your ability to identify potential changes in a client's patterns of behaviour and responses to care require in-the-moment reflection and self-regulation.

### About Skills Used When Acting on Decisions

- The unified process for thinking and decision making (see Figure 5.1) includes a number of skills that can be useful when planning and acting on decisions:
  - Reflect in action.
  - Communicate clearly.
  - Self-regulate performance.
  - Confirm expected outcomes.
  - Demonstrate psychomotor skill.
  - Organize actions in efficient manner.

- Enact client-centred solutions/goals.
- Collaborate on delegation, assignment.
- Coordinate actual care and care delivery.
- Apply professional and ethical perspectives.
- Determine appropriate use of technology in care.
- Monitor external feedback to individualize client care.

### About Barriers to Thinking When Acting on Decisions

- Barriers that the nurse may encounter when thinking and acting on decisions include a lack of clarity about the distinction between an assessment and an action intended to change or improve the client's health; low self-confidence in their ability to carry out a plan; concerns about the environment; and an inability to reflect in the moment because of distractions or other challenges.

### About Helpful Strategies for Acting on Decisions

- Strategies for overcoming barriers can include the use of structured communication tools, building nursing knowledge so that treatments can be anticipated, and mindfulness techniques that enable nurses to focus on nursing practice and the client.

### About Thinking Through Acting on Decisions: NRCE

- This textbook's NRCE framework provides a holistic view of planning and implementing when acting on decisions.

### About a Case Study on Acting on Decisions

- A case study on a community influenza outbreak illustrates the thinking process and how planning and implementation occur in relation to the decisions that have been made.

## CONCLUSION AND THINKING IT THROUGH

Often, nursing students are focused on learning tasks and performing the skills required during the implementation phase of the nursing process. It is very important to understand and appreciate the thinking that must be invested in supporting sound actions. Only with careful assessment and planning that is based on ethical and evidence-informed thinking can competent nursing actions occur. Think before you act, and then act in a reflective manner.

Reflection is embedded throughout the thinking and decision-making process and is a key part of the final step of the process: reviewing actions. This step, discussed in Chapter 6, is a dedicated time for you to revisit, evaluate, and determine whether goals were met. You may also identify if there were unanticipated outcomes or negative effects, not just for the client, but beyond—for the nursing profession or the health care system in general.

## CLASS ACTIVITIES TO CHECK THINKING

### Think-Aloud Pair Problem Solving (TAPPS)

Form pairs. Decide who will be a problem solver and listener for Problem A. The problem solver reads the problem aloud and talks through a response to the problem, while the listener reminds the problem solver to think aloud, asks clarification questions, offers encouragement to keep thinking, but refrains from providing possible answers. Switch roles for Problem B.

For each of these problems, identify what "less optimal" and "most optimal" plans and actions would look like. Jot down your points so that you can compare the responses.

- **Problem A:** An older client reports to the nurse about changes in mood and losing weight after the sudden death of their same-sex partner. The client is depressed and feels socially isolated. The nurse and client set a goal to build coping strategies and other supports.
- **Problem B:** An 8-year-old client was diagnosed with a brain tumour after experiencing severe headaches, vomiting, poor balance and coordination, and seizure activity. Radiation treatment was not successful in reducing the size of the tumour. After continued seizures, the

family, client, and health care team agree to provide end-of-life care at home to the client.

### Activities and Discussion Questions

1. Refer to the decision tree in Figure 5.2. Imagine that you have decided that you must either assign, supervise, or teach a certain procedure. What questions do you ask yourself as you plan for this? What are the advantages of using a decision tree?
2. Review the following situation:
   A 23-year-old client presents to the clinic with a new diagnosis of type 2 diabetes mellitus (DM). The client's pronouns are they/them, was born in India, and has lived in Canada since they were a toddler. They are employed as a freelance writer, sit at a desk during the day, are overweight, are estranged from family members, live on their own, and have been taking antidepressants for a year. They feel that type 2 DM is a milder form of the disease. Blood pressure is 140/85 and a glucometer reading is 11.5 mmol/L. The nurse creates a plan of care. Consider the two conversations that could occur.

---

**Conversation A: Less Optimal Case Planning**

**Nurse:** I see you have a recent diagnosis of diabetes and some risk factors. You need to lose weight now, exercise regularly, and avoid sugars. I will consult with the physician to arrange other tests.

**Client:** Yes, but we can we wait for the tests to come in before I make any changes?

**Nurse:** It is important for you control your blood sugar levels, or you may develop other health problems.

**One year later:** The client has not returned to the clinic and continues to experience health issues.

**Conversation B: More Optimal Case Planning**

**Nurse:** I see that your blood sugar level is high. Has anyone talked to you about how to control your blood sugar?

**Client:** No, but I don't think this is needed. I don't eat much candy or sugary drinks. I like fast food as its easier and cheaper. Can I wait for the tests to come in before I make any changes?

**Nurse:** It helps to be proactive and think about possibilities for changes that can help you live with or improve your diagnosis. We can arrange for you to talk to a dietitian who can help you plan simple, inexpensive healthy meals. What do you think?

**Client:** That makes sense, I guess. Okay.

**Nurse:** Let's follow up on that next week. Are you available to come in? We can also begin to think about your activity level and what your options are for exercise.

**Client:** I am self-conscious about going to a gym.

**Nurse:** We can talk about alternatives next time.

**One year later:** The client has returned to the clinic periodically, has lost 5 kg, and has maintained their health through some dietary changes.

---

In a small group, discuss the following questions:
- What are key differences between the two conversations?
- Is there any aspect of planning this client's care that may require going back and conducting further assessment?
- What other aspects of this client's plan can be individualized?
- How would you conduct a conversation about planning care with this client?

## CASE STUDY REVIEW

Review the case study in Table 5.5.

### Questions

1. What specific plans would you make based on the decision and need to reduce the spread of the disease and treat the individuals with symptoms?

2. Who in the local health care agencies would be able to carry out the identified responses?

3. Review how the case study can be completed. Think ahead—how will you know if the actions are effective and meet the goal(s)?

## EVIDENCE-INFORMED THINKING ACTIVITY

Review the two problems described in the TAPPS activity in this chapter. For the most optimal plans and actions that you identified, what evidence do you have that they are appropriate, relevant and based on research or best practices and nursing standards of care? Find at least two sources of evidence to support your responses.

## QUESTIONS TO ASSESS LEARNING

### Review Questions

1. A nurse is planning a procedure that they have only implemented once before. What activities are most appropriate when planning before acting? Select all that apply.

   a. Aim for efficiency and to complete the task as quickly as possible.
   b. Review policy and procedure steps.
   c. Gather all supplies and bring extra selected items.
   d. Ensure a mentor is available to take over if a step is forgotten.
   e. Choose when the procedure should be implemented.

2. The policy for visiting hours is questioned by a nurse who is caring for a palliative client. The client is dying and would like support from their immediate family to stay late in the evening. What statement by the nurse is an appropriate rationale for supporting the client's goal?

a. "The policy does not apply to this palliative care situation and so can be over-ridden."

b. "Adapting this policy will enable the client to meet their goal and will not risk safety or the care provided to others, with my support."

c. "Policies function as guidelines and can be modified at any time for any reason."

d. "Any client preference is a priority over employer policies and procedures to maintain the trust of the public."

3. A nurse, a psychiatrist, an occupational therapist, and a social worker jointly participate in both the planning and delivery of care to a group of clients at a mental health facility. They identify how their varied scopes of practice and skills will address the client group's goals, and then they provide care. What process does this best describe?

a. Consultation

b. Coordination

c. Consideration

d. Collaboration

## ONE LAST THOUGHT

The importance of acting on decisions is apparent at many levels of health care. One example is illustrated by Jordan's Principle (refer to "Honouring Jordan River Anderson" on the Government of Canada website). Five-year-old Jordan from Norway House Cree Nation in Manitoba passed away in hospital, despite doctors' recommendations for discharge to a special care home, because of government payment disputes over who should provide for his home-based care. The inaction meant that Jordan was deprived of a life outside of a hospital setting. As a result, the Canadian House of Commons passed Jordan's Principle in 2007 to ensure that First Nations children would get the products, services, and supports they need, when they need them, with payments that would be worked out later. This significant example is not a 'last thought' but prepares you for the next chapter about reflecting on actions taken in health care settings.

Reflect on inequities that may be evident when acting on decisions. Can you think of other examples either in your practice or in other parts of Canada where inequities are preventing optimal planning and action? How can you and others advocate for change?

## ONLINE RESOURCES

*2020 National Survey of Canadian Nurses: Use of digital health technology in practice* (2020). Canada Health Infoway. https://www.infoway-inforoute.ca/en/component/edocman/resources/reports/benefits-evaluation/3812-2020-national-survey-of-canadian-nurses-use-of-digital-health-technology-in-practice.

*Delegation to unregulated care providers* (2024). British Columbia College of Nurses & Midwives. https://www.bccnm.ca/RN/PracticeStandards/Pages/delegating.aspx.

Government of Canada. (2024). *Jordan's principle.* https://sac-isc.gc.ca/eng/1568396042341/1568396159824.

ISBAR resource, Lapum, J., St-Amant, O., Hughes, M., et al.. (2020). Resources to Facilitate Interprofessional Communication. In *Communication for the Nursing Professional* (Cdn ed.). 2020; Chapter 3. https://pressbooks.library.torontomu.ca/communicationnursing/chapter/resources-to-facilitate-interprofessional-communication/.

*Resolving ambivalence: A 4-minute technique (can be used by students and nurses)* (2024). NCFDD. https://www.ncfdd.org/makeadecision.

*Self-regulation module* (2024). Nova Scotia College of Nursing. https://www.nscn.ca/professional-practice/practice-support/practice-support-tools/self-regulation/self-regulation-module.

Virtual simulations (available to nurses and students) (2024). In *Essential skills training for health care workers.* CAN-Sim. https://can-sim.ca/hc/.

## REFERENCES

Astle, B., & Duggleby, W. (2024). *Potter and Perry's Canadian fundamentals of nursing* (7th ed.). Elsevier.

Boersma, K., & Freeman, M. (2022). Effective nurse handoffs. *Nursing, 52*(4), 51–54. doi:10.1097/01.NURSE.0000823256.78368.d7.

Booth, R. G., Strudwick, G., McBride, S., et al. (2021). How the nursing profession should adapt for a digital future. *BMJ, 373*(1190). http://dx.doi.org/10.1136/bmj.n1190.

Canadian Interprofessional Health Collaborative. (2010). *A national interprofessional competency framework.* https://phabc.org/wp-content/uploads/2015/07/CIHC-National-Interprofessional-Competency-Framework.pdf.

Canadian Nurses Association. (2017). *Code of ethics for registered nurses*. https://www.cna-aiic.ca/en/nursing/regulated-nursing-in-canada/nursing-ethics.

Canadian Nurses Protective Society. (2021). *INFOLaw: Delegation to other health care workers*. https://cnps.ca/article/delegation-to-other-health-care-workers/.

Cohen, D. J., Davis, M., Balasubramanian, B. A., et al. (2015). Integrating behavioral health and primary care: Consulting, coordinating and collaborating among professionals. *Journal of the American Board of Family Medicine, 28*(Suppl 1), S21–S31. https://doi.org/10.3122/jabfm.2015.S1.150042.

College of Nurses of Ontario. (2022). *Practice guideline: Authorizing mechanisms* [Retired].

College of Nurses of Ontario. (2023). *Scope of practice*. https://www.cno.org/globalassets/docs/prac/49041-scope-of-practice.pdf.

D'Entremont, B. (2009). Clinical pathways: The Ottawa Hospital experience. *Canadian Nurse, 105*(5) https://doi.org/info:doi/.

Ekkens, C. L., & Gordon, P. A. (2021). The mindful path to nursing accuracy: A quasi-experimental study on minimizing medication administration errors. *Holistic Nursing Practice, 35*(3), 115–122. https://doi.org/10.1097/hnp.0000000000000440.

El-Hussein, M. T., & Green, T. (2021). Alphabetical mnemonic to assist in the treatment of an acute ischemic stroke. *Critical Care Nursing Quarterly, 44*(4), 368–378. doi:10.1097/CNQ.0000000000000373.

Kostiuk, S. (2015). Can learning the ISBARR framework help to address nursing students' perceived anxiety and confidence levels associated with handover reports? *Journal of Nursing Education, 54*(10), 583–587. https://doi.org/10.3928/01484834-20150916-07.

Kristoff, T. (2022). Co-constructing a diverse hybrid simulation-based experience on First Nations culture. *Clinical Simulation in Nursing, 67*, 33–38. https://doi.org/10.1016/j.ecns.2022.02.012.

Mackenzie Health. (2023). *Cortellucci Vaughan Hospital*. https://www.mackenziehealth.ca.

Mullin, J., Lee, L., Hertwig, S., et al. (2001). A native smudging ceremony: A young native patient in palliative care teaches his caregivers a lesson in spirituality and cultural diversity. *The Canadian Nurse, 97*(9), 20–22.

Schön, D. A. (1983). *The reflective practitioner: How professionals think in action*. Basic Books.

Starmer, A. J., Spector, N. D., Rajendu, S., et al. (2014). Changes in medical errors after implementation of a handoff program. *The New England Journal of Medicine, 371*(19), 1803–1812. https://doi.org/10.1056/NEJMsa1405556.

Strudwick, G., Jeffs, L., Kemp, J., et al. (2022). Identifying and adapting interventions to reduce documentation burden and improve nurses' efficiency in using electronic health record systems (The IDEA Study): Protocol for a mixed methods study. *BMC Nursing, 21*, 1–8. https://doi.org/10.1186/s12912-022-00989-w.

Tanner, C. A. (2006). Thinking like a nurse: A research-based model of clinical judgment in nursing. *Journal of Nursing Education, 45*(6), 204–211.

Walton, N. A., & Waddell, J. I. (2025). *Yoder-Wise's leading and managing in Canadian nursing* (3rd ed.). Elsevier.

# 6

# Reviewing Actions

## LEARNING OUTCOMES

*After reading this chapter, you will be able to:*
- Describe the links between care outcomes, quality improvement initiatives, and personal reflection.
- Apply the processes of evaluation and reflection to clinical judgement and nursing practice activities.
- Explain when reflection on an action would indicate a need for practice to be adapted or changed.

- Describe clear and collegial strategies for providing feedback and debriefing with others.
- Explain how newly acquired learning from practice experience can help anticipate future client needs.

## GLOSSARY

**Clinical judgement (measurement):** "the observed outcome of critical thinking and decision making; it is an iterative process that uses nursing knowledge to observe and assess presenting situations, identify a prioritized client concern, and generate the best possible evidence-based solutions in order to deliver safe client care" (National Council of State Boards of Nursing, 2019, p. 1)

**Clinical judgement (practice):** the outcome of thinking and decision activities that are focused on and respond to the client's health care needs; also "an interpretation or conclusion about a client's needs, concerns, or health problems, and/or the decision to take action (or not), use or modify standard approaches, or improvise new ones as deemed appropriate by the client's response" (Tanner, 2006, p. 204)

**Evaluation:** a review to determine the effectiveness of nursing care

**Feedback:** giving and responding to information (verbal, written) about nursing care and performance to facilitate professional and personal growth, practical improvements, and optimal care; feedback to the nurse can come from any person involved in care, including the client

**Nursing-sensitive indicators (NSIs):** in clinical care, client outcomes that are influenced by nursing interventions, according to empirical evidence (D'Amour et al., 2014)

**Outcomes:** responses observed as a result of an intervention or action; measurements that relate to the effectiveness and efficiency of an action(s)

**Quality improvement (QI):** a continuous process of improving care delivery and outcomes using a systematic and evidence-informed approach; it includes comparing evaluation results to benchmarks or standards

**Reflection-on-action:** a practice that completes the cycle of reflection; it reveals what nurses gained from their experience and contributes to their ongoing clinical knowledge development and capacity for clinical judgement

The last step of the thinking and decision-making process is to review the nurse's actions and related decisions. Hallmarks of this step are reviewing the outcomes that were achieved and those that were not, and the thinking processes that were applied (i.e., in finding information, deciding what to do, and acting on decisions) along the way. The nurse also evaluates and reflects on their care of the client and their professional practice. As well, they make a final determination—in a final judgement or conclusion—about whether their actions achieved the identified goals.

**TABLE 6.2   Applying the Lasater Clinical Judgment Rubric to Personal Reflection**

| Skill | Beginning | Developing | Accomplished | Exemplary |
|---|---|---|---|---|
| **Noticing**<br>• Focused observation<br>• Recognizing deviations from expected patterns<br>• Information seeking | Is confused; is not organized in gathering data; performs one task at a time; misses patterns; does not seek important information | Is overwhelmed by array of data; misses some important information; sees obvious patterns; makes limited effort to seek more information | Sees general patterns in various data; misses subtle signs or leads; actively seeks subjective information | Focuses on and is assertive in getting relevant information; sees subtle patterns in various data sources; performs consistently |
| **Interpreting**<br>• Prioritizing data<br>• Making sense of data | Has difficulty focusing on important information, and attends to everything; has trouble interpreting simple situations | Attempts to prioritize data but also attends to less relevant data equally; can see patterns in simple situations; requires additional help | Focuses on primary data and follows up on relevant patterns; may attend to less pertinent information | Focuses on most important and relevant information based on evidence; understands patterns in complex situations; makes rational plans |
| **Responding**<br>• Calm, confident manner<br>• Clear communication<br>• Well-planned intervention/ flexibility<br>• Being skillful | Unless very routine, cannot organize care or instill confidence in others; displays confused communication; is task oriented with some monitoring; is unable to perform skills | Shows uncertainty in leadership role; reassures clients in routine situations but can be disorganized; competent but does not consistently display caring; develops interventions based on obvious data; cannot adjust plans; is hesitant in skill performance | Shows general confidence and leadership skills; is stressed in more complex situations; engages in clear and careful communication; has somewhat effective rapport with team; develops interventions that are relevant; sees any changes to care as unexpected issues; displays proficient skills | Assumes responsibility in a team; reassures clients; effectively communicates with appropriate individuals; performs tailored interventions with mastery |
| **Reflecting**<br>• Evaluation and self-reflection<br>• Commitment to improvement | Needs prompting to determine areas for improvement; justifies actions without evaluation; reflects infrequently; is unable to see need to improve | States obvious challenges or errors in practice; has difficulty identifying ways to improve; is defensive; needs external evaluation | Shows desire to improve through reflection on current practice; identifies strengths and weaknesses less systematically | Shows independence in personal performance review; realistically evaluates entire practice; creates active plan to improve weaknesses |

Adapted from Lasater, K. (2007). Clinical judgment development: Using simulation to create an assessment rubric. *Journal of Nursing Education, 46*(11), 496–503.

thinking during your clinical activities and when you evaluate your overall performance. As you review Table 6.2, ask yourself, *During nursing practice activities, how would I evaluate my performance (as a student in a lab or health care setting, or as a new graduate)?* This self-review is particularly helpful when combined with instructor feedback (Lasater & Nielsen, 2024).

Acquiring different experiences is a way for nurses to gain competence in making clinical judgements in practice at an entry level. Your nursing program prepares you for thinking as a nurse and to respond to situations using sound clinical judgement. At a baseline, nursing program graduates are tested for safe clinical judgement using the national registration exam. The National Council of State Boards of Nursing (2019) aims to measure clinical judgement in the exam and defines it as "the observed outcome of critical thinking and decision making; it is an iterative process that uses nursing knowledge to observe and assess presenting situations, identify a prioritized client concern, and generate the best possible evidence-based solutions in order to deliver safe client care" (p. 1). In this measurement-focused definition, note that reflective skills and holistic perspectives are not as evident as in the practice-focused Tanner (2006) model and the Lasater (2007) rubric. However, these skills and perspectives are required for clinical judgement.

Looking back on actions taken when delivering nursing care or addressing health care system issues requires thinking skills and an understanding of evaluation processes. Whether the focus is on improving the client's health or health care systems, these review skills are essential to nursing practice.

---

**KNOWLEDGE CHECK-IN**

- Describe five steps that will help you determine the effectiveness of client care and nursing actions.
- Provide an example of a QI method.
- Explain how reflection is used in clinical judgement.

---

## SKILLS USED WHEN REVIEWING ACTIONS

Clinical judgment supports a holistic perspective of practice. For that reason, and because it explicitly includes reflection and a reflective evaluation stage, this chapter applies the Clinical Judgement Model (Tanner, 2006; see Chapter 2) to illustrate the last step of the thinking and decision-making process. Figure 6.2 presents the unified process for thinking and decision making that incorporates this model. The clinical judgement aspects full of noticing, interpreting, responding, and reflecting are included in the blue centre areas. The related skills needed for *evaluating, reflecting, judging,* and *concluding* are highlighted in the grey-shaded area. Once the review (or reflection) is completed, the results will inform future approaches, leading to a cycle of thinking and decision making as indicated by the arrows. Tanner's Clinical Judgement Model is applied to a case study on reviewing actions, later in this chapter.

### Clinical Reasoning and Other Skills Used When Reviewing Actions

The following reasoning skills are key when reviewing actions in nursing practice. They are applied after client care has been delivered, during evaluation. They are not listed in any specific order.

#### Identify Quality Improvement Approaches and Evidence Gaps

The QI process involves comparing the outcomes of nursing care against standards and benchmarks. Doing so can reveal successes as well as challenges such as errors, missed opportunities, gaps in available information and evidence, systems issues, and low performance satisfaction levels. Identify which QI method you are most familiar with and which QI method(s) are used where you are practising.

*How Can You Develop This Skill?* Select a QI method and apply it consistently at a personal and client level or at a unit or institutional level to enhance ease and efficiency of use. Apply a QI method to various situations to identify evidence gaps and how practice may be improved.

#### Evaluate Effectiveness of Actions and Outcomes

When an action or outcome is evaluated as effective, it has proven to have achieved the intended benefit, which was based on the current available evidence and expectations for care. Often, efficiency is evaluated at the same time as effectiveness to determine whether time, resources, or other services were wasted. Measuring effectiveness requires an understanding of the planned goals and delivery of care. This skill is also integrated in the QI process and the reflective cycle.

*How Can You Develop This Skill?* In addition to using systematic thinking and the QI methods described earlier in this chapter, think about your care as being "nursing sensitive." Ask yourself, *What was within my control to accomplish?; Do I have the resources to compare what was planned to what actually happened?; What information do I need to determine whether an intervention was a success?; How has the client's situation changed, if at all?;* and *How can I improve my care so that best practices are more clearly*

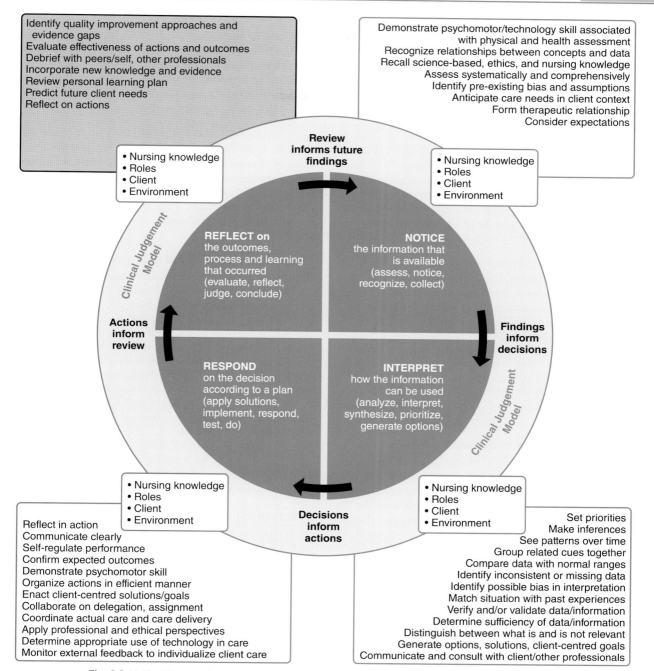

Identify quality improvement approaches and evidence gaps
Evaluate effectiveness of actions and outcomes
Debrief with peers/self, other professionals
Incorporate new knowledge and evidence
Review personal learning plan
Predict future client needs
Reflect on actions

Demonstrate psychomotor/technology skill associated with physical and health assessment
Recognize relationships between concepts and data
Recall science-based, ethics, and nursing knowledge
Assess systematically and comprehensively
Identify pre-existing bias and assumptions
Anticipate care needs in client context
Form therapeutic relationship
Consider expectations

- Nursing knowledge
- Roles
- Client
- Environment

- Nursing knowledge
- Roles
- Client
- Environment

Review informs future findings

Clinical Judgement Model

**REFLECT on** the outcomes, process and learning that occurred (evaluate, reflect, judge, conclude)

**NOTICE** the information that is available (assess, notice, recognize, collect)

**Actions inform review**

**Findings inform decisions**

**RESPOND** on the decision according to a plan (apply solutions, implement, respond, test, do)

**INTERPRET** how the information can be used (analyze, interpret, synthesize, prioritize, generate options)

Clinical Judgement Model

- Nursing knowledge
- Roles
- Client
- Environment

**Decisions inform actions**

- Nursing knowledge
- Roles
- Client
- Environment

Reflect in action
Communicate clearly
Self-regulate performance
Confirm expected outcomes
Demonstrate psychomotor skill
Organize actions in efficient manner
Enact client-centred solutions/goals
Collaborate on delegation, assignment
Coordinate actual care and care delivery
Apply professional and ethical perspectives
Determine appropriate use of technology in care
Monitor external feedback to individualize client care

Set priorities
Make inferences
See patterns over time
Group related cues together
Compare data with normal ranges
Identify inconsistent or missing data
Identify possible bias in interpretation
Match situation with past experiences
Verify and/or validate data/information
Determine sufficiency of data/information
Distinguish between what is and is not relevant
Generate options, solutions, client-centred goals
Communicate and consult with client/other professionals

**Fig. 6.2** Unified Process for Thinking and Decision Making: Applying the Clinical Judgement Model.

*incorporated?* Answering these questions involves reflective and evaluative skills.

## Debrief with Peers/Self, Other Professionals

Debriefing is a process that enables feedback to occur, where giving and responding to information (verbal, written) about nursing care and performance facilitate professional and personal growth, and practical improvements. Debriefing is most effective when it happens right after an event or practice situation and is provided by peers, instructors or colleagues who have direct knowledge so that feedback is more accurate and meaningful. Debriefing can focus on ways to improve and on successes and supports; observable outcomes, rather than personal characteristics, are most useful and objective. It can also occur individually, as self-review and reflection.

*How Can You Develop This Skill?* Seek feedback from others (an instructor, a peer, or a mentor) after a nursing action. Ask questions such as, "Would you be able to offer some comments on my performance?"; "Do you have any practical advice for me?"; and "Is there anything that I did that you would have done differently and why?" Provide others with your feedback in a collegial manner, using comments and rationales such as, "May I share with you some practical advice?"; "I have had similar situations, and have found that I was also challenged by . . ."; and "I can see that you are doing this well."

## Incorporate New Knowledge and Evidence

It is important that new knowledge acquired during the process of care is included in future practice. New evidence can arise during the process of care as well, because nursing knowledge evolves on a regular basis. When the period of an intervention is lengthy, science can change, and the evidence base can look different. For example, consider what was known at the start of the pandemic in March 2020 and what is known now by public health nurses involved in long-term vaccination programs. How nurses provided care and client education changed significantly over time in response to changes in science and nursing knowledge.

*How Can You Develop This Skill?* Keep current by reading and seeking updates about your current area of practice and practice standard changes. Make this a habit. Join a QI committee, listen to other health care professionals' perspectives on the latest care, and discuss how interventions can be improved with your colleagues/peers. Consider becoming a member of your specialty association, which will help you stay up to date with the latest practice initiatives.

## Review Personal Learning Plan

As part of ongoing requirements for registration, provincial and territorial regulatory bodies ask that all nurses engage in regular self-reflection and practice review.

*How Can You Develop This Skill?* Check out the provincial and territorial regulators' websites for templates you can use to develop learning plans for yourself. You can also create your own and keep track of your long-term learning and achievements (see Chapter 8). Ask yourself, *How has my experience this year affected my practice?* and *What has changed in terms of how I do my work?* In the short term, self-reflective exercises as you leave a practice area or complete a shift are helpful. Ask yourself, *What did I learn today that I can apply next time I am with a client?* and *What do I need to look up or read about to develop my knowledge in this area for next time?*

## Predict Future Client Needs

It is important for nurses to understand how to apply what was learned during the experience of delivering nursing care and interventions to future situations. As their nursing knowledge grows, nurses will be able to identify patterns or trends more easily and grasp the overall meaning of a client situation more quickly. The result is that the next time a nurse encounters a similar client situation, they may be able to predict future client needs more accurately and provide more collaborative and effective care.

*How Can You Develop This Skill?* Continue to develop your nursing knowledge. Pay attention to the practice experiences and stories of other nurses and health care professionals. Focus on noticing patterns and trends, grouping cues, and analyzing the meaning of these assessments and how they may appear the same or different in other client situations. Check in with a mentor to confirm your thinking.

## Reflect on Actions

As in other reflective activities, reflecting back on decisions and actions that were taken with clients and in the health care setting can provide an opportunity for professional development. A final reflection is connected to other earlier aspects of the reflective cycle and will lead the nurse to improving future practice. Fully reflective practice is essential for meeting regulatory competencies and standards of nursing care.

*How Can You Develop This Skill?* Review a task, an assigned activity, or a shift, and ask yourself, *Is this the outcome that I expected when I planned and implemented this activity?*; *How do I feel about what I have done?*; and *What feedback or responses have I received from the client and others that can inform my thinking?* Always think ahead to the next time you will encounter a similar situation: What will you change to make your practice better?

**TABLE 6.4   Case Study: Application of the Clinical Judgement Model to Reviewing Actions**

| Client Situation | Nursing Model and Application of Thinking | | |
|---|---|---|---|
| A 60-year-old client had a bowel resection and temporary colostomy 4 days ago to treat an abscess caused by diverticulitis. | **Clinical Judgement Model** | **Clinical Reasoning Skills Used** | **Possible Nursing Responses (Barriers, Strategies)** |
| The client's postoperative recovery has been uneventful. Pain is now managed with nonsteroidal anti-inflammatory drugs every 6 hours. There is a small amount of liquid brown stool in the colostomy pouch. The abdominal surgical site is clean and dry. The client has been prescribed a diet as tolerated. Teaching for colostomy care and diet information was provided. The client indicates they prefer foods from their Caribbean background. They also prefer that the nurse change the colostomy pouch "since you are here anyways—I'll only do it later if I have to." | Noticing | As described in client situation. | |
| | Interpreting | As described in client situation. | |
| | Responding | As described in client situation. | |
| | **Reflecting** | Identify quality improvement approaches and evidence gaps. Evaluate effectiveness of actions and outcomes. Debrief with peers/self, other professionals. Incorporate new knowledge and evidence. Review personal learning plan. Predict future client needs. Reflect on actions. | Consider standard teaching information for colostomy care and clarity of resources. Note that client response to colostomy and stoma care does not fit with self-care goals. Were client goals created collaboratively and clearly? Include clearer communication in future teaching; consult with dietitian as needed about preferred foods. Consider how client learning needs are assessed, and change practice in future. |

The use of the NRCE framework reminds the nurse to look at the whole picture of the client's experience in health care, not just the clinical outcomes. As you have seen, many areas can influence health care and need to be considered by the nurse in every step of thinking and decision making.

## REVIEWING ACTIONS: A CLINICAL JUDGEMENT MODEL CASE STUDY

The process of reviewing actions in nursing practice can involve any of the nursing models described in Chapter 2 (e.g., the clinical reasoning cycle, the ethical decision-making model, and the nursing process). In this section, the Clinical Judgement Model developed by Tanner (2006), with its focus on reflection on action, will be applied to a simple case study, using the example of a client who has received discharge teaching for colostomy care.

The case study in Table 6.4 incorporates key ideas covered in this chapter, including the clinical reasoning skills described earlier. As well, it addresses possible responses to barriers to thinking and strategies to overcome those barriers.

## SUMMARY

This chapter presented the last step of the thinking and decision-making process. As a cyclical activity that does not have a clear end, reflection is an ongoing part of your professional role. Specific clinical reasoning skills are needed to successfully complete this step of the thinking and decision-making process.

It is important to remember that clinical judgement and the culmination of an outcome for the client and the nurse, are very involved and sophisticated activities. As an iterative process, clinical judgement requires the nurse to think back and forth between phases of care, referring to different concepts and information with skill and constant attention.

# KEY POINTS TO REMEMBER

These are the key points to remember from this chapter.

## About Closing the Loop: Looking Back on Actions

- Thinking is a continuous process and does not end once care has been delivered to the client.
- Reviewing your thinking and your clinical performance is necessary to complete the cycle of care, and to continue to provide future nursing practice that is informed, reflective and competent.
- Collaboration with the client about whether outcomes have been met enables client-centred care.
- Evaluating client care involves five steps:
  - Identify the review criteria and standards (such as client goals, expected outcomes, ethical codes, and practice standards or guidelines).
  - Collect and interpret information to evaluate whether the criteria and standards were met.
  - Analyze and summarize results (judge whether the outcomes indicate that the goal was attained or not).
  - Record results and clinical judgements.
  - Close the loop by discontinuing, continuing, or revising care.
- A continuous focus on providing better, safer care, *that always meets or exceeds the minimum standards,* through QI initiatives is a competency required by all nurses.
- Practices can be reviewed and monitored using informal, frequent strategies such as time outs and huddles that emphasize communication.
- Systematic approaches such as the Plan-Do-Study-Act cycle are more formal and can support larger evaluations and change.
- Client outcomes in clinical care that are known to improve with the delivery of high-quality nursing practice are referred to as *nursing-sensitive indicators.*
- The process of reviewing actions involves not only a review of direct care activities and broader health care systems but also reflection on your own thinking processes.
- Reflection-on-action completes the cycle of reflection. It reveals not only how care was delivered but also what nurses gained and learned from the experience.

## About Reflection and Clinical Judgement

- The reflective skills you are learning contribute to your overall capacity to make clinical judgements.
- Clinical judgement is the outcome of thinking and decision-making activities that are focused on and respond to client care needs and result in the formation of a

clinical conclusion. It is important in reviewing interventions, actions, and outcomes of care.
- Tanner's Clinical Judgement Model (2006) and the Lasater Clinical Judgment Rubric (2007) describe the aspects and levels of clinical judgement skill development and ways in which performance may be evaluated.
- When forming clinical judgements, the whole of the nursing care and client situation is considered, not just technical or medical aspects of the care provided.

## About Skills Used When Reviewing Actions

- The unified process for thinking and decision making (see Figure 6.2) includes a number of skills that can be useful when reviewing actions:
  - Identify quality improvement approaches and evidence gaps.
  - Evaluate effectiveness of actions and outcomes.
  - Debrief with peers/self, other professionals.
  - Incorporate new knowledge and evidence.
  - Review personal learning plan.
  - Predict future client needs.
  - Reflect on actions.
- These skills, and the skills described in the previous three chapters, are helpful during clinical reasoning and forming clinical judgements.

## About Barriers to Thinking When Reviewing Actions

- Barriers to thinking when reviewing actions in nursing include a lack of understanding of the context of care and limited information; time restrictions; distractions; a unit culture of blame or fear of reporting errors; and an insufficient personal plan for professional growth.

## About Helpful Strategies for Reviewing Actions

- Strategies for overcoming obstacles to reflection include the use of debriefing frameworks and self-regulation.

## About Thinking Through Reviewing Actions: NRCE

- This textbook's NRCE framework can help guide you to recall the wide range of influences on a client care situation as you review actions and previous decisions.

## About a Case Study on Reviewing Actions

- A case study on discharge teaching and determining whether client needs were met illustrates the decision-reviewing activities of evaluate, reflect, judge, and conclude—the cyclical process for thinking about care.

# CONCLUSION AND THINKING IT THROUGH

The thinking and decision-making process is not step by step or linear in nature. It is cyclical, iterative, and dynamic. Sometimes, nurses may need to return to earlier steps to address issues that arise after responding to the client situation. This is fine—and completely expected. No one, and no process, is perfect. Being mindful and using the NCRE framework to remember what can be included in thinking along the way will help you think about your thinking.

These cognitive processes and a commitment to deeply understand what is involved in practice will help you deliver more holistic care. These processes will be essential in both simple, predictable health care circumstances and more complex, acute situations. Complex decision making is explored in Chapter 7.

# CLASS ACTIVITIES TO CHECK THINKING

## Think-Aloud Pair Problem Solving (TAPPS)

Form pairs. Decide who will be a problem solver and listener for Problem A. The problem solver reads the problem aloud and talks through a response to the problem, while the listener reminds the problem solver to think aloud, asks clarification questions, offers encouragement to keep thinking, but refrains from providing possible answers. Switch roles for Problem B.

For each of these problems, review the outcomes and options for what can be done to improve actions and decisions in a future similar scenario.

- **Problem A:** A nurse working during a night shift on a medical-surgical unit was assigned to a newly admitted client. The client who was recently diagnosed with leukemia was experiencing signs of acute kidney failure. The client reported significant pain and profound fatigue, stating, "I am in so much pain and haven't slept in 5 days – all I want is for the pain to go away and to sleep". Prescribed diuretics and volume expanders were initiated. The client was also treated for pain and fell asleep. The nurse left the client, with fluid infusing, to sleep for the night according to their wishes. At the end of the shift, the nurse evaluated the client as wheezing and short of breath, exhibiting signs of fluid overload. Treatment to address this complication was initiated.
- **Problem B:** While providing care to clients at an urban-based methadone clinic, a nurse was verbally assaulted by a client who used racist and derogatory language towards the nurse. The nurse advocated for themselves and loudly stated, "I am only trying to help you and I don't deserve this treatment!" Eventually, another clinic staff member called police services who arrived and escorted the abusive client from the clinic. The nurse then observed that clients left and some have not returned for their daily methadone dose and counselling appointment since the incident.

## Activities and Discussion Questions

1. In a small group, identify a clinical issue that you have either read about, observed, or directly experienced in nursing practice. How was it addressed? Evaluate the outcome and describe areas for improvement. What are some evidence-informed solutions for future practice?
2. You are assigned to care for a client who has had recent surgery. The care pathway indicates that the indwelling urinary catheter was removed the day after the procedure. It is now day 2, and the client states that they are unable to urinate. What do you do and why? Discuss with a classmate.
3. Self-reflect on how you give and receive feedback. Ask yourself the following questions:
   - *When sharing feedback, am I critical (focusing on negatives) or constructive (focusing on positives)?*
   - *Do I reflect on my approach to giving feedback before I start? How do I want to be seen—supportive or punitive?*
   - *Have I ever let my pride or strong feelings get in the way of what is otherwise good advice and feedback? If yes, How can I overcome this reaction?*
   - *After receiving negative feedback, how can I move forward and include it in a personal development plan?*
4. Think back on a recent clinical activity or laboratory-based simulation experience. Using the Lasater Clinical Judgment Rubric in Table 6.2, self-rate your overall performance as *beginning, developing, accomplished,* or *exemplary*. Provide examples to rationalize your rating.

## CASE STUDY REVIEW

Review the case study in Table 6.4.

### Questions

1. Based on the scenario outcomes, what missing information may be important to review and evaluate? Consider your nursing knowledge, your role in teaching, the client and their context, and the health care environment.

2. Could other individuals or health care professionals be involved to improve client outcomes? If yes, who would they be?

## EVIDENCE-INFORMED THINKING ACTIVITY

Consider the following nursing care situation.

At a long-term care facility, a recurring issue of administering medication to residents outside of the required time frame (missed doses) is attributed to workflow inefficiencies and a high changeover in nursing staff. Family members are concerned that residents are being neglected. The Director of Care wants to apply a quality improvement (QI) method to addressing the issue.

Describe how the steps in the evaluation process are applied when reviewing the identified issue and how improvements to the quality of care can be addressed. Refer to evidence-informed resources as you review this issue.

## QUESTIONS TO ASSESS LEARNING

### Review Questions

1. Which description best explains debriefing in nursing practice?
   a. Provision of feedback to clients about their condition
   b. Post-event intervention to address emotional distress in nurses
   c. Structured discussion to review and analyze a specific event or performance
   d. Technique used to ensure quick feedback to nurses
2. Which are examples of nurse-sensitive indicators? Select all that apply.
   a. Fall
   b. Pressure injury
   c. Surgical bleeding
   d. Postoperative pneumonia
   e. Nosocomial infections
3. A team of nurses examines feedback from a survey of community partners. The nurses decide that the survey questions were not clear and discuss the possibility of repeating the survey and improving their data collection processes. What type of reflection best describes this activity?
   a. Anticipatory reflection
   b. Reflection-in-action
   c. Reflection-on-action
   d. Reflective interpretation
4. Which best defines self-regulation in nursing practice?
   a. Managing one's own thinking, actions, and reactions in a professional setting
   b. Overseeing and regulating the functioning of medical equipment and devices
   c. Adhering strictly to the established nursing protocols and guidelines without assistance
   d. Maintaining a healthy sense of personal well-being

## ONE LAST THOUGHT

Consider the quote by Florence Nightingale (1992):

*"Let us never consider ourselves finished nurses… we must be learning all of our lives."*

Reflecting in action and reflecting on action are critical to competent practice. However, these actions are not enough if results of reflection are not applied to future practice. Ongoing learning supports your professional development and ability to provide increasingly complex care in environments that change in response to new requirements. The next section of this textbook will present how acquired knowledge can be applied in dynamic situations and how a reflective stance on diversity can facilitate better nursing care.

## ONLINE RESOURCES

Accreditation Canada: https://accreditation.ca
Healthcare Excellence Canada: https://www.healthcareexcellence.ca
Patients for Patient Safety Canada: https://www.patients4safety.ca

## REFERENCES

Astle, B., & Duggleby, W. (2024). *Potter and Perry's Canadian fundamentals of nursing* (7th ed.). Elsevier.

Backman, C., Vanderloo, S., Momtahan, K., et al. (2015). Implementation of an electronic data collection tool to monitor nursing-sensitive indicators in a large academic health sciences centre. *Nursing Leadership, 28*(3), 77–91.

Baker, C. (2020). Clinical nursing education in the Canadian context. In K. Page-Cutrara & P. Bradley (Eds.), *The role of the nurse educator in Canada*. Canadian Association of Schools of Nursing.

Benner, P. (2001). *From novice to expert: Excellence and power in clinical nursing practice*. Prentice Hall.

Braithwaite, T. J., Kelly, L. P., & Chakanyuka, C. (2022). File of uncertainties: Exploring student experience of applying decolonizing knowledge in practice. *Quality Advancement in Nursing Education, 8*(3), 1–19. https://doi.org/10.17483/2368-6669.1351.

D'Amour, D., Dubois, C. A., Tchouaket, É., et al. (2014). The occurrence of adverse events potentially attributable to nursing care in medical units: Cross sectional record review. *International Journal of Nursing Studies, 51*(6). https://doi.org/10.1016/j.ijnurstu.2013.10.017.

Harwood, L., & Wilson, B. (2022). All-star quality improvement: Keep it simple. *Nephrology Nursing Journal, 49*(2), 161–163. https://doi.org/10.37526/1526-744X.2022.49.2.161.

Lasater, K. (2007). Clinical judgment development: Using simulation to create an assessment rubric. *Journal of Nursing Education, 46*(11), 496–503.

Lasater, K., & Nielsen, A. (2024). The Lasater clinical judgment rubric: 17 years later. *Journal of Nursing Education, 63*(3), 149–155. https://doi.org/10.3928/01484834-20240108-05.

National Council of State Boards of Nursing. (2019). *Next Generation NCLEX news: Clinical judgment measurement model*. https://www.ncsbn.org/public-files/NGN_Winter19.pdf.

Nightingale, F. (1992). *Notes on nursing: What it is, and what it is not*. Lippincott Williams & Wilkins.

Singh, M., & Thirsk, L. (2022). *LoBiondo-Wood and Haber's nursing research in Canada* (5th ed.). Elsevier.

Stewart, D., MacLure, K., Pallivalapila, A., et al. (2020). Views and experiences of decision-makers on organisational safety culture and medication errors. *International Journal of Clinical Practice, 74*(9). https://doi.org/10.1111/ijcp.13560.

Tanner, C. A. (2006). Thinking like a nurse: A research-based model of clinical judgment in nursing. *Journal of Nursing Education, 45*(6), 204–211.

Walton, N. A., & Waddell, J. I. (2025). *Yoder-Wise's leading and managing in Canadian nursing* (3rd ed.). Elsevier.

# PART C

# Thinking It Through in Nursing Practice

This third and last section of the textbook will provide further context for thinking and making decisions in Canadian nursing practice. Thinking through complex client or health care issues is frequently required by nurses who care for clients experiencing multiple health concerns or communities that are affected by more widespread social or structural determinants of health. Development as a reflective practitioner requires the nurse to embrace contemporary nursing practice standards and actively reflect on diversity, knowledge of Indigenous populations, planetary health, and ways to grow as a professional nurse.

Chapter 7 addresses complexity in nursing practice and how thinking it through is applied in challenging circumstances. Differences between simple and complex situations and examples of types of complex decisions are described. Specific concepts such as stability, predictability, and ambiguity are discussed for their role in clinical decision making. Organizing thinking and the use of intuition and experience are presented as ways that nurses can manage complex care and health care issues.

Chapter 8 offers a final review of thinking it through as a nurse and covers the development of reflection. Recalling the cycle of reflection and critical thinking skills, various ways to apply reflection are presented in the context of professional development and practice and when incorporating contemporary nursing requirements. Suggestions for planning your own professional growth as a reflective practitioner are included.

**Part C will help you answer the questions,** *how can I adapt my thinking to make decisions in more complex client or nursing practice situations, and how can I use reflection as a tool to grow professionally and incorporate nursing practice requirements into my thinking and decision making?*

# Complex Decision Making

## LEARNING OUTCOMES

*After reading this chapter, you will be able to:*

- Identify factors that increase the complexity of decision making in nursing practice.
- Describe ways to organize thinking when making complex client and health care decisions.
- Apply decision-making processes to more complex client situations.
- Explain the role of intuition in nursing practice and when forming clinical judgements.

## GLOSSARY

**Ambiguity:** a situation that has more than one possible meaning or interpretation; an unclear choice in the given context

**Cognitive load:** the relative demand on thinking required by a particular task or tasks

**Cognitive overload:** the result of too much mental demand on the decision-maker from too much information or activity at any one point in time

**Complex decision:** in nursing, one in which the nurse must make a choice about a client or health care situation that has no obvious immediate answer; it may involve multiple client(s) factors or other concerns that are present simultaneously in a single clinical situation

**Complexity:** "the degree to which a client's condition and care requirements are identifiable and established; the sum of the variables influencing a client's current health status; and the variability of a client's condition or care requirements" (College of Nurses of Ontario, 2018, p. 5)

**Intuition:** the immediate understanding of the meaning of a clinical situation, without the need for conscious reasoning, and is a function of experience with similar situations; often occurs with recognition of cues and patterns (Benner, 2001; Tanner, 2006)

**Predictability:** the degree to which client outcomes and care requirements can be anticipated; it is future focused

**Stability:** a current client or health care situation that is not changing and is unlikely to change based on what is known at the time; it is present focused

How does simple decision making differ from complex decision making? This chapter explores this question and presents practical information on thinking through more complicated client and health care situations. It also introduces some factors that can make a situation more complicated, unpredictable, or unstable. Recognizing these factors is important in analyzing information, determining appropriate nursing care and making sound clinical judgements.

Novice nurses often think that every circumstance they encounter is complex. This perception may be due to a lack of familiarity with different care situations or with a lack of proficiency in using the decision-making processes needed to address challenges in practice. Every situation a nurse encounters for the first time may appear complicated, but with knowledge and experience, this view can change. This chapter includes case studies on simple and complex situations to further support students and novice nurses in *thinking it through*.

## A CLOSER LOOK AT DECISION MAKING IN COMPLEX SITUATIONS

This textbook has focused mainly on thinking and decision making about a single client or clinical situation where one client issue is present. However, such simple scenarios do not reflect the reality of nursing practice in many health care settings. More often than not, clients have complex needs, and health care situations involve clinical, professional, and administrative challenges. It is not enough to know how to manage only one problem while providing care. Although a nurse can physically accomplish one activity at a time, they must understand how several problems are connected and how the response to a number of issues can be coordinated to meet various outcomes.

For simpler problems, the goal and the plan to achieve that goal are well defined, with few factors that could potentially influence care implementation. In simple situations, the care process is more predictable. Predictability is the degree to which client outcomes and care requirements can be anticipated; it is future focused. On the other hand, stability refers to a current client or health care situation that is not changing and is unlikely to change according to a reasonable interpretation of the available information; it is present focused. For a client situation that is stable, the perceived risk of complications is lower. At times, for simpler problems, even if the plan and approach to care are not tailored exactly to the specific client need or preference, the client will still be able to reach the established goals.

Simple tasks require fewer cues to be processed than complex tasks, so they place a lower cognitive demand on the decision-maker (Muntean, 2012). This means that providing care for a stable client or a single, specific health concern involves fewer factors and will lead to fewer intervention options. It may be easier to make decisions in such situations.

So far, deciding what to do has been applied to a single point of client care. When considering the overall approach to the process of client care (the *BIG* picture), know that there is always a main decision point in that process. That stated, nurses make multiple decisions throughout the entire thinking and decision-making process (Table 7.1). They select options and make choices *all the time*. Remember that this thinking also applies to nonclinical situations such as health policy development or public health initiatives. Refer to the Appendix for examples of what thinking and decision making can look like in different nursing scenarios.

In nursing programs, students are often presented with well-defined problems. For example, they are given assignments on a certain topic, and specific answers are expected. However, in real-world health care settings—in any nursing practice area—nurses often face more complex problems and challenging situations or practice environments that are less defined. Students may encounter these situations towards the end of their program to prepare them for practice. Let's take a closer look at what complex decision making can look like.

## WHAT IS A COMPLEX DECISION?

In nursing, a complex decision is one in which the nurse must make a choice about a client or health care situation that has no obvious immediate answer. Here, the "client or health care situation" refers to the issue, condition, concern, or clinical presentation that falls within the nurse's scope of practice, and one where the nurse or client identifies that a change or improvement is necessary. A complex decision can include risk, uncertainty, or ambiguity, and have few precedents. A decision often becomes difficult when multiple client factors or too much data are present. At times, a complex decision may involve more than one client, each with their own competing needs, that require the nurse's attention (i.e., the question becomes, *Which client should I respond to first?*). Alternatively, complex decisions may arise during a public health crisis when many institutions and service groups each contribute a significant amount of data and analyses (i.e., the question becomes, *How can I make sense of this information and prioritize responses?*).

For complex problems, the goal and the path to that goal are not as clear as they are with simple, straightforward problems. Each client is unique, and some may have numerous physical, social, emotional, spiritual, and situational challenges. In these circumstances, the range of possible actions and interventions tends to be greater.

"The complexity of a client's condition influences the nursing knowledge required to provide the level of care the client needs. A more complex client situation and less stable environment create an increased need for consultation" (College of Nurses of Ontario, 2018, p. 3). They also require the nurse to evaluate a number of care requirements.

In a complex situation, certain circumstances influence how care is planned and implemented. The client situation may be unstable (e.g., changing and dynamic), and the perceived risk of complications may be high. The outcome of managing care may be less predictable (e.g., difficult to accurately anticipate), and the process of providing care may more likely require adaptation. Also, the nurse may find it difficult to apply nursing models effectively to more challenging issues due to insufficient experience or expertise. Flexibility may be needed when using nursing models in practice. As well, the likelihood that the nurse will need to move back and forth between the steps of a model when thinking and decision making is greater in complex situations; for example, the nurse may need to more frequently return to assessment—or finding information—if a decision could not be reached.

Have you ever asked an expert nurse about a client concern that you were having difficulty resolving, and they replied, "Well, it depends ..."? Complex decision making and its outcomes are dependent on the context of care. As a result, the care the nurse plans and implements in complex circumstances must account for more variables and cues, the possibility for change, and include interactions with other health care professionals.

## TABLE 7.1  Decisions Throughout the Thinking and Decision-Making Process

| Activities Where Decisions Can Occur | Examples of Decisions |
|---|---|
| **Assessment:** figuring out what new information is needed and how to obtain it in relation to available resources; recalling most relevant clinical manifestations | Selecting a screening tool for depression or cognitive decline<br>Responding to the client's direct concerns of shortness of breath with a focused assessment of the respiratory system |
| **Analysis:** considering the clinical manifestations or presentation of a situation and its meaning; deciding what is a priority | Deciding whether anxiety or pathophysiology is the possible cause of a client's high blood pressure measurement<br>Choosing what action is critical to perform/cannot wait |
| **Coordination:** choosing a time that is appropriate for the client's needs and based on the availability of other health care professionals' services and resources | Selecting the most appropriate timing for client education when other health care professionals need to also provide timely client care |
| **Consulting/collaborating:** deciding to seek or not seek other information before deciding what to do | Choosing to contact a physician about the deterioration of a client's chronic abscess |
| **Planning:** selecting and weighing options to include in future action | Anticipating the best approach to care for a client's rise in blood glucose levels (monitoring/observing, acting, informing others) |
| **Communication:** selecting an appropriate strategy to send and receive information between people<br>• *Applying therapeutic approaches*<br>• *Supporting information exchanges* | Determining how to relate to a grieving family member who experienced sudden loss<br>Choosing how to deliver client education to a neurodiverse youth who has been prescribed a new medication |
| **Intervention:** selecting from identified activities in the established plan of care, based on priority, effect, or prevention of future harm | Choosing which order/medication prescribed by the physician should be administered first<br>Deciding how to efficiently use resources to reduce waste and duplication of effort |
| **Evaluation:** determining whether future actions should be adapted or revised to correct errors or improve outcomes | Continuing to monitor client's weight loss over a period of a week while on a new diet<br>Advocating for a new prescription for an analgesic to address unresolved postsurgical pain |

---

### REFLECTIVE PRACTICE MOMENT

Recall situation awareness (Endsley & Jones, 2012) from Chapter 3. Being aware of what is happening around you and understanding the significance of that information is important. A large amount of information is more challenging to deal with.

Think back on a practice experience that you found challenging.

- **Perception:** *What was the client concern and the purpose of the nursing activity?*
- **Comprehension:** *Were there multiple sources of information and environmental pressures, and how were they understood?*
- **Projection:** *Did you incorporate the necessary information into your decision making? If not, why?*

Having an awareness of the scope of a client concern and the relationship among multiple sources of information will help you generate options and find solutions in more complex decision-making scenarios.

Complex decision making can be anticipated when certain factors are present. Factors that make thinking and decision making complex include:

- *Apparent contradiction:* The data or information is inconsistent or confusing, and systemic or individual beliefs and values are opposing or diverse.
- *Ambiguity:* Not enough information is available to clearly form a goal and a plan of care that will meet identified needs.
- *Never-before-experienced situations:* A truly unique situation that has not been seen before provides no basis on which to act decisively.
- *Requirement for multiple consultations:* Various health care professionals' knowledge is needed to make a decision. Consultants who are involved in the provision of care may need to debate.
- *Outcomes that are unclear until actions are implemented:* The effects or responses to the intervention are not immediately known.

- *No way to evaluate or measure outcomes:* No measure of success exists, or success may take a long time to determine.
- *A known multistep process:* Many steps will be needed to achieve an identified goal, and each step may change or affect the overall circumstances and plan.

The presence of these factors requires the nurse to conduct more analyses, consider various interpretations, and synthesize more information before making a decision on what is occurring and what can be done.

## TYPES OF COMPLEX DECISIONS

Factors that make thinking challenging are evident in the following types of complex decisions: decisions with time limitations, multiple goals and too much data, and conflicting information (Thompson et al., 2004).

### Decisions With Time Limitations
#### "I Don't Have Time to Think!"
A lack of time can affect decision making and increase its perceived complexity. Even a relatively simple decision can be challenging if little time is given to make a choice. For instance, time limitations can affect decision making in circumstances such as the following:

- A client's condition changes and requires urgent care to prevent significant injury or further deterioration ("we need to decide *now*").
- Intervention is dependent on the timely completion of another essential care activity that is complex or interprofessional in nature ("we can't decide until we see what happens next").
- Less time for decisions is available due to competing demands and a set time frame in which to complete care ("we have too much to do in too little time").

Some situations require fast or rapid decision making, where there is little opportunity to find additional information other than what is immediately available. Other situations involve a perceived pressure to quickly complete care but allow some time for further analysis and interpretation of information. *It is important to be able to identify these situations correctly, because you always want to ensure that you have appropriate and adequate data.*

At times, the decision about what to do for a client may be clear. For example, in an emergency or critical situation, there may be only one obvious goal, option, and plan. In fact, in such a situation, it may be necessary to skip a long analysis, interpretation, and synthesis of information because delaying a known evidence-informed action could further harm the client. You will be most familiar with this approach in a situation where a client is assessed as pulseless and not breathing. If the environment is safe enough that health care can be provided, codes, algorithms, or decision trees that break down and prioritize activities are employed. A code in hospital that triggers action in a complex situation (e.g., Code Blue for a myocardial infarction) helps with some aspects of decision making and saves time based on scientific and clinical evidence. Even in these very specific situations where care is delivered quickly, health care providers, including nurses, *always need to ensure that the plan they are following is appropriate for the client*. A nurse never stops thinking it through.

### Decisions With Multiple Goals and Too Much Data
#### "My Brain Is Full!"
The complexity of thinking and decision making increases when multiple goals must be achieved. What should be done first, and is there overlap between the actions to achieve each goal? The nurse may be faced with these and other questions, when issues such as the following arise in the health care setting:

- Several clients have similar concerns that all need to be addressed right away.
- One client has many issues that are high priority, in addition to strong personal preferences.
- A number of prescriptions and orders are presented at once, for one or more clients.
- A particular aspect of care or a procedure has multiple steps that occur over time and that must be coordinated with other activities.

The steps associated with the thinking and decision-making process and the evidence that informs decisions can be challenging to apply when multiple goals must be met. When the client's preferences or needs, other health care professionals' goals, and the aim of efficiency in the health care system are present, the nurse must find a balance between respect for the client's preferences and ensuring evidence-informed practice. For example, when advocating for the client and deciding to provide care that differs slightly from the goals of care in a general clinical practice pathway, the nurse must have a strong rationale for doing so and must be sure to deliver safe care. Consultation and collaboration are often needed before such a decision is made.

When a nurse is caring for multiple clients, prioritizing client needs and related nursing actions introduces additional challenges. When clients have similar issues, decisions about who to prioritize can be difficult. This is often the case on a specialty unit where clients are admitted for similar conditions.

The biggest challenge nurses face when dealing with multiple goals is having too much data. Your working memory, or what you can remember in the short term, can only hold so much information. You may have heard of the "magic number 7," which represents the number of pieces of data a person can successfully hold in short-term memory (Miller, 1956). When cognitive load—the relative demand on thinking required for a particular task or tasks—is not balanced with your knowledge and experience, you may feel overwhelmed (Rogers & Franklin, 2021). You may experience cognitive overload if a lot of information is available at once; too little information is not enough, and too much information cannot be filtered through to make a decision. In these circumstances, the ability to prioritize cues and sort data become important.

## Decisions With Conflicting Information

### "Nothing Makes Sense!"

At times, decisions can seem complex because a difference or apparent contradiction exists between a standard of nursing practice or a policy, client preferences, and another health care professional's practice or way of proceeding with care. For instance, circumstances may involve:

- Professional requirements that differ from the client's specific preferences or needs.
- Environmental conditions that do not support the care that is indicated.
- Another health care professional's recommendations or actions that affect the nurse's ability to plan and provide nursing care.

In situations with conflicting information, the nurse must confirm whether the information is correct. The nurse applies nursing knowledge and evidence-informed thinking when doing so. However, it is important to bear in mind that two pieces of information that appear contradictory can sometimes both be correct. In these circumstances, the nurse may need to continue to find more information and uncover cues that can explain and confirm what is happening. Strategies to make sense of conflicting information may include shared decision making with the client, Two-Eyed Seeing, or an understanding of cultural relativism. These and other approaches can help the nurse understand different views, preferences, and interpretations.

Recall situations where ethical issues were involved and where a nursing model (see Chapter 4) was used to explore options in clinical dilemmas. Often, if information is varied and solutions are unclear, a compromise can be found among the options, and a safe plan and client agreement can be reached.

---

**KNOWLEDGE CHECK-IN**

- *What is the difference between a simple and a complex problem?*
- *Identify factors that can make thinking and decision making complex. Why do they have this effect?*
- *Describe an emergency situation and explain what makes it complex.*
- *Why is it that too many options can present a problem in decision making?*

---

At times, different types of complex decisions overlap. For example, too little time and too much conflicting information may be part of a single situation on which a decision must be made, which increases complexity further. No matter the type of complexity involved, the nurse must choose an option and determine a course of action.

## KEY CONTRIBUTORS TO COMPLEXITY IN NURSING PRACTICE

Complexity is "the degree to which a client's condition and care requirements are identifiable and established; the sum of the variables influencing a client's current health status; and the variability of a client's condition or care requirements" (College of Nurses of Ontario, 2018, p. 5). Nurses must be able to recognize complexity to provide appropriate care and make informed clinical judgements. Key contributors tend to be the presence of instability, unpredictability, and ambiguity in a clinical situation.

### Instability and Unpredictability

Complex circumstances in which a client's condition is unstable (their condition is changing) and unpredictable (their outcomes cannot be clearly anticipated) require the nurse to make care decisions more frequently (Yee, 2023). The practice setting can also contribute to instability and unpredictability and affect decision making. The general practice environment, which includes defined resources and a certain level of busyness, can directly influence the ease with which decisions are made. For example, poorly resourced settings where multiple, unrelated care activities are occurring simultaneously are complex and potentially unstable (setting is changing and dynamic) and unpredictable (setting is unreliable and resources cannot be anticipated). In a more complex situation that is less stable and predictable, the nurse must consider their scope of practice, professional designation, role, level of competency and qualifications to ensure that they are able to make the required decisions and practise safely.

A higher level of consultation and collaboration is required when caring for clients with unpredictable and unstable conditions. Registered nurses and registered or licensed practical or psychiatric nurses need to consult and collaborate with other health care professionals to clarify information or aspects of care outside the nurse's scope of knowledge or practice and communicate plans to ensure the safest, most efficient, and appropriate care is provided. Figure 7.1 depicts how clients with conditions that are unstable and unpredictable may require more collaboration and consultation, which effects the overall complexity of care and decision making.

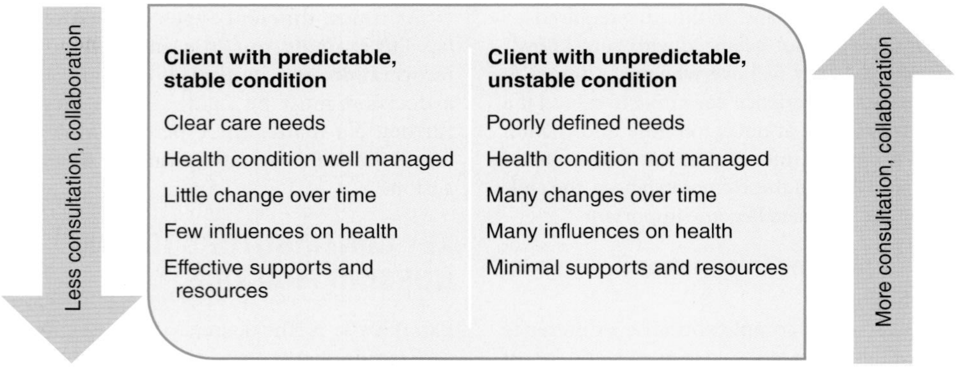

| Less consultation, collaboration | Client with predictable, stable condition | Client with unpredictable, unstable condition | More consultation, collaboration |
|---|---|---|---|
| | Clear care needs | Poorly defined needs | |
| | Health condition well managed | Health condition not managed | |
| | Little change over time | Many changes over time | |
| | Few influences on health | Many influences on health | |
| | Effective supports and resources | Minimal supports and resources | |

**Fig. 7.1** Changing predictability and stability.

## Ambiguity

Ambiguity makes thinking and decision making complex and is part of forming clinical judgement. According to Tanner (2006), clinical judgement is complex and "required in clinical situations that are, by definition, underdetermined, ambiguous, and often fraught with value conflicts among individuals with competing interests" (p. 205). Ambiguity occurs when there is more than one possible meaning or interpretation in a situation, or when a choice is unclear in the given context.

During your education, you have learned that many rules, facts, best practices, standards, and policies and procedures are available to guide practice. However, they may not always apply. All nurses, even expert nurses, deal with ambiguity. Sometimes, the information you have on hand produces options that are ambiguous in terms of how they will affect care now and in the future. Other times, the information you have on hand appears incomplete, and you may question if or what you should further assess. As a novice nurse, you may think best when following the rules and recalling facts. As you develop more experience, the client care situation or context will have more meaning for you, which will inform and improve your decision making process in practice.

Analyzing cues can be challenging and create ambiguity in more complex situations. For example, if a client has a blood pressure reading of 162/96 mm Hg, but is very anxious and upset, is this elevated measurement significant? Alternatively, if a client shows signs and symptoms that are "borderline" between normal and abnormal, should you act or not? How would you respond if a client loudly expresses significant pain but exhibits vital signs in the normal range, or a client with a blood pressure of 190/100 mm Hg develops blurry vision but insists they are feeling fine? Your response to each of these scenarios will likely require more information based on further assessment, the environment, other influences, or consultation with others. Additional information may reduce ambiguity and your uncertainty about what to do next and what client care should be prioritized.

### TOOLBOX FOR THINKING

Working with ambiguous information is a challenging reality. Consider a few examples of strategic questions that may help clarify how to respond in an uncertain situation:

- If you can't decide based on the data that you have now, what change in data would prompt you to make a decision and intervene?
- At what point in the care of the client would you feel confident in acting?
- How long are you prepared to wait in this circumstance? Is the current status of the client acceptable or are there risks?
- What is the recent trend showing? Will waiting result in a decline in the client's condition?

Ambiguity also occurs in nursing practice when the client's preferences or goals are unclear and can be interpreted in several ways. In such situations, consultation and collaboration with the client, family, or other health care providers can help make choices and determine the best goal and response. On the other hand, conflict with other health care professionals or a lack of role clarity can contribute to ambiguity and increase stress and anxiety.

How do you make a decision with little information? Get more information seems to be the obvious answer. It is important to pursue information that is known to be missing. However, having too much information to sort through can also be a problem. For example, it may lead you to miss, and, thus, overlook relevant cues. Information overload can affect your decision-making performance.

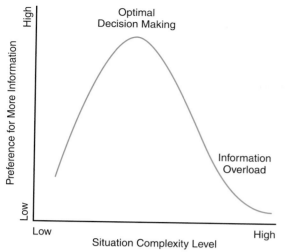

**Fig. 7.2** Decision-making performance. (Adapted from Levitin, D. (2015). The organized mind: Thinking straight in the age of information overload (p. 309). Penguin Canada.)

The optimal situation for decision-making performance is to have not too much complexity that you cannot reach a decision and just enough information to make a reasonable and safe choice. Think of optimal decision making as an upside-down U shape (Figure 7.2). The U-shaped curve describes decision-making performance. When you have little information and low situation complexity, decision making may be ineffective. If you have information overload and high situation complexity, decision making may be equally ineffective. Processing too much information in a high-need situation can result in information overload (Levitin, 2015). As the figure shows, optimal decision making performance (and less ambiguity) occurs when the preferred amount and type of information is available and a manageable amount of complexity is present.

Finding your own "optimal" performance in decision making will depend on your knowledge, scope of practice, level of experience, and confidence.

## WAYS TO ORGANIZE YOUR THINKING IN COMPLEX SITUATIONS

When clinical and health care situations are complex, applying a systematic approach to decision making through the use of nursing models will help ensure that rationales and evidence are considered. The clinical reasoning and critical thinking skills presented in this textbook are also important to making sound decisions in complex situations.

This section examines ways to organize your thinking about more complex client and health care situations. The NRCE framework is used to present a wide range of strategies that will help you address some of the challenges of complexity.

### Nursing Knowledge

Think *N,* and use nursing knowledge and theory to organize data that you gather.

### Visual Representation

Visual representation is one way to analyze and interpret a problem and various solutions. Strategies for sorting data visually and comparing possible solutions include:
- ***Writing it down in a list***:
  What do you know about the issue? Do all the items in the list point to a single solution?
- ***Applying the ABCDs***:
  Using *a*irway, *b*reathing, *c*irculation, and *d*isability cues can help sort out data, prioritize options, and focus on what to do first. Not all cues will be equally applicable in every situation. In a complex situation, this strategy helps narrow the nurse's focus and visualize a process.
- ***Creating a pros-and-cons table***:
  What are the advantages of a solution? What are the disadvantages? Are there more pros than cons? Are the cons "deal breakers" and indicate such unsafe options that a new solution will be needed?
- ***Drawing a diagram, flowchart, or map***:
  Drawing what you are observing and thinking can enhance your ability to understand complex relationships (Alfaro-Lefevre, 2020). Can you see an upward trend? Are you able to include everything in one map or diagram? Is something missing or not connected to other data?

### Cognitive Strategies

Other cognitive strategies involve thinking through options step by step:
- ***Using a means-ends analysis***:
  This is a forward-thinking strategy. It means that you look at stages of a plan (its subgoals) and tackle each on its own to reach a larger end goal (Halpern, 2014). How does this problem-solving strategy work? Define your initial state, and then consider your desired end goal and the means needed to reach it. Break down the means into subgoals and take action to solve each, one at a time. Consider a situation in which the end goal is providing discharge teaching to a client and their family who all speak a language other than English. First, the nurse must identify the preferred language and how best to communicate. A translator is then found. Also, teaching materials in that language are gathered. The nurse then works with the translator to assess client needs and teach the required information, and so on. Puzzles can

---

### BOX 7.1   Tower Puzzle

In the figure, move the three pieces from A to C so they appear at C in the same configuration (smallest on top, largest on bottom). Follow these rules: only move one piece at a time onto either A, B, or C, but never place a larger piece on top of a smaller piece. You can simulate this game using a quarter, nickel, and dime, and three spaces to represent A, B, and C. Try to do this in only seven moves!

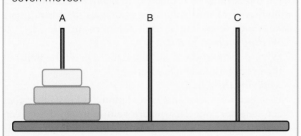

You must set up and complete subgoals—moving pieces back and forth to temporary locations—before you achieve the end goal of this puzzle.

Pierce, R. (2023). *Tower of Hanoi.* https://www.mathsisfun.com/games/towerofhanoi.html

---

### BOX 7.2   Water Lily Brain Teaser

Water lilies double in the area they cover in a lake every 24 hours. The time from the first water lily appearing to time that the lake is completely covered is 48 days. On what day is the lake *half* covered by water lilies?

To answer this question, think about what the lake looks like on day 48, the last day. What does it look like on day 47, based on how the water lilies replicate?

---

help you practise thinking step by step with an end goal in mind. See Box 7.1 for an example.

- ***Working backwards***:
  This is a backward-thinking strategy (Halpern, 2014). If your goal is clear, but you are not sure how to get there, start at that end goal and work back through to the initial problem. This works when there are fewer paths *from* the goal than *to* the goal. For example, a single step may need to be taken immediately before the end of an activity, and one or two steps may need to take place before that step (and so on). Consider a situation in which the nurse is required to independently insert a urinary catheter in a client who is immobile. The nurse must identify what is needed by the end of the procedure before beginning the insertion. The nurse helps the client into the best position for ease of access to the insertion area *before* setting up the sterile field, because they will *not be able to assist the client after donning sterile gloves to begin the insertion.* In addition to communicating with the client, the nurse prepares the urinary drainage system so it can be easily accessed for final connection to the indwelling catheter. Also, they must prepare all of the nonsterile equipment for each step of the procedure and ensure access to sterile supplies before they begin and don sterile gloves. A brain teaser that can help you practise working through a problem backwards appears in Box 7.2 (Fixx, 1978; Halpern, 2014).

- ***Using trial and error***:
  This process involves experimenting with several options until you find one that works. Nurses who use clinical reasoning skills and thinking processes do not use trial and error as an overall strategy for care. This strategy can be useful *only* if the best method to achieve a desired outcome is unclear *and* the risk of any type of harm, damage, or significant waste is *very low.* Otherwise, this strategy is not advisable, and consultation with other, more experienced health care professionals is necessary to explore options. Consider a situation in which the nurse must apply knowledge during a dry dressing change to a simple wound in a client's joint area. They may need to apply and reapply it several times to safely protect the wound and achieve a good fit with the client's pattern of movement. The nurse would ask themselves, *If I do this, what could happen as the client moves, and what would be the outcome?* and *If that doesn't work, what would be the next option?*

## Professional Roles

Think *R* when understanding other health care professionals' roles that are critical to finding solutions in complex situations. When more professionals are involved in the decision making and care of a client, complexity increases. However, consultation and interprofessional collaboration on knowledge and options offers benefits. Strategies for working with other health care professionals include:

- ***Brainstorming***:
  You may have heard that the best way to produce good ideas is to have a lot of ideas. Brainstorming, which is the process of generating as many reasonable solutions as possible, can be done individually or in groups. Different professionals contribute varied perspectives. Then, options can be sorted through, using visual representation or cognitive strategies.

- ***Consulting an expert***:
  Seeking an expert's opinion on a complex situation takes advantage of their role, experience and acquired knowledge. Novice nurses often use this strategy.

Resources such as standards and legal requirements for the profession act as guides for any care provided or actions performed.

- **Crowdsourcing:**
  This strategy takes advantage of multiple expert and other opinions, often using the Internet. Nurses who are looking for options using this strategy need to be able to accurately identify credible online sources.

## Client Context

Think *C* to recall that the client context can offer solutions in complex situations. In client-centred care, further assessments and collaborations with the client (or significant others or families) about appropriate options can be useful. Strategies to consider include:

- **Taking hints:**
  Additional information or extra cues (think about these as hints) that are provided by the client to the nurse, even after planning and implementing care has occurred, can facilitate better solutions. Such added detail may change how the problem is viewed and, when analyzed, can produce more options and influence decisions, actions and outcomes.

- **Referring to Maslow's hierarchy of needs:**
  Prioritizing a client's basic needs is another strategy for identifying what to do first (see Chapter 4). When faced with trying to meet multiple goals, start with goals that address basic needs. Clients provide specific input on their interpretation of their needs. This input reflects their preferences, culture, experiences in health care, and past trauma. Keep in mind that Maslow's hierarchy of needs may not work for all clients because, at times, their preferences or needs will not align with the hierarchy's order (Lapum & Hughes, 2021). Ensure that you ask the client the right questions and apply your nursing knowledge and safe client-centred perspectives.

- **Analyzing trends:**
  More data from the client can be obtained by looking at changes in the client's condition or at the evolution of a health care situation over time. Compare the current data to initial or baseline data. The nurse can ask themselves, *What is the client's status?*; *Is it different from yesterday or from the initial assessment?*; and *Does the client's condition change frequently and require monitoring?*

Of course, the whole of the client situation needs to be considered. When the client is seen holistically, ambiguity and the possibility for error in decision making can decrease. Consider the following examples:

- A client has a low resting heart rate of 55 bpm. Although this rate may be problematic for certain clients, for an athlete, it may be normal and make physiological sense.

- A client with chronic obstructive pulmonary disease (COPD) is concerned about sudden changes in their shortness of breath, so immediately following up on that cue is important. To gain a more holistic view, the nurse would ask themself, *What other factors besides the baseline COPD are affecting the client's situation?*

- A client from a vulnerable group has distrust of the health care system because they were never included in decision making about their own health. As a result, they may need more time to engage and communicate with health care providers, which may necessitate different approaches to their care.

## Health Care Environment

Think *E* to remember to consider the health care environment in complex decision making. In busy health care settings, many built-in strategies can assist with decision making. These strategies are aimed at ensuring safety for clients and health care providers, and a judicious use of supplies, resources, and time. Employers have a vested interest in providing tools for nurses and other health care professionals to use when deciding what to do in complex situations.

The environment is a very broad area to consider. Start by thinking about the direct setting that the client, group, or population is in, and move outwards from there. A number of resources in the health care environment help organize the response to complex situations and decision making, including:

- **Knowing emergency codes and procedures:**
  Recalling the colour codes used to denote types of emergencies helps narrow your focus on what to do. Understanding the related policies and procedures to follow prepares you with the necessary knowledge to make decisions in these complex situations.

- **Following internal communication processes:**
  Complex situations create complex communication problems. Recall ISBAR-R, or introduction/identify, situation, background, assessment, recommendation, and repeat back/receive (see Chapter 5). ISBAR-R provides clarity in communication between individuals, in guidelines for family meetings, and in formal team collaborations with other health care professionals or committees. Communication processes and documentation can help reduce confusion and make decisions that reflect many needs and experiences.

- **Nursing in teams:**
  A nursing work environment that supports a team approach can be leveraged to make complex decisions. Mentorship, collaboration, and consultation are good strategies for nurses working in teams (especially novice nurses) when addressing tough problems.

## To Sum Up

Organizing your thinking in complex situations can be a challenge. Applying a nursing model, the NRCE framework used in this textbook, and approaches to thinking BIG and *small* at the same time can seem overwhelming and takes practice. You will need to use critical thinking and clinical reasoning skills to do this and to understand how all aspects of a complex health care situation are integrated. For instance, the impact on clients of a pandemic, contemporary political and economic challenges, and the social and structural determinants of health should be in the back of your mind when providing nursing care.

Be aware that the strategies discussed in this section can be combined. For instance, the nurse may be more confident about the discharge decisions they make with a client experiencing multiple chronic illnesses and who has complex dietary requirements by writing them down; identifying the end goal and subgoals to reach it; taking hints from the client; consulting with an expert; prioritizing key client needs; considering the client's food insecurity and income level; and ensuring the necessary community supports and resources are in place to meet the client's desired health goal.

It is a good idea to practise applying these and any other types of strategies to complex situations when developing your nursing practice. All of these strategies can be applied to the nursing models presented in this textbook.

## APPLYING SOLUTIONS TO SIMPLE AND COMPLEX SITUATIONS IN NURSING PRACTICE

This section presents two case studies (one on a simple situation and the other on a complex situation) to illustrate how a nurse can think through and make decisions in those situations. A different nursing model and the NRCE framework are used in each case study.

### Simple Decision Making Case Study

The situation in this case study (Box 7.3) has a few clear variables and facts. Therefore, when applying nursing knowledge and clinical reasoning skills, the options for care are straightforward. No additional information arises as care proceeds that would prompt changes to thinking and decision making. This case study applies the nursing process to think through the simple situation. Note that the nursing process can also be used to ensure optimal outcomes for acute and complex situations (Ead, 2019). This case study also applies the NRCE framework to help clarify variables to think about in each stage of the nursing process. Recall that not all components of the framework will necessarily apply at each stage of the nursing process.

It is essential to understand that simple decision making does not mean that the decisions themselves are less important or essential. In this case, the main respiratory concern must be addressed in a timely manner, the plan is fairly clear and care proceeds without alteration.

### Complex Decision Making Case Study

In contrast to the preceding case study, the situation in this case study (Box 7.4) has multiple variables and facts that relate to different client concerns. As a result, when applying nursing knowledge and clinical reasoning skills, the options for care are less clear. This case study applies the Clinical Judgement Model (Tanner, 2006) to think through the situation. It also applies the NRCE framework to help clarify variables to think about in each aspect of the model. Compare the complexity of this case study with that of the preceding one.

As this more complex case study shows, sometimes you must return to an earlier point in the thinking process to find more information and reset a plan of care. It is important to observe that it is not the age of the client that necessarily increases the complexity; be aware of bias and ageism in thinking. Instead, the focus is on the additional information that must be considered altogether.

## THE ROLE OF INTUITION AS EVIDENCE

Nursing **intuition** is the immediate understanding of the meaning of a clinical situation, without the need for conscious reasoning or apparent logic, and is a function of experience with similar situations; it often results from recognition of cues and patterns (Benner, 2001; Tanner, 2006). Intuition is more than a "gut feeling," a "sixth sense," or a "hunch," as it is often described in common conversation. In nursing practice, it is the ability to see parts of a client situation as a whole and to make a reasonable, competent decision with limited information (Melin-Johansson et al., 2017). Intuition can support rapid, effective decision making and clinical performance in response to complex client needs or conditions (Rosciano et al., 2016).

Intuition is developed based on nursing knowledge and a significant amount of nursing experience in similar client or health care situations and is a characteristic of expert practice; however, more research is needed to confirm this point (Rosciano et al., 2016). Recall Chapter 1's description of fast thinking. Fast thinking, or *System 1 thinking*, is intuitive, reflexive, and seemingly effortless—a hallmark of an experienced nurse. However, even expert nurses use models and thinking processes in new situations or when they need to explain their decisions. For expert nurses, a situation presents a cue that opens up access to a large amount of information in their memory, and an answer presents

## BOX 7.3 Thinking Through Simple Decision Making: Respiratory Condition in an Adult

### Scenario

A 41-year-old client arrives at the urgent care centre and reports difficulty breathing, a productive cough, and congestion for the last 3 days. The client states, "I'm usually active but can't catch my breath when I walk across a room now. I must sit down." The client is resting in a tripod position and cannot complete a sentence without taking several breaths.

### Assess

- **N:** *Respiratory rate is 34 breaths/min, chest movement is symmetrical, sounds are diminished bilaterally in lower lung fields, and sputum is yellow and thick. Pulse oximetry is 86% on room air. Heart rate is 96 bpm and regular, and capillary refill is less than 3 seconds. The client denies chest pain, dizziness, or blood in sputum. Peripheral radial pulses are 3+ bilaterally. Temperature is 38.2°C (100.8°F), and the skin is warm and pink. Lips are grey, and mucous membranes are moist. Bowel sounds are active in all four quadrants, and the abdomen is soft and nontender. Last bowel movement was this morning, with no diarrhea. The client denies any frequency or burning with urination. The client is alert and oriented to person, place, time, and situation. Pupils are equal, round, and reactive to light and accommodation.*
- **R:** *Consultation with other nurses and health care professionals is available in the urgent care centre.*
- **C:** *The client is contributing to the assessment discussion. The client reports no reported history of smoking or respiratory conditions, no known exposure to pollutants or other irritants, and no allergies.*
- **E:** *The urgent care centre provides guidelines and support for the provision of nursing care that align with provincial standards; and staff will support any decisions for delivery of care.*

### Analyze

- **N:** *Begin to identify the problem. Most of the assessment results outside of the anticipated range relate to the respiratory system. These are all respiratory changes that have occurred in the last 3 days. Grey lips could relate to circulation, but they could relate to poor oxygenation and the pulse oximetry reading. You may consider that shortness of breath could reflect poor physical fitness, but the client indicates they are physically active.*
  - *How severe is it?* Recall the ABCD survey. The airway is patent, but secretions are thick. Breathing is significantly compromised, as indicated by the pulse oximetry reading and the shortness of breath when sitting and speaking. The client's circulation and level of consciousness (i.e., disability) are within expected ranges at this time.
  - *What could this mean?* The client has a temperature and feels warm, which may indicate an infection. Urinary and gastrointestinal systems present normally, so they may not be the source of infection. Therefore, an infection in the respiratory system, such as pneumonia, may be most likely.
  - *What is the main decision point that will guide nursing activities?* The goal is to address the perfusion issue related to difficult breathing and secretions, and the underlying cause.
- **R:** *Identify the goal and needs collaboratively with other health care professionals.*
- **C:** *Confirm whether additional information or client changes are observed, and whether other preferences or culturally based requests are identified by the client as the goal is created.*

### Plan

- **N:** *Anticipate immediate care needs that will meet the goal.*
- **R:** *Communicate and consult with the appropriate health care professionals for prescriptions and orders to respond to a diagnosis of pneumonia; that is, oxygen, X-ray, fluid administration, antibiotics and other medications, bloodwork, and sputum collection for culture and testing.*
- **C:** *Confirm whether the client agrees with the plan.*
- **E:** *Ensure that all appropriate supplies are available to proceed.*

### Implement

- **N:** *Carry out the planned interventions. Results of the ABCD survey confirm that airway and breathing are the priority over circulation and disability at this time: apply oxygen, administer fluids, collect sputum sample, administer antibiotics and other medications, and arrange for further diagnostic testing.*
- **R:** *Check whether the appropriate level of nursing staff can provide care. Assignment/supervision occurs.*
- **C:** *Note at this point in the situation whether any further changes are observed.*

### Evaluate

- **N:** *Return to the goal to monitor (reassess) and compare results to baseline and anticipated normal values. Consider any new information that is found during the evaluation of outcomes.*
- **R:** *Reflect on the efficiency and coordination of care delivery.*
- **C:** *In this case, note that the client responds to supplemental oxygen, increased fluids, and continuing antibiotics upon discharge home. They are better able to clear their airway and steadily improve.*

## BOX 7.4    Thinking Through Complex Decision Making: Respiratory Condition in an Older Adult

### Scenario

A 74-year-old client arrives at the urgent care centre, dropped off by their neighbour, and reports difficulty breathing, a productive cough, and congestion for the last 6 days. The client states, "I can't catch my breath when I'm sitting." The client is resting in a tripod position and cannot complete a sentence without taking several breaths.

### Notice

- *N: Respiratory rate is 34 breaths/min, chest movement is symmetrical, sounds are diminished bilaterally in lower lung fields with crackles, and sputum is yellowish green and thick. Pulse oximetry is 82% on room air. The client has a history of smoking. They are allergic to codeine. Heart rate is 110 bpm and irregularly irregular, and capillary refill is greater than 3 seconds. The client denies chest pain, dizziness, or blood in sputum. Bilateral peripheral edema is noted in lower legs, and pulses are 1+ bilaterally. Temperature is 37.9°C (100.2°F), and the skin is warm and pink. Lips are grey, and mucous membranes are moist. Bowel sounds are active in all four quadrants, and the abdomen is soft and nontender. Small bowel movement was this morning, with no diarrhea. The client reports small amounts of amber urine, with no burning. The client is alert and oriented to person, place, time, and situation. Pupils are equal, round, and reactive to light and accommodation.*
- *R: Consultation with other nurses and health care professionals is available in the urgent care centre.*
- *C: The client is contributing to the assessment discussion. The client reports that they have COPD and congestive heart failure (CHF), and they last visited the clinic a month ago with the same respiratory issues. The client does not drive.*
- *E: The urgent care centre provides guidelines, codes, and support for the provision of nursing care that align with provincial standards; and staff will support any decisions for delivery of care.*

### Interpret

- *N: Begin to identify the problem. Many of the assessment results outside of the anticipated range relate to the respiratory system. Grey lips could relate to circulation, or poor oxygenation and the very low pulse oximetry reading. You may consider that shortness of breath is normal in a client with COPD or CHF. The respiratory changes occurred in the last week.*
  - *How severe is it? Recall the ABCD survey. The airway is patent, but secretions are thick. Breathing is*

significantly compromised as indicated by the pulse oximetry reading and the shortness of breath when sitting and speaking. The client may experience increased fatigue and not be able to move secretions. Heart rate is higher and irregularly irregular which indicates circulation may be affected. The level of consciousness (i.e., disability) is within expected ranges at this time.
- *What could this mean? The client has a borderline temperature and feels warm, which may indicate an infection. Gastrointestinal systems present normally, and dark urine may indicate dehydration. Therefore, an infection in the respiratory system, such as pneumonia or an exacerbation of COPD, may be most likely. The presence of CHF may also affect the client's response to a respiratory infection or to prescribed care.*
- *What is the main decision point that will guide nursing activities? The goal is to address the perfusion issue related to difficult breathing and secretions, and the underlying cause, and not worsen other health conditions.*
- *R: Identify the goal and needs collaboratively with other health care professionals.*
- *C: Note at this point in this situation, there are questions about reliability of transportation provided by neighbours, and what the outcome was for this same concern last month. The client can verify some information which will help respond to their needs.*

### Respond

- *N: Anticipate immediate care needs that will meet the goal. Plan ahead for what is known. There may be a concern about fluid administration and CHF. How will fluid overload be monitored? What other issues can be foreseen? Carry out the planned interventions. Use the ABCD survey to identify which orders to implement first. Airway and breathing are the priorities at this time, so apply oxygen, administer fluids at an appropriate rate, collect sputum sample, administer antibiotics and other medications, and arrange for further diagnostic testing. However, given the presence of CHF, it is reasonable to closely monitor for further changes in circulation and disability.*
- *R: Communicate and consult with the appropriate health care professionals for prescriptions and orders to respond to a diagnosis of pneumonia; that is, oxygen, X-ray, fluid administration, antibiotics and other medications, bloodwork, and sputum collection for culture and testing.*

---

**BOX 7.4  Thinking Through Complex Decision Making: Respiratory Condition in an Older Adult—cont'd**

- **C:** Observe client responses and reflect-in-action. When antibiotics are discussed, the client shares that after the last clinic visit a month ago, they did not take the full prescription of antibiotics when they started feeling better, and they have so many other pills to take (client educational needs are assessed at this point to support medication adherence). The client indicates that they live alone and does not often leave the house (social supports need to be assessed). This is an additional decision point that will return you to noticing and guide possible revisions to nursing activities.
- **E:** Ensure that resources for accessing transportation and community supports through the urgent care centre are available and activated for the client.

**Reflect**
- **N:** Return to the goal to monitor (reassess) and compare results to baseline and anticipated normal values. Consider any new information that is found during the evaluation of outcomes. Recall the importance of acting on hints or cues, even at this point.
- **R:** Reflect on the efficiency and coordination of care delivery and any nursing knowledge area that requires development (i.e., CHF and fluid administration, and client teaching about medication regimens).
- **C:** In this case, note that the client responds to supplemental oxygen, increased fluids with additional monitoring of CHF, and continuing antibiotics upon discharge home after teaching is provided. They are better able to clear their airway and steadily improve.

---

itself. The rationale for action is there, but it is automatically recognized and matched with the clinical situation. To a novice nurse, it may seem that the expert nurse "skipped a step" in thinking, but the expert nurse is simply adept at engaging in nonlinear, holistic thinking about a situation.

For the expert nurse, intuition can be a source of evidence in clinical judgement. A nurse who draws on years of practice experience will use scientific and theoretical knowledge, and the intuition that develops from deep familiarity with cues and patterns, as part of the body of evidence when making decisions and judgements. However, even for experts, intuition should not be the sole basis of decision making in complex situations because relying on intuition only can lead to biased, less informed decisions (Spurlock, 2018). It is important to underscore that all nurses rely on clinical reasoning and evidence-informed rationales in practice. It is unlikely that newer nurses will have nursing intuition in complex clinical situations until they have acquired meaningful experience over a long period of time.

## SUMMARY

This chapter explored decision making in more complex client and health care situations. As well, it applied ways of thinking and the critical thinking and clinical reasoning skills introduced in previous chapters.

"Complex decision tasks place a much higher cognitive load on the decision-maker. They must attend to more cues and process them relationally to reach an appropriate decision" (Muntean, 2012, p. 19). When faced with a lot of information or cues, the nurse must decide which are more important and which should be attended to first. As discussed in the chapter, the nurse can use various strategies to effectively think through challenging client care situations or situations in which there is a lot of information.

## KEY POINTS TO REMEMBER

These are the key points to remember from this chapter.

### About a Closer Look at Decision Making in Complex Situations

- For simpler problems, the goal and the plan to achieve that goal are well defined, with few factors that could potentially influence care implementation.
- Predictable and stable client conditions and situations present a low risk for any complications or changes to the expected path of care.

- Simple decision-making tasks require fewer cues to be processed than complex tasks and so there is a lower cognitive demand on the decision-maker.
- The nurse makes decisions at all points in the thinking process.

### About What Is a Complex Decision?

- A complex decision is one in which the nurse must make a choice about a client or health care situation that has no obvious immediate answer, few precedents, and more risk, uncertainty, or ambiguity.

- For complex problems, the goal and the path to that goal are not as clear as they are in simple, straightforward problems. The range of possible answers to a given concern is greater. Also, there may be multiple concerns.

- Unpredictable and unstable client conditions or situations present a higher risk of complications and unanticipated changes.

- Flexible and iterative thinking processes are required when applying nursing models to complex situations.

- Factors that make a decision complex may include apparent contradiction; ambiguity; never-before-experienced situations; requirement for multiple consultations; outcomes that are unclear until actions are implemented; no way to evaluate or measure outcomes; and a known multistep process.

## About Types of Complex Decisions

- Types of complex decisions can include: time limitations, multiple goals and too much data, and conflicting information characterize complex decisions.

## About Key Contributors to Complexity in Nursing Practice

- When a client's condition is unstable (their condition is changing) and unpredictable (their outcomes cannot be clearly anticipated), nurses are required to make decisions more frequently.

- Complex practice settings can also contribute to instability and unpredictability and affect decision making.

- Ambiguity is part of forming clinical judgements.

- Ambiguity, when there is more than one possible meaning or interpretation in a situation, or when a choice is unclear in the given context, is faced by all nurses (even expert nurses).

- Ambiguity can occur in nursing practice when the client's preferences or future outcomes are unclear and can be interpreted in several ways.

- The optimal situation for decision-making performance is to have not too much complexity that you cannot reach a decision and just enough information to make a reasonable choice. Finding your own "optimal" performance in decision making will depend on your knowledge, scope of practice, level of experience, and confidence.

## About Ways to Organize Your Thinking in Complex Situations

- Writing it down in a list; applying the ABCDs; creating a pros-and-cons table; drawing a diagram, flowchart, or map

- Using a means-end analysis; working backwards; using trial and error

- Brainstorming; consulting an expert; crowdsourcing

- Taking hints (from the client); referring to Maslow's hierarchy of needs; analyzing trends

- Knowing emergency codes and procedures; following internal communication processes; nursing in teams

- Keep in mind that simple decisions are not unimportant.

## About Applying Solutions to Simple and Complex Situations

- It is essential to understand that simple decision making does not mean that the decisions themselves are less important or essential.

- In complex cases, sometimes you must return to find more information and reset a plan of care.

- Not all components of the NRCE framework may apply at each stage of a selected nursing model.

## About Intuition

- Intuition is developed based on nursing knowledge and a fair amount of nursing experience in similar client or health care situations and is a characteristic of expert practice.

- For the expert nurse, the use of intuition is a source of evidence in their use of clinical judgement.

- Not all nurses will become expert nurses.

## CONCLUSION AND THINKING IT THROUGH

Continue to think about your own client interactions and experiences and how complexity is determined. Listen to others' stories about clients and the multiple challenges they have faced. Expanding your nursing knowledge and understanding of how pieces of this knowledge are connected is a continual activity in professional practices and will build your capacity for making decisions in complex situations. Find your "aha!" moment with each experience and conversation you have.

Professional and personal confidence is one of the last, elusive components to thinking it through in clinical and nursing-related practice situations. Chapter 8 will revisit the idea of reflection and why it is so important to safe practice and to your own growth and development as a nurse.

# CLASS ACTIVITIES TO CHECK THINKING

## Think-Aloud Pair Problem Solving (TAPPS)

Form pairs. Decide who will be a problem solver and listener for Problem A. The problem solver reads the problem aloud and talks through a response to the problem, while the listener reminds the problem solver to think aloud, asks clarification questions, offers encouragement to keep thinking, but refrains from providing possible answers. Switch solver and listener roles for Problem B.

For each problem, decide if there is enough information, available options, or feedback to progress to the next step. Apply the identified nursing model to approach the problem.

- *Problem A (nursing process):* A 78-year-old client with a history of coronary artery disease and hypercholesterolemia is brought to the clinic by a family member who reports that over the past year they have noticed their parent's mental capacity deteriorate. At times alert and other times disoriented and agitated, the client misplaces common items (places milk in the cupboard and sugar in the refrigerator) and was recently found by a neighbour on the street unable to remember where they were. Testing was conducted and a diagnosis of Alzheimer's disease was made. The family member prefers to keep the client in their own home, in the environment they have lived in for 35 years.
- *Problem B (clinical reasoning cycle):* A 23-year-old client is living in a First Nations community in remote area of Manitoba. The client is 30 weeks pregnant and has gestational diabetes that is managed well. They have been advised by the physician who regularly visits the community that they should transfer to Winnipeg for labour and delivery because they are "at risk." The client is upset and does not want to travel to a large and unfamiliar city without the support of older family members who cannot travel with them.

Discuss with each other how stability, predictability, and ambiguity are present when making decisions in these situations. What is the role of the nursing models in helping to organize your thinking when information is missing?

## Activities and Discussion Questions

1. An expert nurse observes a client's reaction to medication and decides not to conduct further assessments; they proceed with meeting other assigned client needs. A novice nurse requires more information about the same client situation and cannot decide on how to proceed. The novice nurse feels pressured to move forward with the timely care of other clients. Discuss in pairs:
   - What may be the rationale behind the thinking of the expert nurse? What could be the concerns of the novice nurse?
   - What could be suggested to the novice nurse in this situation?
2. In each of the following circumstances, provide a strategy for approaching a solution:
   - The problem is ill defined.
   - Few options exist to a well-defined problem.
   - The problem is complex, and many health care professionals are involved.
   - More information is needed to clarify the problem.
   - A lack of options exists at this time.

# CASE STUDY REVIEW

Refer to Boxes 7.3 and 7.4. What makes one case study simple and the other more complex? What would further increase the complexity of the case study in Box 7.4?

Pair up with a classmate and further develop the case presented in Box 7.4. Fill in details that increase complexity and fit with the case presentation (include more vital signs, lab tests and results, and suggest a change in the client condition or living situation that would require different decision making, etc.). How would the changes you suggest affect goals and decision making in the case study?

# EVIDENCE-INFORMED THINKING ACTIVITY

Formal decisions in health care delivery require evidence. Evidence that informs decisions comes from science, best practices, policy and procedure, or past experiences that have been based on these types of evidence. However, the intuition that is more prominently featured in the thinking of expert nurses is not as obviously evidence informed. Or is it?

Although you may not be an expert nurse, you have likely had the experience of an immediate understanding of a clinical situation but haven't been able to state why at the time. Think back to that example and find the evidence for your intuitive response. Where did the evidence come from? Was it accurate and up to date? How can this realization that your "hunch" was evidence-informed be applied in future practice?

## QUESTIONS TO ASSESS LEARNING

### Review Questions

1. A 34-year-old who identifies as nonbinary arrives in the emergency department (ED) and reports abdominal pain, difficulty breathing, and a fever. For the last 3 days, they have experienced nausea and vomiting and fatigue. Further information indicates the client has been urinating frequently and is very thirsty, asking for some ice water. The client is upset because one of the unit staff addressed them as "she."

   - *Vital signs:* T 38.9°C (102°F), P 96 bpm and weak, R 26 bpm, and BP 88/60 mm Hg. The urine reagent strip results show pH 6.9, protein 2+, glucose 1+, and ketones 3+.
   - *Past medical history:* includes type 1 diabetes mellitus and hypothyroidism.
   - *Current medications:* include levothyroxine 25 mcg daily, insulin glargine (U-300) 12 units subcutaneously daily, and acetaminophen 650 mg q4h PRN for temperature above 38.5°C (101.3°F).
   - Lab results:
     - Hemoglobin: 130 g/L
     - Hematocrit: 40%
     - Platelets: 300 × 10⁹/L
     - RBC: 4.8 × 10¹²/L
     - WBC: 1.8 × 10⁹/L
     - Potassium: 3.0 mmol/L
     - Serum glucose: 17 mmol/L
     - Serum pH: 7.3
     - Serum ketones: 3.4 mmol/L

   The client has been in the ED for 3.5 hours and has had no urine output. The nurse notes that the client is increasingly restless, and their breathing is becoming deeper with apparent dyspnea. The nurse communicates the latest assessment findings to the care team using ISBAR-R. Complete the following diagram by selecting from the options provided in the table: one potential condition most likely experienced, two actions the nurse should take, and two parameters the nurse should monitor and continue to review.

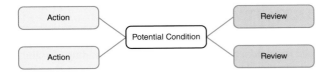

| Actions to Take |
| --- |
| Address their concern about being disrespected |
| Initiate IV fluid 0.9% NaCl |
| Administer IV insulin |
| Administer IV potassium |

| Potential Conditions |
| --- |
| Hypoglycemia |
| Diabetic ketoacidosis |
| Hyperosmolar hyperglycemic state |

| Parameters to Monitor/Review |
| --- |
| Breath sounds |
| pH, potassium, and glucose |
| Abdominal pain |
| GI functioning |

*GI,* Gastrointestinal; *IV,* intravenous; *NaCl,* sodium chloride

2. A new parent with a 2-week-old infant meets with the visiting nurse. They report that they are having difficulties in their relationship with their partner because of the adjustments in the home since the birth, and they are very upset and feel isolated. The parent is very tired and only getting 3 to 4 hours of sleep a night. What is the priority for the nurse in this particular case?

   a. Sleep deprivation
   b. Isolation from partner
   c. Infant's physical health
   d. Adjustments in the home

3. A nurse is assigned the care of two clients. The first client, a 70-year-old adult, is recovering from a hiatal hernia repair and requires assistance with activities of daily living (ADL). The second client, also 70 years old, has abdominal pain not yet diagnosed and has had occasional periods of confusion. What is the most appropriate rationale for the nurse's decision to assess the second client first?

   a. The second client has many complicating conditions.
   b. The first client needs to learn how to care for themself.
   c. The second client has a health condition that is not controlled or defined.
   d. The first client had a very common surgical procedure.

## ONE LAST THOUGHT

Complexity in client care situations is challenging because there are many issues for the nurse to consider that may seem to be unrelated to each other. To resolve issues, the nurse needs to understand how they are, or are not, connected. As you complete this chapter and the learning activities, ask yourself the following questions:

- When I make decisions, do I usually understand how a client's multiple concerns are related? Or do I just focus on one issue without considering the impact of others?

- How do I recognize when it is time to make a decision in a complex situation?
- How confident do I feel in my decisions in these situations, and what contributes to my confidence (or what does not)?

In the next chapter, more information will be presented for you to include in decision making when considering client care and professional issues as a reflective practitioner.

## ONLINE RESOURCES

*Application of the nursing process in a complex health care environment*—Canadian Nurse (2019): https://www.canadian-nurse.com/dev-cn-en/blogs/cn-content/2019/09/16/application-of-the-nursing-process-in-a-complex-he
Clinical judgement, priorities and Maslow's hierarchy of needs: Lapum, J., & Hughes, M. (2021). Introduction to health assessment for the nursing professional—Part I: Priorities of care: https://pressbooks.library.torontomu.ca/assessmentnursing/chapter/priorities-of-care/

## REFERENCES

Alfaro-Lefevre, R. (2020). *Critical thinking, clinical reasoning, and clinical judgement: A practical approach* (7th ed.). Elsevier.
Benner, P. (2001). *From novice to expert: Excellence and power in clinical nursing practice.* Prentice Hall.
College of Nurses of Ontario. (2018). *RN and RPN practice: The client, the nurse and the environment.* https://neltoolkit.rnao.ca/sites/default/files/RN%20and%20RPN%20Practice_The%20Client,%20the%20Nurse%20and%20the%20Environment.pdf
Ead, H. (2019, September 16). Application of the nursing process in a complex health care environment. *Canadian Nurse.* https://www.canadian-nurse.com/dev-cn-en/blogs/cn-content/2019/09/16/application-of-the-nursing-process-in-a-complex-he
Endsley, M. R., & Jones, D. G. (2012). *Designing for situational awareness: An approach to user-centred design* (2nd ed.). CRC Press.
Fixx, J. F. (1978). *Solve it.* Doubleday.
Halpern, D. (2014). *Thought and knowledge: An introduction to critical thinking* (5th ed.). Psychology Press.
Lapum, J., & Hughes, M. (2021). *Introduction to health assessment for the nursing professional—Part I.* https://pressbooks.library.torontomu.ca/assessmentnursing/front-matter/introduction/

Levitin, D. (2015). *The organized mind: Thinking straight in the age of information overload.* Canada: Penguin.
Melin-Johansson, C., Palmqvist, R., & Rönnberg, L. (2017). Clinical intuition in the nursing process and decision-making—A mixed-studies review. *Journal of Clinical Nursing, 26*(23–24), 3936–3949. https://doi.org/10.1111/jocn.13814.
Miller, G. A. (1956). The magical number seven, plus or minus two: Some limits on our capacity for processing information. *Psychological Review, 63*(2), 81–87. https://doi.org/10.1037/h0043158.
Muntean, W. (2012). *Nursing clinical decision-making: A literature review.* https://www.ncsbn.org/research-item/nursing-clinical-decisionmaking-a-literature-review
Pierce, R. (2023). *Tower of Hanoi.* https://www.mathsisfun.com/games/towerofhanoi.html
Rogers, B., & Franklin, A. E. (2021). Cognitive load experienced by nurses in simulation-based learning: An integrative review. *Nursing Education Today, 99.* https://doi.org/10.1016/j.nedt.2021.104815
Rosciano, A., Lindell, D., Bryer, J., et al. (2016). Nurse practitioners' use of intuition. *The Journal for Nurse Practitioners, 12*(8), 560–565. https://doi.org/10.1016/j.nurpra.2016.06.007.
Spurlock, D. (2018). Cautious certainty: Not easy, but nearly always necessary. *Journal of Nursing Education, 57*(12), 703–704. https://doi.org/10.3928/01484834-20181119-01.
Tanner, C. A. (2006). Thinking like a nurse: A research-based model of clinical judgment in nursing. *Journal of Nursing Education, 45*(6), 204–211.
Thompson, C., Cullum, N., McCaughan, D., et al. (2004). Nurses, information use, and clinical decision making—The real world potential for evidence-based decisions in nursing. *Evidence-Based Nursing, 7*(3), 68–72. https://doi.org/10.1136/ebn.7.3.68.
Yee, A. (2023). Clinical decision-making in the intensive care unit: A concept analysis. *Intensive & Critical Care Nursing, 77.* https://doi.org/10.1016/j.iccn.2023.103430

# 8

# Thinking It Through as a Reflective Practitioner

## LEARNING OUTCOMES

*After reading this chapter, you will be able to:*
- Identify characteristics of a reflective practitioner.
- Develop ways to improve mindfulness during nursing care delivery.
- Describe how reflective skills are used to incorporate sustainable development goals, equity, diversity and inclusion, and reconciliation in nursing practice.
- Apply reflection to a personal plan that supports thinking and decision making in nursing practice.

## GLOSSARY

**Anticipatory reflection:** a future-focused reflection; reflection on what may occur next, based on past experiences and learning

**Deliberate practice:** focused, repeated activities that are aimed at improving optimal performance, with feedback from a skilled practitioner

**Emotional intelligence (EI):** the ability to perceive, appraise and assess emotions (in yourself and others), access and process emotional information, generate feelings, and regulate emotions for professional growth

**Mindfulness:** the quality of mind that notices what is present in the moment, without judgement or interference

**Reflective practitioner:** someone who lives reflection naturally in their everyday, mindful practice; pays attention to their experiences and is self-aware of their own and others' responses to those experiences

**Resilience:** the ability to remain agile and effective amidst stress and bounce back quickly from difficult situations (Advisory Board, 2018, p. 11)

The information presented in this textbook has provided you with a foundation for *thinking it through* in nursing practice. The concept of reflection and how reflective practice can support clinical reasoning skill development are revisited in this last chapter.

Reflection is a learning activity on its own. It helps you discover what you know and what you do not know and is an essential part of thinking as a nurse. Nursing knowledge and professional practice roles, and the context of the client and the health care environment are considered by the nurse during reflective practice. In Canada, understanding how these essential components contribute to decision making in dynamic and contemporary health care settings enables nurses to meet provincial and territorial practice standards and competencies.

Pulling together all the information that you have learned and regularly applying it in your future practice is a habit that will facilitate lifelong learning. In this last chapter, focused approaches and examples for building reflective and clinical reasoning skills are presented. The nurse as a skilled reflective practitioner can make informed decisions, form clinical judgements, meet diverse client needs, and navigate professional issues that arise in an increasingly challenging health care environment.

## WHAT IS A REFLECTIVE PRACTITIONER?

Reflection and reflective skills have been discussed in this textbook as both a professional competency and a way of thinking through nursing practice situations. Recall the reflective model that was presented in Figure 2.5 in Chapter 2. Gibbs's Reflective Cycle (Gibbs, 1988) was offered as a method for noticing what had happened, making sense of the feelings and situation that were experienced, and then drawing conclusions that may be applied in the future. You may have been exposed to other reflective theories. However, theories and models are not prescriptive tools to be followed blindly but are mechanisms used to change and improve practice (Johns, 2022).

Reflective practice uses systematic reflection and reflective skills to enable you to learn from your experiences and develop as a professional. A **reflective practitioner** is someone who lives reflection naturally in their everyday, mindful practice (Johns, 2022). Reflective practitioners in nursing pay attention to experiences as they happen and are self-aware of their own and others' responses to those experiences. They make a conscious effort to look at a situation with an awareness of their own beliefs, values, and practice (Patel & Metersky, 2022) and incorporate situation awareness when perceiving and comprehending what is going on around them (see Chapter 3). Therefore, reflective practitioners not only *do* reflection, but fully engage in *being* reflective. What does this mean? Using reflection as a tool is a good place to start, but the aim is to adopt a naturally, continually reflective posture. These practitioners learn through reflection on nursing experiences.

Because thinking and decision making can sometimes be problematic and difficult in professional situations, it makes sense that, in addition to one's physical performance, thoughts and cognitive processes are a focus of reflection.

Health care practitioners are continually thinking and reflecting on what they do and why they do it.

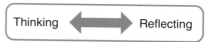

How is reflection in practice developed? Draw on your critical thinking skills for this, and review traits that were presented in Chapter 2. According to Fay (1987), curiosity, commitment, and intelligence are key requirements for developing a reflective attitude. Here is a closer look at each requirement:

- *Curiosity:* focusing on self-inquiry; the exploration of possibilities; and deep interest in finding out something new.
- *Commitment:* actively engaging in new and challenging situations that develop and strengthen professional skills and making a promise to oneself to face and learn from difficulties.
- *Intelligence:* being open to new knowledge and their value to practice. Reflection can nurture processing and acquiring new knowledge.

When interacting with clients, these three key requirements can strengthen reflective practices. When continually applied, your practice can develop from *doing* reflection to *being* reflective (Johns, 2022). Refer to Figure 8.1. Note that this image shows how being reflective can develop, which is different from the reflective cycle. As the figure shows, reflection becomes more advanced and intuitive with more experience.

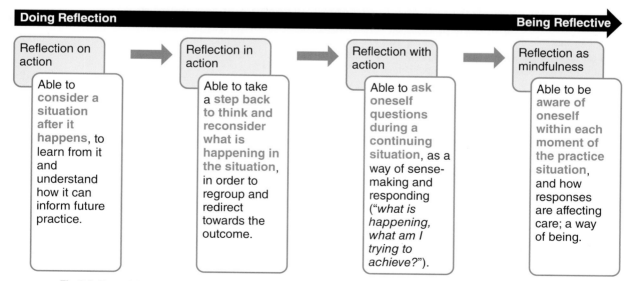

**Fig 8.1** From doing to being reflective. (Adapted from Johns, C. (2022). *Becoming a reflective practitioner* (6th ed.). Wiley-Blackwell.)

A nurse's reflective abilities develop over time. A novice reflective practitioner begins by thinking about what happened after they have performed venipuncture on a client, for example. You are familiar with this as *reflection-on-action*. A more experienced nurse may think about what is happening by taking a step back or pausing in the process of inserting a venous cannula to adjust their approach. Recall that this is *reflection-in-action*. An even more experienced nurse may start asking themselves questions during insertion (without pausing) about whether the angle of insertion is too steep or the client is tolerating the procedure to adapt the care being provided. Finally, an expert practitioner will be fully aware of their thinking from moment to moment and intuitively respond to anatomy and the feel of the insertion, the client's perceived discomfort, and the overall context of care in a smooth and seamless fashion. Reflection begins as an external reflective activity and develops into an internalized, intuitive activity.

Reflection and reflective skills are associated with other actions such as mindfulness, anticipatory reflection, and deliberate practice. Your understanding of these actions and how they apply to nursing practice will help you become a reflective practitioner.

## MINDFULNESS

Mindfulness can be described as a quality of mind that helps an individual notice what is present in the moment, without judgement or interference (Johns, 2022; Kabat-Zinn, 2006). Being mindful enables you to be more aware of patterns of thinking and responding to situations. Refer to Box 8.1 for a comparison of two approaches to mindfulness. With consistent application, mindfulness enables you to reduce the influence of distractions in practice, and increase reflection during the provision of care. Using mindful practices may also reduce the effects of burnout and attrition in the nursing workforce in Canada (Burkett, 2020).

*Being mindful enables good decision making and clinical judgement in nursing practice because a clearer and focused understanding of the situation is achieved.*

What does mindfulness involve? Being present in the moment during any nursing activity can serve to focus attention and reduce unhelpful thoughts. Valuing social resources, professional supports, and mentoring opportunities also support mindful practice in nursing. Practising mindfulness can include a short daily meditation or a time-out to let challenging thoughts go. Take a mental break and focus your attention on how stress or distraction can affect your physical and mental state. Calming videos and apps are readily available online that can suit your preferences and schedule. Other activities such as walking, exercise, yoga, seated stretching (ParticipACTION, 2024), or focusing on soothing music can also provide opportunities to practise mindfulness.

---

### BOX 8.1   Mindfulness: A Comparison

A nurse has been working in the same clinical unit for 10 years. The complexity of care and the workload on the unit has increased. The nurse frequently worries about not completing planned client care and, as a result, continues to think about work after the shift is over. This affects quality of sleep and results in fatigue, anxiety, and an overall inability to relax. The nurse commits to addressing the issue and decides to employ a more mindful approach to practice.

#### More Mindful Practice

Being present in the moment, the nurse realizes the negative impact of the increased workload. They refocus their attention on the care at hand, organize client needs based on priority, and communicate their actions clearly to others. The nurse responds when colleagues need assistance and accepts others' offers of help. This perspective helps them achieve realistic work goals for each shift. After work, the nurse dedicates a defined time for a final reflection on the day during a short walk or sometimes writes thoughts down in a personal journal. The nurse sleeps well and feels more rested and less anxious. The nurse is motivated to provide the best care to clients.

#### Less Mindful Practice

The nurse recognizes the negative effects of the stressful and busy work environment. Talking with other colleagues during the shift about shared challenges seems to increase feelings of anger and anxiety. The nurse is distracted by all client issues and tries to address each of them without assistance because others are overworked. After the shift, they adopt some calming practices such as yoga class, meditation, or reading before bed, but thoughts of the long shift and unmet client needs continue to worry and frustrate them. The nurse does not continue with yoga or meditation and accepts that this is how nursing practice has changed.

## BOX 8.2 Mindfulness Strategies for Nursing Practice

**To foster organization in nursing work:**
- Gain insight into current stressors.
- Participate in flexible work schedules.
- Increase personal autonomy in practice.
- Seek out work in interesting roles (e.g., leadership, specialization).
- Access coping resources as needed.

**To foster work–life balance:**
- Exercise regularly.
- Set emotional boundaries between work and personal activities.
- Engage in recreational activities outside the work environment.
- Nurture practices to promote well-being.
- Avoid overinvolvement with clients.

Badu, E., O'Brien, A., Mitchell, R., et al. (2020). Workplace stress and resilience in the Australian nursing workforce: A comprehensive integrative review. *International Journal of Mental Health Nursing, 29*, 5–34. https://doi.org/10.1111/inm.12662

**Resilience** is a skill that can be developed through mindfulness (Sieg, 2020). To be resilient means to be agile and effective during a stressful period and to recover quickly from difficult situations (Advisory Board, 2018). A resilient person is self-confident and optimistic, maintains good relationships with others, keeps things in perspective, and sets and tries to attain goals. Mindful strategies such as organizing nursing practice work and focusing on work–life balance can build resilience (Box 8.2). Mindfulness can also support self-reliance, positive thinking, emotional intelligence (discussed later in this chapter), and the development of a passion for nursing practice (Harwood et al., 2021).

## ANTICIPATORY REFLECTION

Reflection is not only "thinking about thinking" in the moment, while performing an intervention or nursing action, or once that specific activity has been completed. Reflection on one's own actions can inform how you plan your care and make decisions.

**Anticipatory reflection** is a future-focused reflection, or "reflection *for* action" (Schön, 1987; van Manen, 1991). This reflective activity is aimed at thinking about what may occur next based on past experiences and learning. Questions to ask yourself at the start of care, *before a nursing activity,* can include:

- From the information that I received during the client hand-off, do I need to review a nursing procedure or practice standard before providing care?
- Based on my previous clinical experiences, what do I think may be most important when engaging in care with this client?

- What possible issues may arise in this clinical situation?
- Is there any information that I may need to focus on when I meet the client?
- If I approach the client in this way, what do I see happening as a result?

Remember, anticipatory reflection happens before you provide any care. It is part of getting mentally ready for the thinking and decision-making processes that you will use. It does not replace the process of finding information or assessment activities.

## DELIBERATE PRACTICE

**Deliberate practice** is purposeful, repeated activities that are aimed at improving optimal performance (Ericsson & Harwell, 2019; Ericsson et al., 1993). Meaningful feedback from a skilled practitioner is essential to focus the learner on aspects of knowledge and skill that require development and mastery. Deliberate practice requires mindfulness and the ability to think forward and back. This process is reflective and looks different for everyone—all learning takes time, and some take longer to achieve mastery of a skill than others.

Deliberate practice is a learning strategy. Students and new graduates need to practice in a relevant or reality-based context to promote learning and augment decision making skills. You have the opportunity in your nursing program to seek and receive feedback on your performance. This feedback can include reflection, self-assessment, and (importantly) feedback directly to you from instructors and practising nurses on how you can improve your skills and thinking. If you practise your skills in a busy lab and then complete a self-checklist without an instructor to comment on your performance, you are not engaging in deliberate practice (Gonzalez & Kardong-Edgren, 2017).

## ✳ TOOLBOX FOR THINKING

Feedback about your behaviour that indicates areas for improvement can be used as a reflective learning opportunity, even if you are initially surprised or upset by what you hear. Consider responding:
- "I hear what you are saying."
- "Thank you for telling me. Can you provide more details?"
- "How can I make this better?"
- "I recognize that I still have work to do."
- "I never thought of it that way and have to give this some more thought."

Strategies for addressing feedback involve identifying biases, considering your effect on others, and making plans to change behaviours in future experiences or encounters.

Reflective actions—mindfulness, anticipatory reflection, and deliberate practice—all contribute to focused decision making. They are needed to be able to simultaneously look forward and back, which is characteristic of more experienced nurses exhibiting clinical judgement (Benner et al., 1995; Tanner, 2006). Thinking *BIG* and *small* at the same time is required to be able to "see" the whole of the client or practice situation. Reflection is also needed to apply nursing models for thinking and decision making in practice.

Clinical reasoning skills that have been presented in earlier chapters can help with reflection and with becoming a reflective practitioner. These skills include:

- Recognizing relationships between concepts and data
- Recalling science-based, ethics, and nursing knowledge
- Identifying pre-existing bias and assumptions
- Anticipating care needs in client context
- Considering expectations
- Making inferences
- Seeing patterns over time
- Grouping related cues together
- Identifying possible bias in interpretation
- Matching situation with past experiences
- Reflecting in action
- Self-regulating performance
- Incorporating new knowledge and evidence
- Reviewing personal learning plan
- Predicting future client needs
- Reflecting on action(s)

---

**REFLECTIVE PRACTICE MOMENT**

Think back on the last clinical experience you had, and identify which skills you used.

- Did you take any time to reflect before providing care?
- Were you thinking about what you were doing while doing it (BIG and small)?
- Did you think about what you did, on your own or with another (mentor, instructor) after providing care?

---

Nursing programs offer ways for you to apply reflective and clinical reasoning skills through case studies, in-person or virtual clinical simulations, role-play with standardized actors, and supervised clinical experiences, to name a few. Practising reflection takes time and personal focus. Take advantage of the chances early in your education to apply your developing reflective skills. Remember, the more you practise, the better you can become at thinking it through and making meaningful decisions.

## THE ROLE OF REFLECTION IN CANADIAN NURSING

Reflection is a competency required for entry into nursing practice in Canada. It is a skill needed to meet the provincial and territorial standards of nursing care. For instance,

the College of Nurses of Ontario (2019) requires that a registered nurse entering the profession "demonstrates self-awareness through reflective practice and solicitation of feedback" (p. 7) and "engages in self-reflection to interact from a place of cultural humility and create culturally safe environments where clients perceive respect for their unique health care practices, preferences, and decisions" (p. 8). Such competencies are included in most jurisdictions in Canada.

Similarly, licensed practical nurses' national entry-level competencies specify that they engage in "self-reflection and continuous learning to maintain and enhance competence" (Canadian Council for Practical Nurse Regulators, 2019, p. 5). Regardless of your area of practice or your designation as a nurse in the profession, reflection is essential.

### Reflection and Clinical Judgement

Reflection and reflective skills—which are also very similar to critical thinking skills (refer to Chapter 1)—are important for developing clinical reasoning skills and clinical judgement in nursing. Recall that the registration exam for registered nurses in most jurisdictions in Canada focuses on measuring clinical judgement. Several aspects of the Clinical Judgement Model (Tanner, 2006) and other nursing models require reflection. Therefore, the contribution of reflection to competency and safe, regulated practice is clear.

When thinking through each step of a nursing model, the nurse reflects on their *n*ursing knowledge, professional *r*oles and those of other health care professionals or workers, the *c*lient as a whole, and the health care *e*nvironment (NRCE) as represented by the framework used in this textbook. For example, in Canada, depending on where a nurse is practising, there may be specific disease prevalence, variability in practitioner availability (i.e., few physicians or nurse practitioners), different client cultural or language influences, or particular determinants of health (social or structural) that require reflection and reflective skills when finding information, deciding what to do, acting on decisions, and reviewing actions.

---

**KNOWLEDGE CHECK-IN**

- What does it mean to be a reflective practitioner?
- Describe an example of mindful practice in nursing.
- How is anticipatory reflection helpful in thinking and decision making?
- Explain how deliberate practice can help with thinking in nursing practice.

---

Reflective skills have value in developing other competencies which require significant reflection to apply information in nursing practice situations. The next sections of this chapter outline the areas in which a reflective stance can contribute to competent, safe, professional, and contemporary nursing practice.

## REFLECTION AND MEETING CLIENT NEEDS IN CONTEMPORARY PRACTICE

Thinking beyond the immediate practice setting and recognizing the world involving the client is part of what thinking BIG is all about. The lived contexts of clients and the health care system in which they are cared for are important to assess, analyze and interpret, respond to, and evaluate to provide complete and meaningful nursing care.

Reflection is a foundation for thinking in nursing and helps recognize and address clients' needs. In Canada, client contexts that change or become part of contemporary practice must be acknowledged and acted on by the reflective practitioner. Sustainability of the planet is important for continued healthy living for all. A lens on equity, diversity, and inclusion (EDI) can support fair and safe health care for everyone. Acknowledging the Calls to Action from the Truth and Reconciliation Commission of Canada (2015) will lead to meaningful responses in nursing practice.

Without active reflection, these important areas may be overlooked. When they are recognized and acknowledged as a critical need, they can be addressed and incorporated in nursing practice. Nurses advocate for the client when they act on the client's identified needs and incorporate knowledge about the contexts in which they live. When a nurse adopts this stance of reflection and advocacy based on client needs, *better decision making can occur.*

### Sustainable Development Goals

The United Nations (2015) produced an agenda to achieve Sustainable Development Goals (SDGs) which were adopted by countries to attain a more sustainable and prosperous state of being for the planet. Like the social determinants of health, these goals directly and indirectly influence how nurses work and think in practice. There are 17 goals:

1. No poverty
2. Zero hunger
3. Good health and well-being
4. Quality education
5. Gender equality
6. Clean water and sanitation
7. Affordable and clean energy
8. Decent work and economic growth
9. Industry, innovation and infrastructure
10. Reduced inequalities
11. Sustainable cities and communities
12. Responsible consumption and production
13. Climate action
14. Life below water
15. Life on land
16. Peace, justice and strong institutions
17. Partnerships for the goals

All nurses have a role in attaining the SDGs through their thinking in practice; the International Council of Nurses (2017) stated that "nurses, as the primary providers of healthcare to all communities in all settings, are key to the achievement of the SDGs" (p. 3).

Global nursing professional organizations have reported that SDGs 2, 3, and 4 have received the highest levels of attention (Chiu et al., 2022). Organizing food drives and collecting for food banks can help address hunger, especially for vulnerable client populations. Activities to promote good health include running health fairs and clinics, conducting health teaching, donating medical or hygiene supplies, raising funds to support and increase awareness of disease prevalence and social issues, and ensuring delivery of excellent care. Increasing access to education and meals for school-age children is a focus for supporting quality education. Know that all SDGs are closely linked and relate to the social and structural determinants of health that nurses reflect on before, during, and after the provision of care. Understanding these connections can help you analyze, interpret, and synthesize information that you assess in nursing practice.

Over the last few years, the SDGs have been included in nursing curricula and research and health care agencies' strategic plans and practices. In your own practice, you can also think about how your work can contribute to planetary health. Think about the following actions:

- Limiting waste in medical supplies
- Advocating for equitable application processes and gender equality when hiring nurses
- Paying attention to possible inequities in the way that health care is delivered
- Becoming involved in committees where decision making occurs and how policy and procedure are created

These actions and others support the SDGs in practice through reflection on what is happening around you.

Reflecting on the larger impact of your own practice may seem daunting and less important to your daily activities. However, remaining curious, asking questions, and advocating for health for all can get you started. Becoming a member of a local or provincial or territorial nursing organization is also a way to broaden your perspective and increase your awareness of the potential of nursing practice for positive change. Being exposed to new ways of thinking will inform and enrich your practice. Refer to Table 8.1 for examples of thinking competencies that are crucial to advancing SDGs. Notice how they resemble those required by nurses in decision making.

**TABLE 8.1   Examples of Thinking Competencies for Sustainability**

| Competency | Examples of Thinking in Practice |
|---|---|
| Anticipatory | Analyze multiple futures; create a vision for the future; assess the consequences of possible actions; and manage risk and change. |
| Collaboration | Learn from others; understand and respect the needs, perspectives, and actions of others (empathy); be sensitive to others (empathic leadership); navigate group conflict; and facilitate problem solving with others. |
| Critical thinking | Question norms, practices, and opinions; reflect on one's own values, perceptions, and actions; form an evidence-informed viewpoint. |
| Integrated problem solving | Apply different problem-solving frameworks to complex sustainability problems, and develop viable, inclusive, and equitable solution options that promote sustainable development, integrating all of these competencies. |
| Self-awareness | Reflect on one's own role in the local community and (global) society; continually evaluate and further motivate one's actions; deal with one's feelings and desires. |
| Systems thinking | Recognize and understand relationships; analyze complex systems; think about how systems are connected; and deal with uncertainty. |

Adapted from UNESCO. (2017). *Education for Sustainable Development Goals: Learning objectives.* https://unesdoc.unesco.org/ark:/48223/pf0000247444

## Equity, Diversity, and Inclusion

In Chapter 3, unconscious bias was identified as unrecognized assumptions or ideas that a nurse may have about someone or something that influences their decision making and behaviours. Practising self-reflection and taking feedback from others on your own interpretations of a given situation is a first step toward equitable and inclusive nursing practice and thinking.

The ability to self-reflect is essential for antiracist and nondiscriminatory culturally safe health care delivery for Black and South Asian clients and other racialized populations. Activities that develop your skills of reflection are included in your nursing education. For example, the Canadian Association of Schools of Nursing's (2022) National Nursing Framework highlights that baccalaureate graduates must "demonstrate cultural humility, cultural safety, anti-racist, and anti-discriminatory nursing practice" (pp. 14–15).

Self-assessment can help you reflect on your responsibility for achieving EDI in practice. Draw on information learned in your nursing program and through your professional and personal interactions with others, and consider the following questions (Danda et al., 2022):
- What does the term *racism* mean to you? What has shaped your understanding of this term? Has your understanding of the term changed over time? If so, how?
- Do you believe that racism exists in health care? What examples from your nursing practice inform your answer? Have you had the opportunity to listen to Black clients and other racialized people, their advocates, or experienced health care providers who can share their thoughts on health care delivery in Canada from this lens?
- What is your role in practising antiracism in health care? How is your role the same or different from the role that Canadian nursing professional associations play in addressing these issues?

All nurses have an important role in antiracist practice in Canadian health care. It is not a role for "other" nurses or policymakers to address—you need to be a part of this action. Incorporating this perspective and nursing knowledge into your work enables you to practise more informed, equitable, and inclusive decision making.

## Truth and Reconciliation Commission Calls to Action

Reflection and action are necessary for nurses to participate in activities that decolonize health care and nursing practices. It can be a challenge to deeply and critically reflect on something you do not know enough about. Your learning and actions should reflect the intentions in the Truth and Reconciliation Commission of Canada (2015) Calls to Action and articles of the United Nations Declaration of the Rights of Indigenous Peoples (United Nations, 2007), and focus on a stance of self-reflection for cultural humility (First Nations Health Authority et al., 2021).

Decolonization is the process of deconstructing colonial ideologies of ownership, superiority, White privilege and Western thought, and acknowledging, valuing, and supporting Indigenous knowledge (Bourque Bearskin, 2023).

In nursing and health care, colonization is still evident in the removal and exclusion of Indigenous knowledge from health care sites and practices. In the same way that this textbook on thinking through clinical decisions does not fully cover details of specific clinical nursing practice information, it does not fully address aspects of Indigenous and other individual cultures because of the depth and breadth of description that would be required. You must draw on information learned in other courses and from contacts or experiences to reflect on how thinking processes can support the application of critical knowledge and decolonization activities. You may find many other resources in territories and Indigenous communities that are local to you.

Questions that you can ask yourself about your understanding of Indigenous knowledge and culture are *Am I basing my understanding on knowledge that comes from Indigenous sources?* and *Have I had the opportunity to hear from or speak with someone who has lived experiences with Indigenous culture?* Box 8.3 provides an example of how identifying client need through reflection and collaboration can begin to change policy and procedure in health care institutions. Reflection on this example and others can acknowledge and initiate ways to address Calls to Action such as #22 to #24 (Truth and Reconciliation Commission of Canada, 2015). Consider reflection in this instance as an overarching and ongoing activity and not one that only occurs at one point in time.

---

### BOX 8.3 Reflecting on Client Needs for Indigenous Healing Practices

By reflecting on gaps in knowledge and practice, nurses can address client needs. For example, if a client identifies a need for smudging, a traditional practice that is part of some Indigenous cultures in Canada, standard operating procedures can be collaboratively created to ensure that all clients can be supported.

As one health care provider reflected, "Smudging was a part of the patient's normal practice. When she learned she would be able to smudge in the hospital even though she couldn't leave her room, there was a sense of relief."

Reflection is essential, but it is not enough. Decision making for both clients and health care providers is facilitated by meaningful collaboration on plans and actions that address clients' identified needs. Acting on what is needed creates a culturally respectful and safe health care environment for clients.

The Ottawa Hospital. (n.d.). *Smudge procedure gives comfort to Indigenous patients and families.* https://www.ottawahospital.on.ca/en/healthy-tomorrows/smudge-procedure-gives-comfort-to-indigenous-patients-and-families/

---

Think about the following in the context of your nursing practice:

- Identify a topic related to Indigenous healing practices that would be important to know more about. Who holds this information?
- What concrete steps can you take to learn about this topic?
- Explain how knowing more about Indigenous healing practices can help you improve as a professional nurse and in collaborative decision making.
- Find individuals in the local community who may be willing to help you acquire Indigenous perspectives.
- Be open to listening and responding to others' feedback.

Using reflective skills can create knowledge and build understanding that supports respect, reconciliation, and trust. When a nurse appropriately reflects on their care of a client and approaches care planning from the client's point of view, decision-making power can be reframed, redistributed, and shared.

## APPLYING REFLECTIVE SKILLS TO EVERYDAY NURSING PRACTICE AND DECISION MAKING

Being a reflective practitioner has the potential to translate into better client care outcomes (Burkett, 2020). Therefore, reflecting on what you know and do should be a continual, never-ending activity to improve client care. Contemporary nursing practice offers many opportunities to apply reflective skills. Engaging in time management and conflict management, learning from your mistakes, navigating the practice environment, and preparing for registration or licensing exams are all areas that require reflection and decision-making skills.

### Time Management

Time management skills are important tools to achieve personal and professional goals. "Time management is the appropriate use of tools, techniques, and principles to control time spent on low-priority needs and to ensure that time is invested in activities that lead toward achieving desired, high-priority goals" (Walton & Waddell, 2025, p. 534). It is the ability to spend your time on the things that matter to you, your client, and the organization in which you practice. Identifying resources to manage time requires reflection and the application of thinking processes. It is part of *E* in the NRCE framework used in this textbook.

Managing time that prioritizes activities requires critical thinking, clinical reasoning, and reflective skills (many of these skills are similar, as you have discovered). The nurse must understand what is occurring in a situation and why and be able to discern its relevance in relation to what needs to be done at any given time.

Your time, and everyone else's time, is very valuable. Once it is gone, you can never get it back. Reflect on your use of time and strategies you can employ to address any challenges you may have:

- **Do you say "yes" to everyone?**
  Learn to say "no" if the activity would delay your own time-sensitive assigned work or goals for the day, or if it does not contribute to a team effort or a shared workload; be polite and suggest someone else who could assist; if the activity can be done later, discuss how you can take it on once you have completed your own work. Find a balance between collaboration and your own workload.
- **Are you taking on more than you can do in any given time period?**
  Prioritize what you need to do, based on your goals; consider delegating or assigning work to another who is available to assist; and recognize that tasks can be reprioritized based on changing client needs and circumstances in the health care setting.
- **Do you procrastinate and put off tasks because they are too hard to do or too complex?**
  Create a list, number the tasks, and stick to it; assign a certain amount of time to each task; break complex tasks down into smaller activities (e.g., "arranging for a client's discharge from hospital" involves reviewing physician's order and prescriptions, confirming transportation and follow-up appointments, conducting a client needs assessment, teaching).
- **Are you always interrupted?**
  If others are interrupting you during the provision of nursing care, determine if the request is critical. If it is, adjust your work and provide assistance promptly. If it is not, or if your own work is critical (e.g., medication administration), ask that they come back later. Avoid working in busy areas where there are constant distractions, if possible; use mindful practices to focus your attention; turn your phone to "silent"; and communicate your busy times to others, so they will know not to disturb you.
- **Do you take too long to complete something because "it's not perfect yet"?**
  Identify what needs to be done, and finish the task when it is completed safely and competently. Recognize that a "less-than-perfect job" can be very adequate and meet the required outcomes. Move on!
- **Are you disorganized, stopping and starting multiple tasks without a plan?**
  Create a plan or list and follow it; minimize distractions; focus on completing each task from start to finish unless there is a critical incident that requires you to step away from it; and return to the last task you were doing and finish the work.

Organizing notes to use during a clinical shift can be based on time, to help plan your client care for the day. The way you keep your notes should reflect your own thinking processes. This can help reinforce habits of thinking and how you make decisions on what to do next. Create your own template for shift notes or adapt one that already exists. Remember that notes containing confidential client information should be kept safe or destroyed after use.

Reflect on what consumes your time during nursing practice by writing down your activities in the order in which you did them, at a break or after a shift. Looking at your notes later can help you be more objective. Determine whether your activities were driven by goals and priorities and if they occurred in a logical, efficient order.

## Conflict Management

Conflict is a "difference in the preferred strategies, actions, or beliefs within a person (i.e., inner conflict) or between people" that causes, or has the potential to cause, harm (Walton & Waddell, 2025, p. 432). Situations involving conflict occur daily. Unresolved conflict can result in increased dissatisfaction with work, absenteeism, and poorer client outcomes.

What is your natural reaction to conflict? Reflecting on your own approach to managing conflict in both personal and professional interactions is an important first step. You may recognize your approach in this list (Walton & Waddell, 2025, pp. 439–443):

- *Avoidance*: withdrawing from others and not cooperating in a solution to conflict; this may prolong or worsen a disagreement
- *Accommodation*: sacrificing your own values and needs to satisfy others'; disappointment and resentment may result if this repeatedly occurs
- *Competition*: pursuing your own needs and wants at the expense of others; this may force defensive reactions from others and disrupt collegial relationships
- *Compromise*: using assertive and cooperative thinking will help meet others halfway and more negotiation can result in a win-win outcome; it is effective in balancing power
- *Collaboration*: working together with others requires creativity and cooperation to analyze and identify solutions for areas of conflict; it is time-consuming but more effective in achieving a common goal

Refer to therapeutic communication practices learned in your nursing program. Finding out more information and understanding your own past experiences, assumptions, and biases in challenging situations are critical to approaching conflict. From there, deciding what to do and acting on that decision may be clearer to you.

Steps in thinking that appropriately manage conflicts in health care situations can include:

- Gather more information before analyzing (keep calm and do not jump to conclusions).

- Take a moment to view the situation from everyone's perspective (not just your own).
- Focus on the goal for client care (remember the BIG picture).
- Take time to explore solutions (collaborate, do not rush, and take breaks to think if needed).
- Look for options that can meet the needs of most people involved.

These steps are very similar to the thinking processes that you have already read about in this textbook.

## Emotional Intelligence

Emotional intelligence (EI) is a concept that can significantly affect your ability to clinically reason, be sensitive to others' emotions, and work through situations of conflict. EI is described as the ability to perceive, appraise, and assess emotions (in yourself and others), access and process emotional information, generate feelings, and regulate emotions for professional growth (Smith et al., 2009). It promotes effective communication, empathy, conflict resolution, and reduction of anxiety. When collaborating with other professionals about clinical decisions in situations that are ethical, chaotic, and bound by codes of practice, emotions can affect health care practitioners and consequently, client care. Refer to Box 8.4 for an example of how EI is demonstrated in nursing practice.

Nursing students who develop EI are better able to endure pressures of practice and make better clinical decision (Raghubir, 2018; Smith et al., 2009). Factors that support EI include:

- *Motivation to achieve empathy:* this is a strong desire to understand another person's emotions, thoughts, and perspectives, and to act on that desire.
  - My colleague is upset, and I should offer support or find out why they feel that way.
  - Is the client acting fearful of this treatment because of a past experience or because they are not understanding what is happening?
- *Self-awareness and self-regulation:* discussed earlier in this textbook, these are crucial factors for maintaining well-being of nurses and clients, and for appreciating the impact of emotions on others (positive or negative).
  - Am I upset because I am feeling criticized?
  - I need to remain as calm as I can so that I can provide reassurance to the client.
  - How can I present my different idea so that others are not feeling disrespected?

More reflection after a conflict will summarize the thinking process and build your skills and knowledge for managing future challenging situations.

---

> ### BOX 8.4  Example of Emotional Intelligence in Nursing Practice
>
> A nurse working with the cardiac team in an emergency room is involved in the admission of a 40-year-old client who had a myocardial infarction at home. The client's partner called 911. Cardiopulmonary resuscitation (CPR) was not immediately initiated until paramedics arrived, and spontaneous circulation did not return for 45 minutes. Given this delay, the nurse understands that an anoxic brain injury may have occurred and that prognosis would be poor. Although no diagnosis has been made, the nurse anticipates that the client's partner will also require care and support. The nurse then thinks of their own partner who is a similar age to the client and is overwhelmed with emotion, in addition to feeling frustration as to why the client's partner could not initiate CPR. The nurse becomes aware of their own feelings, anticipates that these may be different from the partner's feelings and needs, further assesses the partner's experiences, and is able to provide supportive care.

Adapted from Raghubir, A. (2018). Emotional intelligence in professional nursing practice: A concept review using Rodgers's evolutionary analysis approach. *International Journal of Nursing Science, 5*, 126–130. https://doi.org/10.1016/j.ijnss.2018.03.004

## Learning From Mistakes

Everyone makes mistakes. Reflective practice allows nurses to focus on the competent performance of a clinical skill. Studies have shown that reflective and mindful behaviours can minimize errors during skill performance by increasing overall attention to tasks and being present in the moment with clients (Ekkens & Gordon, 2021).

Nurses have a responsibility to the public to maintain trust in the profession and safety in health care delivery. Because some errors are foreseeable and because we are aware of risks in how a skill is performed, we can use anticipatory reflection and focus on avoiding mistakes. One critical skill example is medication administration. Sentinel events (errors resulting in unexpected death or physical or psychological harm such as an in-hospital suicide or wrong-site surgery) and near misses (clinical situations that result in no harm but reveal a serious problem to correct such as some medication administration errors) are examples of error types (Waddell & Walton, 2025, p. 398). Near misses can provide useful lessons for reducing risk.

Mistakes and client safety issues can occur because of miscommunication, incompetence, policy violation, or poor decision making. Some of the strategies named in this textbook can help: communicating with ISBAR-R (introduction/identify, situation, background, assessment, recommendation, and repeat back/receive); engaging in deliberate practice; understanding the environment you are working in; applying mindfulness; and using decision-making frameworks.

If you make a mistake, do this:

- Find out more information through assessments and determine the nature and extent of the error.
- Take immediate steps to prevent or reduce further harm and *seek assistance* as needed.
- Report the error according to *policy and procedure.*
- Document the client reaction, what was done, and actions that were taken to address the error.
- Reflect on what occurred—the circumstances that contributed to the error and decisions that led to the error.
- Engage in ways to prevent similar situations in the future.

You will improve and grow when you learn from mistakes that were made, no matter how small. The Healthcare Excellence Canada (2023) website has a number of tools and resources to support safe practice in health care settings and facilitate reflection-on-action.

## Navigating the Practice Environment

Integrating into the practice environment can be difficult for nursing students and new graduates. Time limitations, conflict, errors, and the requirement of incorporating diverse client needs into goals for nursing practice can be overwhelming. So too can ethical care dilemmas, microaggressions, unfamiliar situations, and new health care trends. Such challenges can lead nurses to feel guilty, devalued, lonely or isolated, or unsure, which can interfere with thinking, making decisions, and caring for clients. Effective strategies that employ reflective and clinical reasoning skills are essential to confront these issues and maintain a supportive and inclusive health care environment for clients and nurses.

In Canada, nursing students and new graduates may be pressured by an ethical commitment to contribute to client care in a meaningful way and to do their part (McMillan et al., 2023). Guilt often arises in nursing practice when making difficult decisions that impact client outcomes. For example, dealing with minimal resources and making tough decisions because of this can result in a feeling that while you are giving one client what they need, you are depriving another of quality care. Begin to navigate feelings of guilt by doing the following:

- Engaging with ethical decision-making frameworks, and referring to such as the *Code of Ethics* of the Canadian Nurses Association (2017).
- Seeking advice and guidance from colleagues, supervisors, or instructors.

- Building a community of support with other health care professionals.
- Communicating clearly about expectations, rationale, and the need to address system limitations.

In addition, adopting a reflective stance can provide clarity and support in navigating ethical challenges through self-assessment and awareness of the health care context.

Racial microaggressions may be experienced in practice settings and are defined as "brief and commonplace daily verbal, behavioral, or environmental indignities, whether intentional or unintentional, that communicate hostile, derogatory, or negative racial slights and insults towards people of color" (Sue et al., 2007, p. 271). These may be experienced during interactions with clients and their families, or other health care providers. In such situations, nurses may feel devalued, harassed, and dismissed which can affect their abilities to clinically reason, form clinical judgements, and make decisions. Education about and awareness of microaggressions can prepare health care professionals to respond. Also, reflection and debriefing with a supervisor or instructor can begin to address the effects of an instance of microaggression. To respond to a client's microaggression while prioritizing safety, follow these six steps (Overland et al., 2019):

1. Ensure the client is stable.
2. Address the comment and name the behaviour as inappropriate.
3. Refocus the conversation on the client's health goals.
4. Share your perspectives.
5. Remind the client of the health care team's roles.
6. Temporarily step away from the client to reflect, regroup, or consult with others.

Loneliness or isolation is a common experience among new nurses, particularly when facing new environments with high workloads and emotional demands. Students who regularly find themselves in these circumstances may feel ignored by other nurses and that they are without support from a team that they do not know (O'Mara et al., 2014). Some approaches to address loneliness or isolation include:

- Gradually establish a support network within the health care team and with trusted peers.
- Participate in professional organizations and committees that can help you alleviate feelings of general isolation.
- Reflect regularly on your key accomplishments and areas for growth.

Opportunities for nurses to reflect and share experiences, seek advice, and cultivate resilience in challenging times can reduce feelings of being alone.

For novice nurses, feeling unsure and lacking confidence can also result from trying to learn new tasks and deciding what is needed in client care situations. In addition to reaching out to others (do not be afraid to ask

student completed the procedure with the last experience and learning in mind. The activity was completed competently by the student. Debriefing was again conducted, and additional feedback was given.

- List the key strategies used to support deliberate practice in this student learning activity.

- Why do you think this student learned from this deliberate practice experience?
- How can you seek out similar feedback opportunities in your learning?

## EVIDENCE-INFORMED THINKING ACTIVITY

The issue of time management is often a focus of students and new nurses. Explore the evidence related to time management in nursing practice. Conduct a brief literature search on this topic in peer-reviewed articles that explore, describe, or support efficient and effective practice. Can you find any? Reflect on other related concepts that are often associated with time management, and modify your search. What are the influences on time management in nursing practice? Think about how influences that you read about in the literature affect your own time management strategies, and consider ways to address these.

## QUESTIONS TO ASSESS LEARNING

### Review Questions

1. A nurse has just administered an oral medication to a client and then realizes that they have miscalculated the dosage. What is the nurse's first step?
   a. Assess the client.
   b. Report to the manager.
   c. Call the physician.
   d. Reflect on the error.
2. Reflection is a nursing skill that facilitates what aspect(s) of care? Select all that apply.
   a. Decision making
   b. Clinical judgement
   c. Clinical reasoning
   d. Communication
   e. Cultural sensitivity
3. Which action most directly demonstrates antiracism in the nursing profession?
   a. Exclusion of individuals from health care services based on their racial background
   b. Advocacy for equality in treatment and opportunity for racialized people in practice and education
   c. Proposing policy changes that address racial discrimination in provincial law
   d. Acceptance and perpetuation of unconscious bias in nursing practices

## ONE LAST THOUGHT

Hopefully you have made the connections between the sections of this textbook. Theoretical concepts, frameworks, and models in Part A can be applied to nursing practice situations described in Part B. In Part C, you have seen how everything can be pulled together to think in more complex situations and as a reflective practitioner who must navigate contemporary practice environments. Refer to the Appendix for more examples of how thinking and concepts in this textbook work together in various nursing practice situations.

Thinking is hard work. This textbook has guided you to use clinical reasoning skills, form clinical judgements and make clinical decisions through the introduction of a unified process of thinking and decision making. This process reflects several nursing models and is described, in part, using the textbook's NRCE framework.

Not all of what a nurse needs to consider when thinking and making decisions is covered in this textbook. But the essentials of *how* you need to consider thinking and decision making have been introduced. You will have a full career to adapt your systems for thinking and to develop and grow as you think it through.

## ONLINE RESOURCES

*Anti-racism primer: Self-reflect*—George Brown College (2024): https://www.georgebrown.ca/anti-racism/primer/self-reflect

Healthcare Excellence Canada: https://www.healthcareexcellence.ca
Healthy Minds Innovations: https://hminnovations.org
*How to identify and overcome your implicit bias*—Maryville University (2021): https://online.maryville.edu/blog/addressing-implicit-bias/

*Indigenous cultural safety, cultural humility and anti-racism: Practice standard companion guide*—British Columbia College of Nurses & Midwives (2022): https://www.bccnm.ca/Documents/cultural_safety_humility/ps_companion_guide.pdf

*Mindfulness exercises*—Mayo Clinic (2022): https://www.mayoclinic.org/healthy-lifestyle/consumer-health/in-depth/mindfulness-exercises/art-20046356

National Council of State Boards of Nursing (NCSBN): https://www.ncsbn.org

*Northern and Indigenous health and healthcare*—Open Press (n.d.): https://openpress.usask.ca/northernhealthcare/

ParticipACTION: https://www.participaction.com

*Practice resources: Cultural competence*—Registered Practical Nurses Association of Ontario (n.d.): https://www.werpn.com/education/practice-resources/cultural-competency-resources-for-nurses/

*SDGs in the classroom toolkit*—York University (2024): https://www.yorku.ca/unsdgs/toolkit/and https://www.yorku.ca/unsdgs/toolkit/teaching-the-17-un-sdgs/discipline-specific-material-for-the-sdgs/health/

*What is mindfulness?*—Smiling Mind (2023): https://www.smilingmind.com.au/mindfulness

## REFERENCES

Advisory Board. (2018, August 2). *Global Centre for Nursing Executives. Research report. Rebuild the foundation for a resilient workforce.* https://www.advisory.com/research/nursing-executive-center/white-papers/2018/rebuild-the-foundation-for-a-resilient-workforce

Badu, E., O'Brien, A., Mitchell, R., et al. (2020). Workplace stress and resilience in the Australian nursing workforce: A comprehensive integrative review. *International Journal of Mental Health Nursing, 29,* 5–34. https://doi.org/10.1111/inm.12662.

Benner, P., Stannard, D., & Hooper, P. L. (1995). A "thinking-in-action" approach to teaching clinical judgment: A classroom innovation for acute care advanced practice nurses. *Advanced Practice Nursing Quarterly, 1*(4), 70–77.

Bourque Bearskin, M. L. (2023). Decolonization the what, why and how: A treaties on Indigenous nursing knowledge. *Nursing Philosophy, 24,* e12430. https://doi.org/10.1111/nup.12430.

Bradley, C. S., Dreifuerst, K. T., Johnson, B. K., et al. (2022). More than a meme: The Dunning-Kruger effect as an opportunity for positive change in nursing education. *Clinical Simulation in Nursing, 66,* 58–65. https://doi.org/10.1016/j.ecns.2022.02.010.

Burkett, J. (2020, December 7). How mindfulness could slash healthcare costs by reducing burnout and attrition. *Canadian Nurse.* https://community.cna-aiic.ca/dev-cn-en/blogs/cn-content/2020/12/07/how-mindfulness-could-slash-health-care-costs-by-r.

Canadian Association of Schools of Nursing. (2022). *National nursing education framework.* https://www.casn.ca/wp-content/uploads/2022/12/National-Nursing-Education-Framework_2023_EN_FINAL.pdf

Canadian Council for Practical Nurse Regulators. (2019). *Entry level competencies for licensed practical nurses.* https://www.clpna.com/wp-content/uploads/2023/08/CCPNR_Entry-Level_Competencies_LPNs-ID-104799.pdf

Canadian Nurses Association. (2017). *Code of ethics for registered nurses.* https://www.cna-aiic.ca/en/nursing/regulated-nursing-in-canada/nursing-ethics

Chiu, P., Hawkins, J., Eviza, K., & Gray, S. (2022). Nursing and the sustainable development goals: Scaling up and measuring our impact during the decade of action. *Journal of Nursing Scholarship, 54*(6), 664–667. https://doi.org/10.1111/jnu.12791.

College of Nurses of Ontario. (2019). *Entry-to-practice competencies for registered nurses.* https://www.cno.org/globalassets/docs/reg/41037-entry-to-practice-competencies-2020.pdf

Danda, M., Key, J., & Pitcher, C. (2022, May 16). Hearing our voices (part 1): Facilitating nurses' reflection on taking anti-racist action. *Canadian Nurse.* https://www.canadian-nurse.com/blogs/cn-content/2022/05/16/hearing-our-voices-part-1-facilitating-nurses-refl.

Diekelmann, J., & Diekelmann, N. (2009). *Schooling learning teaching.* iUniverse.

Ekkens, C. L., & Gordon, P. A. (2021, May/June). The mindful path to nursing accuracy: A quasi-experimental study on minimizing medication administration errors. *Holistic Nursing Practice,* 115–122. https://doi.org/10.1097/HNP.0000000000000440.

Ericsson, K. A., & Harwell, K. W. (2019). deliberate practice and proposed limits on the effects of practice on the acquisition of expert performance: Why the original definition matters and recommendations for future research. *Frontiers in Psychology, 10,* 2396. https://doi.org/10.3389/fpsyg.2019.02396.

Ericsson, K. A., Krampe, R. T., & Tesch-Römer, C. (1993). The role of deliberate practice in the acquisition of expert performance. *Psychological Review, 100,* 363–406. https://doi.org/10.1037/0033-295X.87.3.215.

Fay, B. (1987). *Critical social science.* Polity Press.

First Nations Health Authority, First Nations Health Council, & First Nations Health Director's Association. (2021, April 21). *Anti-racism, cultural safety & humility framework.* https://www.fnha.ca/Documents/FNHA-FNHC-FNHDA-Anti-Racism-Cultural-Safety-and-Humility-Framework.pdf

Gibbs, G. (1988). Learning by doing: A guide to teaching and learning methods. Further Education Unit. Oxford Polytechnic.

Gonzalez, L., & Kardong-Edgren, S. (2017). Deliberate practice for mastery learning in nursing. *Clinical Simulation in Nursing, 13*(1), 10–14. https://dx.doi.org/10.1016/j.ecns.2016.10.005.

Harwood, L., Wilson, B., Crandall, J., et al. (2021). Resilience, mindfulness, and self-compassion: Tools for nephrology nurses. *Nephrology Nursing Journal, 48*(3), 241–249. https://doi.org/10.37526/1526-744X.2021.48.3.241.

Healthcare Excellence Canada. (2023). *Resources.* https://www.healthcareexcellence.ca/en/resources/

International Council of Nurses. (2017). *Nurses: A voice to lead—Achieving the SDGs.* https://www.icnvoicetolead.com/wp-content/uploads/2017/04/ICN_AVoiceToLead_guidance-Pack-9.pdf

Johns, C. (2022). *Becoming a reflective practitioner* (6th ed.). Wiley-Blackwell.

Kabat-Zinn, J. (2006). Mindfulness-based interventions in context: Past, present and future. *Clinical Psychology: Science and Practice, 10*(2), 144–156. https://doi.org/10.1093/clipsy.bpg016.

Kruger, J., & Dunning, D. (1999). Unskilled and unaware of it: How difficulties in recognizing one's own incompetence lead to inflated self-assessments. *Journal of Personality and Social Psychology, 77*(6), 1121–1134. https://doi.org/10.1037/0022-3514.77.6.1121.

McMillan, K., Akoo, C., & Catigbe-Cates, A. (2023). New graduate nurses navigating entry to practice in the COVID-19 pandemic. *Canadian Journal of Nursing Research, 55*(1), 78–90. doi :10.1177/08445621221150946journals.sagepub.com/home/cjn.

O'Mara, L., McDonald, J., Gillespie, M., et al. (2014). Challenging clinical learning environments: Experiences of undergraduate students. *Nurse Education in Practice, 14*, 208–213. http://dx.doi.org/10.1016/j.nepr.2013.08.012.

The Ottawa Hospital. (n.d.). *Smudge procedure gives comfort to Indigenous patients and families.* https://www.ottawahospital.on.ca/en/healthy-tomorrows/smudge-procedure-gives-comfort-to-indigenous-patients-and-families/

Overland, M. K., Zumsteg, J. M., Lindo, E. G., et al. (2019). Microaggressions in clinical training and practice. *PM&R: The Journal of Injury, Function and Rehabilitation, 11*, 1004–1012. https://doi.org/10.1002/pmrj.12229.

ParticipACTION. (2024). *Mindfulness.* https://www.participaction.com/the-science/explore-benefits/mindfulness/

Patel, K. M., & Metersky, K. (2022). Reflective practice in nursing: A concept analysis. *International Journal of Nursing Knowledge, 33*(3), 180–187. https://doi.org/10.1111/2047-3095.12350.

Raghubir, A. (2018). Emotional intelligence in professional nursing practice: A concept review using Rodgers's evolutionary analysis approach. *International Journal of Nursing Science, 5*(2), 126–130. https://doi.org/10.1016/j.ijnss.2018.03.004.

Schön, D. A. (1987). *Educating the reflective practitioner: Toward a new design for teaching and learning in the professions.* Jossey-Bass.

Sieg, D. (2020). *7 habits of highly resilient nurses.* https://nursingcentered.sigmanursing.org/features/top-stories/Vol41_1_7-habits-of-highly-resilient-nurses

Smith, K. B., Profetto-McGrath, J., & Cummings, G. (2009). Emotional intelligence and nursing: An integrative literature review. *International Journal of Nursing Studies, 46*, 1624–1636. https://doi.org/10.1016/j.ijnurstu.2009.05.024.

Sue, D. W., Capodilupo, C. M., Torino, G. C., et al. (2007). Racial microaggressions in everyday life: Implications for clinical practice. *American Psychologist, 62*(4), 271–286. https://doi.org/10.1037/0003-066X.62.4.271.

Tanner, C. A. (2006). Thinking like a nurse: A research-based model of clinical judgment in nursing. *Journal of Nursing Education, 45*(6), 204–211.

Truth and Reconciliation Commission of Canada. (2015). *Truth and Reconciliation Commission of Canada: Calls to Action.* https://publications.gc.ca/collections/collection_2015/trc/IR4-8-2015-eng.pdf

UNESCO. (2017). *Education for Sustainable Development Goals: Learning objectives.* https://unesdoc.unesco.org/ark:/48223/pf0000247444

United Nations. (2007). *United Nations Declaration on the Rights of Indigenous Peoples.* https://www.un.org/development/desa/indigenouspeoples/wp-content/uploads/sites/19/2019/01/UNDRIP_E_web.pdf

United Nations. (2015). *Transforming our world: The 2030 Agenda for Sustainable Development.* https://sdgs.un.org/2030agenda

van Manen, M. (1991). *The tact of teaching: The meaning of pedagogical thoughtfulness.* SUNY Press.

Walton, N. A., & Waddell, J. I. (2025). *Yoder-Wise's leading and managing in Canadian nursing* (3rd ed.). Elsevier.

# Putting It All Together: Thinking *BIG* and *Small*

It can be challenging to understand how multiple cognitive processes are applied directly to nursing practice. The use of frameworks, models, concepts, and decision making may be less obvious in the practice environment because they are often considered invisible, internal processes. Consider how your thinking can be made more explicit and evident to others when acting as a nurse and applying the concepts and skills introduced in this textbook. How will other nurses, health care professionals, and clients "see" your thinking and the evidence for your decisions and actions?

The information in this appendix further illustrates how and where concepts in this textbook can be applied and made obvious to others through action. Three different nursing activities are used as examples to demonstrate this application: a clinical shift, a nursing policy review, and a personal development exercise. The unified process of thinking and decision making (finding information, deciding what to do, acting on a decision, and reviewing actions) and examples of concepts and skills from the textbook are shown in each of these activity descriptions. Recall that the unified process offers a summary of a variety of nursing models in its four steps. Alternatively, you can apply a nursing model of your choice to these activities in a similar way.

When you review each example, think *BIG* as you consider the activity *in its entirety*. Thinking *BIG* enables you to see the following familiar steps over a whole clinical shift, for instance. Consider the **entire thinking process** in this way:

- **finding information** about what is occurring at the start of an activity (e.g., assessing and gathering data on the full client assignment for a particular shift)
- **deciding** how to generally approach and engage in the activity (e.g., analyzing, interpreting, synthesizing, and prioritizing goals for a clinical shift)
- **acting on the decision** by establishing and implementing a specific plan (e.g., formulating a plan for organizing and performing nursing work that meets the priorities)

- **reviewing** the overall success of the activity (e.g., evaluating whether priorities for the shift were met or not).

You will also think *smaller* at the same time. This means that the same familiar steps will be applied during shorter-term actions that happen throughout these larger activities. Consider the first step of **finding information** about required nursing policies (before proceeding to deciding what to do in the actual review of the policy itself) in this example:

- **finding information** about the nursing policy and its related topics (e.g., understanding the scope and availability of resources, materials, and evidence)
- **deciding** how to organize the available information and data (e.g., analyzing, interpreting, synthesizing, and prioritizing what was found)
- **acting on a decision** to focus on and examine a key resource (e.g., establishing and implementing a plan and timeframe to study that resource)
- **reviewing** the key resource and overall value of the available information found (e.g., evaluating the information to use in the next steps of policy review).

Many concepts and skills described in this textbook are applied repeatedly during both short- and long-term nursing activities and do not occur discretely as shown in the examples in this appendix. Note how using these concepts and skills in a flexible manner can contribute to your ability to think it through in diverse nursing situations.

## A CLINICAL SHIFT

The timeframes and nursing actions in Table A.1 represent the general experience of a nurse during a 12-hour shift. A clinical shift is a **complex** activity based on the multiple-step processes involved, consultations required and unpredictable nature of its outcomes. Note the process for BIG thinking about the shift (finding information about what the shift will involve, deciding how to approach workload

**TABLE A.2    Application of Thinking and Decision Making to Nursing Policy Review—cont'd**

| Nursing Actions | Think BIG: Unified Process | Think Small: Examples of Steps in Unified Process and NRCE[+] | Examples of Applied Concepts and Skills |
|---|---|---|---|
| **April–May** Draft revisions to orientation policy and procedure; incorporate new feedback | Acting on decisions | • Acting on decisions to prioritize new nurse feedback and revise documents (*N:* apply subject matter expertise and writing and communication skills; *C:* emphasize client safety outcomes; *E:* include occupational health resources) | • Critical thinking and clinical reasoning skills |
| **May–June** Send to leadership; note scope of work and schedule summer implementation if revisions approved | Reviewing actions | • Reviewing actions for achievement of goal | • Reflection-on and beyond-action<br>• Self-regulation<br>• Self-reflection |

[+]NRCE: *N*ursing knowledge, professional *r*oles, *c*lient context, health care *e*nvironment.

## A PROFESSIONAL DEVELOPMENT EXERCISE

The nursing actions in Table A.3 illustrate key processes and concepts evident when a nurse attends an afternoon workshop on a new video communication technology for remote health care settings. A personal development activity is often considered a **simple** activity because it is focused on an individual's specific needs, competence, and goals and is structured, predictable, and measurable. In this education activity, the client is considered indirectly in the context of the nurse's professional development (the future provision of better client care is an outcome of this activity). As in the other examples, note the iterative (back and forth) nature of thinking by the nurse. Examples of the NRCE are included, and various concepts and skills are associated with each of the nursing actions.

**TABLE A.3    Application of Thinking and Decision Making to a Professional Development Exercise**

| Nursing Actions | Think BIG: Unified Process | Think Small: Examples of Steps in Unified Process and NRCE[+] | Examples of Applied Concepts and Skills |
|---|---|---|---|
| **13:00–14:00** Receive new information on aspect of video communication technology during workshop | • Finding information | • Finding information on function and application of technology (*N:* note modes of communication; *R:* identify competence and scope of practice) | • Anticipatory reflection<br>• Critical thinking skills |
| | • Deciding what to do | • Deciding what to do in personal nursing practice (*N:* compare current and new knowledge on technology; analyze gap in professional knowledge; *C:* interpret client health and education needs; *E:* prioritize timely care and increased access) | • Emotional intelligence<br>• Cognitive overload<br>• Critical thinking, clinical reasoning skills |

*Continued*

**TABLE A.3    Application of Thinking and Decision Making to a Professional Development Exercise—cont'd**

| Nursing Actions | Think BIG: Unified Process | Think Small: Examples of Steps in Unified Process and NRCE[+] | Examples of Applied Concepts and Skills |
|---|---|---|---|
| **14:00–14:15** Discuss application of technology with other workshop participants during question-and-answer period | • Deciding what to do | • Deciding what to do to address confidentiality (*N*: incorporate ethical principles; *C*: recognize video and privacy needs, and cost of mobile devices to clients; *E*: ensure secure access to Internet/Wi-Fi in remote areas) | • Sustainable development goals<br>• Structural determinants of health<br>• Client access<br>• Critical thinking, clinical reasoning skills |
| **14:15–14:30** Confirm unclear functions of the technology with workshop leader at break | | • Finding information on functionality (*E*: use technology for sharing images without personal video option)<br>• Deciding what to do for practice area (*N*: modes of communication; synthesize new ways for clients and nurses to apply this in remote areas) | • Self-reflection<br>• Mindfulness<br>• Self-efficacy |
| **14:30–15:30** Demonstrate knowledge in hands on practice time with video technology | • Acting on decisions | • Acting on decision to adopt technology (*N*: plan for including in own practice; *C*: plan for how clients will use to improve communication of their health) | • Deliberate practice<br>• Self-efficacy<br>• Self-regulation<br>• Mindfulness<br>• Critical thinking, clinical reasoning skills |
| Receive feedback on demonstration | • Reviewing actions | • Reviewing use of technology (*N*: evaluate value of workshop to personal practice; reflect on changes to nurse's own thinking) | • Deliberate practice<br>• Professional communication |
| **15:30–16:00** Complete quiz and earn certificate | • Reviewing actions | • Reviewing of personal development and advancement of practice (*N*: project use in next client interaction; *R*: anticipate which colleagues will be able to use new technology; *C*: client engagement opportunities; *E*: embed procedures for using technology in practice setting) | • Reflecting on actions<br>• Mindfulness<br>• Self-regulation<br>• Self-reflection<br>• Confidence |

[+]NRCE: *N*ursing knowledge, professional *r*oles, *c*lient context, health care *e*nvironment.

# GLOSSARY

**Acronym** a word, pronounced as such, that is created from the initial letters of other words; it is used to describe something in an abbreviated way; a type of mnemonic

**Acrostic** a saying, phrase, rhyme, or some other composition taken from letters in a group of words in order used to improve recall; a type of mnemonic

**Ambiguity** a situation that has more than one possible meaning or interpretation; an unclear choice in the given context

**Analysis** the process of uncovering patterns and trends in information; the second phase of the decision-making or judgement process, where data is used to determine key issues and relationships about a client's status, situation, and environment

**Anticipatory reflection** a future-focused reflection; consideration of what may occur next, based on past experiences and learning

**Assessment** the first step of the nursing process, which involves comprehensive data collection; recognition of the client's status, situation, and environment; and of the nurse's and others' knowledge and role

**Clinical judgement** the outcome of thinking and decision-making activities that are focused on and respond to the client's health care needs; also, "an interpretation or conclusion about a client's needs, concerns, or health problems, and/or the decision to take action (or not), use or modify standard approaches, or improvise new ones as deemed appropriate by the patient's response" (Tanner, 2006, p. 204)

**Clinical judgement (measurement)** "the observed outcome of critical thinking and decision making; it is an iterative process that uses nursing knowledge to observe and assess presenting situations, identify a prioritized client concern, and generate the best possible evidence-based solutions in order to deliver safe client care" (National Council of State Boards of Nursing, 2019, p. 1)

**Clinical judgement (practice)** the outcome of thinking and decision activities that are focused on and respond to the client's health care needs; also "an interpretation or conclusion about a client's needs, concerns, or health problems, and/or the decision to take action (or not), use or modify standard approaches, or improvise new ones as deemed appropriate by the client's response" (Tanner, 2006, p. 204)

**Clinical reasoning** a goal-oriented and purposeful process for thinking about a client's care

**Cognitive load** the relative demand on thinking required by a particular task or tasks

**Cognitive overload** the result of too much mental demand on the decision-maker from too much information or activity at any one point in time

**Collaboration** the process whereby a client or family member participates in the development and delivery of a plan of care, or when professionals interacting in real time discuss a client's presenting symptoms, describe their views on treatment, and jointly develop a plan of care

**Complex decision** in nursing, one in which the nurse must make a choice about a client or health care situation that has no obvious immediate answer; it may involve multiple client(s) factors or other concerns that are present simultaneously in a single clinical situation

**Complexity** "the degree to which a client's condition and care requirements are identifiable and established; the sum of the variables influencing a client's current health status; and the variability of a client's condition or care requirements" (College of Nurses of Ontario, 2018, p. 5)

**Consultation** the process of confirming or checking information with a client or family, or seeking advice, validating plans of care, or corroborating perceptions of a client's needs with another professional

**Coordination** working together with a client or client family for a common goal; at least two professionals communicating and working in parallel or in a back-and-forth fashion to achieve a common client-centred goal, while delivering care separately

**Critical thinking** the purposeful, informed, and self-regulated thinking about connected ideas to increase the likelihood of a desired outcome; a particular attitude, thinking skills, and knowledge are needed to think critically

**Cultural safety** a critical awareness, where health care professionals and organizations engage in ongoing self-reflection and hold themselves accountable for providing culturally safe care, as defined by the client themself and as measured through progress toward achieving health equity

**Decision making** selecting the best option from the alternatives that are available; in nursing, a process that requires the use of both critical thinking and clinical reasoning

**Deliberate practice** focused, repeated activities that are aimed at improving optimal performance, with feedback from a skilled practitioner

**Emotional intelligence (EI)** the ability to perceive, appraise and assess emotions (in yourself and others), access and process emotional information, generate feelings, and regulate emotions for professional growth

**Evaluation** a review to determine the effectiveness of nursing care

**Feedback** giving and responding to information (verbal, written) about nursing care and performance to facilitate professional and personal growth, practical improvements, and optimal care; feedback to the nurse can come from any person involved in care, including the client

**Framework** a basic structure that describes (but does not fully explain) a system or concept; it helps connect many big ideas about a topic to a method or process of doing something related to that topic

**Generating options (or solutions)** identifying expected outcomes and using hypotheses to define future interventions; highlighting desired outcomes and what should be avoided

**Implementation**    initiation and completion of planned actions or nursing interventions; it includes documenting or recording the care provided

**Interpretation**    the process of assigning meaning to information; it relies on analysis of the data

**Interprofessional collaboration**    "a partnership between a team of health providers and a client in a participatory, collaborative and coordinated approach to shared decision-making around health and social issues" (Canadian Interprofessional Health Collaborative, 2010, p. 24)

**Intuition**    the immediate understanding of the meaning of a clinical situation, without the need for conscious reasoning, and is a function of experience with similar situations; often occurs with recognition of cues and patterns (Benner, 2001; Tanner, 2006)

**Metacognition**    the ability to reflect on and become aware of what we know and what we do not know and to use this understanding when continuing to learn (Halpern, 2014)

**Mindfulness**    the quality of mind that notices what is present in the moment, without judgement or interference

**Mnemonic**    a device—such as a pattern of letters, ideas, or associations—for remembering facts and information more easily

**Model**    a simplified description of a process that can facilitate its understanding and application to different situations; it is a more concrete representation of an abstract idea (Halpern, 2014)

**Nursing-sensitive indicators (NSIs)**    in clinical care, client outcomes that are influenced by nursing interventions, according to empirical evidence (D'Amour et al., 2014)

**Outcomes**    responses observed as a result of an intervention or action; measurements that relate to the effectiveness and efficiency of an action(s)

**Planning**    a description of how client-centred outcomes will be achieved, which is developed once priorities and outcomes for addressing a problem are identified; planning involves collaborating, consulting, and communicating, and can address several client issues at once

**Predictability**    the degree to which client outcomes and care requirements can be anticipated; it is future focused

**Prioritization**    the ranking of client or nursing-related issues using criteria for urgency or importance, so that a sequence of nursing actions can be determined

**Problem solving**    a process for generating reasonable options to overcome identified barriers that are preventing the attainment of a goal or outcome

**Professional communication**    communication that conveys a role of responsibility and accountability for one's actions and is clear, courteous, individual, trustworthy, and assertive; with other health care professionals, follows evidence-informed frameworks

**Quality improvement (QI)**    a continuous process of improving care delivery and outcomes using a systematic and evidence-informed approach; it includes comparing evaluation results to benchmarks or standards

**Reflection-in-action**    the ability of a nurse to observe ("read" or notice) the client and their response to a nursing intervention, and to adjust the interventions as needed based on that observation (Tanner, 2006)

**Reflection-on-action**    a practice that completes the cycle of reflection; it reveals what nurses gained from their experience and contributes to their ongoing clinical knowledge development and capacity for clinical judgement

**Reflective practitioner**    someone who lives reflection naturally in their everyday, mindful practice; pays attention to their experiences and is self-aware of their own and others' responses to those experiences

**Resilience**    the ability to remain agile and effective amidst stress and bounce back quickly from difficult situations (Advisory Board, 2018, p. 11)

**Risk**    the probability or likelihood that something may occur; in nursing, it is associated with the severity of any anticipated consequence of that risk; it is represented by a situation where there is a possibility of loss or injury, or a situation that may create a hazard

**Self-efficacy**    the overall belief in one's ability or competence to manage challenges or changes in life

**Self-reflection**    when the nurse clearly identifies, explores, and analyzes their thinking to develop knowledge and an appreciation of their performance in the context of professional practice learning

**Self-regulation**    the ability to reflect on thinking and identify one's learning needs, set goals, select useful resources, and self-evaluate accomplishments and subsequent development that is required to improve

**Situation awareness**    being aware of what is happening around you and understanding what that information means, now and in the future (Endsley & Jones, 2012); the focus or context of awareness is related to the specific purpose of the activity, such as caring for a client

**Stability**    a current client or health care situation that is not changing and is unlikely to change in the foreseeable future; it is present focused

**Synthesis**    the combining or mixing of everything that is known to form a whole idea or a new perspective; interpretation and synthesis are closely related

**Taking action**    carrying out the solutions that address the highest priorities; similar to intervention, it includes the most appropriate activities and the tasks/skills required to perform the intervention (administering, communicating, teaching, documenting, coordinating, etc.)

**Thinking**    a cognitive activity that can include many elements, including feelings and emotions

**Unconscious bias**    also called *implicit bias*, it refers to unrecognized stereotypes and ideas that one has about cultures or people that influence one's decision making and behaviours; occurs outside of conscious awareness

This section provides selected answers to the end-of-chapter learning activities. When responding to any question, think about what you have learned in your program and nursing practice. Consider how you will apply your knowledge in the responses and adapt your answers to further understand your specific learning circumstances and the client groups that you care for in your jurisdiction.

## CHAPTER 1

### Notes on the Case Study Review

Consider the many possible client situations that this scenario presents. Seek more information from the client (e.g., conduct physical and cognitive or mental health assessments, elicit feelings, make note of recent activities and nutritional intake), staff, family, other nursing colleagues, and from recent documentation from other professionals, as applies. Possibilities that relate to this scenario and what the nurse may do next relate to potential urinary tract infection, head injury from an undocumented fall, changes in blood pressure or blood glucose levels, stroke, etc. Reflect on your thinking and rationale for what you consider could be happening in the scenario. Check your assumptions and biases.

### Answers to Review Questions

1. b

*Rationale:* At the bedside, critical thinking is referred to as *clinical reasoning*. A judgement or decision has not been demonstrated in this example.

2. d

*Rationale:* In this situation, the nurse analyzed the information and selected an option for action—a *decision*. Later, the outcome of the decision and a holistic view of care, which would include an evaluation, would demonstrate clinical judgement.

3. a

*Rationale: Critical thinking* that is not at the bedside reflects purposeful, informed activity so that a decision can be made.

4. c

*Rationale:* The outcome of thinking and decision activities that was focused on and responded to the client's health care needs was demonstrated in this situation as *clinical judgement*.

## CHAPTER 2

### Notes on the Case Study Review

This case study requires the application of a specific nursing model to organize your thinking. Each question addresses finding information, deciding what to do, acting on a decision, and reviewing actions.

1. When describing the client situation, assess the client situation, collect cues, and notice what information is available in the scenario description. This may include:
   - Recent surgical repair of fractured femur; slow to respond; incision healing; leg pain reported at 4/10 and chest pain with deep breaths; dyspnea for 1 hour with dry cough and crackles on left side of chest; vital signs as described

2. Understanding the client situation requires analysis, processing information, and interpreting data. Consider any gaps in what is known. Will more information be helpful, based on what you think may be happening? Consider:
   - Baseline vital signs for comparison, further neurological assessment, irregular heart rate, blood work
   - Possibility of pulmonary embolism, or other respiratory conditions such as pneumonia, can be explored through consultation with other health care providers

3. Actions include planning based on decisions made and goals set. A rationale for how you implement care, take action, or respond to the client situation and needs will be required. Consider:
   - Collaboration with other health care providers to treat the client for a pulmonary embolism, based on clinical manifestations of elevated heart rate, anxiety, cough, and decreased oxygen saturation, and further diagnostic testing (e.g., radiological testing, D-dimer, electrocardiogram)
   - Delivery of anticoagulant or related therapy, oxygen administration, and cardiovascular support

4. Evaluating and reflecting on outcomes will help determine whether care was effective in meeting the established goals. Outcomes may include:
   - No reported shortness of breath; normal oxygen saturation levels; no reported pain; appropriate responses to questions; and diagnostic test results within normal ranges (Tyerman & Cobbett, 2023, pp. 622–624)

## Notes on the Evidence-Informed Thinking Activity

To create the NCSBN Clinical Judgement Measurement Model (NCJMM), researchers at NCSBN reviewed nursing literature, cognitive psychology, psychological assessments, and science related to decision making in nursing practice and clinical judgement. NCSBN researchers also conducted studies involving nurses and exam writers.

## Answers to Review Questions

1. a
*Rationale: Mnemonics* help nurses understand and recall care and interventions that may be required. Theories, a client's past experiences, and self-care practices do not directly inform nursing practice knowledge of care and intervention options.

2. d
*Rationale: Available policies and procedures* relate to the health care environment, while the other response options relate to knowledge, nursing roles, and the client context.

3. b
*Rationale:* Client goals are incorporated in the client context, while external distractions, best practices, and current evidence do not relate directly to the client.

4. b
*Rationale:* Professional roles and *scope of practice* are related; knowledge of skills, inclusive client care, and hospital policy do not relate to professional roles and responsibilities.

## CHAPTER 3

### Notes on the Case Study Review

With reference to Table 3.6, consider the following points in your group discussion. Base your thinking on the clinical reasoning cycle (Levett-Jones et al., 2010) and the information that was discovered. Consider the client situation, collect cues and information, and recall knowledge using the clinical reasoning skills associated with finding information. What will you do next? How will the clinical scenario continue? How could it conclude?

- Consider the situation and information from the case study included: presentation of chest pain at 7/10 at rest; client history of dyslipidemia and obesity; vital signs as described on oxygen; and reported restlessness, anxiety, and diaphoresis.
- Process this information, which requires interpretation and inference. A client's report of chest pain requires health care providers to address the possibility of a myocardial infarction (MI) first, and then other potential conditions. The damage that occurs to cardiac muscle is irreversible. Further testing that supports the diagnosis of an MI would occur collaboratively with others.
- Identify the problem of an MI through confirmation of results from an electrocardiogram (ECG), blood work, cardiac markers, and other assessments.
- Focus goals primarily on preventing damage to the cardiac muscle and addressing chest pain.
- Take action following critical pathways for care of clients experiencing a diagnosed MI. The nurse works with others and initiates orders/prescriptions to meet the goal of care.
- Evaluate outcomes by confirming that chest pain is resolved and that follow-up diagnostic testing reflects positive changes or no worsening results.
- Reflect on the process of care, decision making, collaboration, and learning. How has this case study activity expanded your knowledge and thinking?

## Answers to Review Questions

1. c
*Rationale:* Unconscious bias is not deliberate, conscious, and does not reflect intentional favouritism; it is a bias that is unintended and that we are unaware of. It must be exposed through reflection and overcome.

2. b
*Rationale:* Situation awareness enables the nurse to assess the client in a more complete, holistic manner that includes the entirety of the client's circumstance. It does not relate to multitasking, does not necessarily augment accurate medication administration, and is not limited to complex care settings.

3. a
*Rationale:* As a cognitive strategy, mnemonics allow quicker retrieval of learned information. They are not used when communicating to clients, are not always alphabetical, and must be used in an informed way because they do not often include a rationale.

## CHAPTER 4

### Notes on Think-Aloud Pair Problem Solve (TAPPS)

In Problem A, there are more data to consider. Pain, vital signs, and fetal heart rate and strip description (decelerations) are all relevant to analyze. They can be interpreted as outside of normal ranges and described as possible placental insufficiency leading to problems with fetal perfusion. It is important to recognize that fetal compromise could occur if the possible conditions and decision making are not prioritized (Keenan-Lindsay, 2022, pp. 434, 479).

Problem B describes a situation that includes comparably minimal data: a visible piece of protruding bowel. This can be clearly analyzed, interpreted with further assessment of vital signs and pain, and synthesized as wound dehiscence. Surgical follow-up is a priority (Tyerman & Cobbett, 2023 pp. 225, 421).

## Notes on the Case Study Review

Reflect on the information in this case study individually and with others. With reference to Table 4.5, review how the case study can be completed and consider the steps to take. The steps you identify and the supporting rationale for them may be specific to information available in your jurisdiction. Deciding on an action requires an understanding of the situation and involves a determination of what to do based on choices made from available options. This process often necessitates communication with others. In this ethical scenario, communication is required. The ideal outcome in this case study is for the client requesting MAID and the nurse with a conscientious objection (CO) to be equally supported in their desires and needs.

Consider the following: If the client and MAID practitioner are able to arrange the death after the nurse with CO is off duty (who is on the next shift), all needs may be met, but the client may feel judged. Allow for someone to take over from the objecting nurse and enable the process per the client's wishes; however, in rural areas or with limited staffing, this may be a challenge.

Once an action is selected, all health care providers engage in the ethical action. Reflection on and review of the actions would involve a confirmation with all involved that the goals of the client were met and that the health care providers and nurse were supported in their own professional needs. A possible solution would be to create an opt-in versus opt-out approach to MAID and this type of care in the future. That is, those wanting to participate could make themselves known—similarly to how nurses must currently make their objection known—and be part of a consult service (Panchuk & Thirsk, 2021, pp. 771–772). Burnout may be a risk.

## Answers to Review Questions

1. b
*Rationale:* The nurse has found patterns and begun to assign meaning to the information, and is thus analyzing and interpreting the client data. No prioritization or synthesis were demonstrated in this example. Also, the nurse went beyond data recognition and identification.

2. a
*Rationale:* Physiological changes of increased confusion require follow-up. The client's preference to call their

daughter can be addressed once the client condition is assessed more fully. A client calling their daughter is not an issue of confidentiality, and personal values of family do not play a role here.

3. c
*Rationale:* Actively answering questions from clients or others during a task does not illustrate mindful action. Examples of attending to one's own thought processes and mental state include focusing and minimizing distracting questions and noise.

4. d
*Rationale:* It may be erroneous to attribute truth or correct thinking to a source solely because of their authority. Other fallacies relate to either/or options, the thinking of the majority, and jumping to conclusions without evidence.

# CHAPTER 5

## Notes on Activities and Discussion Questions

1. The advantages of using a decision tree include reduced complexity; increased ease of interpretation through a visual presentation of data, rules, and processes; a combination of options in a single presentation; and better consistency in decision making in situations defined by the decision tree. Do you find there are other advantages for you personally?
2. In your discussion, think about the effects of establishing therapeutic relationships and applying communication strategies. Consider other possible aspects of a client's life and lifestyle that could influence plans of care. What language would you choose when communicating with a client about goals in this situation?

## Notes on the Case Study Review

With reference to Table 5.5, consider the following:
1. Specific plans to reduce the spread of influenza include an understanding of how spread is occurring, a reinforcement of handwashing policy, vaccination, use of contact/droplet precautions as needed, treatment of those clients who are symptomatic, requiring staff self-monitoring of symptoms, and confirming communication strategies on changes in case data.
2. Local health care agencies and health care providers who would be involved could include care staff and nurses at the retirement community, physicians caring for residents, public health nurses, educators, officials, and those responsible for provincial analysis and reporting of influenza cases and outbreaks.
3. Actions are effective and meet the goal(s) if antiviral therapy results in reduced symptoms in clients;

compliance with handwashing increases; ongoing monitoring shows reduced incidence of new cases; surveying shows reduced incidence of illness in staff; and vaccination rates are high.

## Answers to Review Questions

1. b, c, e

*Rationale:* Appropriate planning activities include ensuring that institutional policy and procedures are reviewed, and supplies and equipment are gathered. Speed is not an appropriate strategy and is not the same as efficiency. The nurse should know how to troubleshoot or self-correct any problems instead of relying on another colleague to complete work and base the implementation and timing of the procedure on client need.

2. b

*Rationale:* Reasons for adapting a policy can be client based and should not involve risk to the safety of others. The nurse accepts and supports the decision and can provide a rationale to others. Policies are respected and not arbitrarily overridden or disregarded based on any client preference.

3. d

*Rationale:* Collaboration occurs when at least two or more health care providers interact in real time to discuss the order of care, a client's presenting symptoms, or their views on treatment to jointly develop a plan to deliver care.

# CHAPTER 6

## Notes on Think-Aloud Pair Problem Solve (TAPPS)

In Problem A, fluid overload could have been avoided with frequent monitoring of the client's condition overnight. Acute kidney failure indicates a potential risk for fluid overload with fluid administration. Review various resources you have for this condition. The client's wish to sleep could have been respected while meeting goals for maintaining their physical condition and delivering necessary treatment. The client could have been included in decision making and planning care.

Problem B requires you to review resources for best practices in communication and de-escalation of conflict. Safety of the nurse and others in the environment is paramount. Respect for the client and their health is also important. The client's context and actions rather than expression of the nurse's feelings in that moment may have refocused the client's attention. Discuss how a nurse's familiarity with policy and procedure may support this situation. Afterwards, incident debriefing with the clinic team could help understand what occurred, necessary legal processes,

and any revisions that could be made to procedure, safety protocols, and training.

## Notes on the Case Study Review

With reference to Table 6.4, consider the outcomes.

1. Client teaching on care of a colostomy and diet was provided. The client feedback on the teaching was that they had specific food preferences and that they did not want to care for their colostomy at this time. Review and evaluation of this outcome may involve drawing on *nursing knowledge:* alternative ways of teaching, the effects of body stigma; *professional roles:* consultation with other health care providers, such as a dietitian or stoma nurse who has specific expertise; *client context:* motivation to learn, adherence to self-care practices, learning and diet preferences, client autonomy; and *health care environment:* privacy of teaching environment, and appropriateness of discharge teaching policies and procedures.

2. Other health care providers may be involved who can help improve outcomes. Dietitians and wound or stoma care nurses have specific knowledge to further support the client. The client's family physician can be made aware to support longer term follow-up care. If body image is found to be a concern, psychological support can be provided as needed. Other options for support include family members and community groups.

## Answers to Review Questions

1. c

*Rationale:* Broadly, debriefing is a structured activity that enables review and analysis of a learning or practice event. It is not necessarily quick, nor does it specifically involve clients or emotional distress.

2. a, b, d, e

*Rationale:* Nurse-sensitive indicators are those that can be affected by nursing care. Falls, pressure injuries, postoperative pneumonias, and infections acquired in hospital are events on which nursing actions can have an effect. Surgical bleeding is not directly related to nursing care.

3. c

*Rationale:* Reflection after an activity occurs is referred to as reflection-on-action (looking back on an action to further understand). This example does not show anticipation (happening before an event, based on past experience) and it does not occur during the survey activity. The term *reflective interpretation* has not been presented in this textbook.

4. a

*Rationale:* Self-reflection involves managing one's own thinking as a professional activity. It does not relate specifically to equipment or protocols and is not limited to personal well-being.

## CHAPTER 7

### Notes on Activities and Discussion Questions

2. Answers:
   - The problem is ill defined? Restate the problem or goal in different ways.
   - Few options exist to a well-defined problem? Consider trial and error, if safe to do so.
   - The problem is complex? Use means/end analysis and simplify the steps.
   - More information is needed to clarify the problem? Consult or crowdsource with other health care professionals.
   - A lack of options exists at this time? Brainstorm.

### Notes on the Case Study Review

Reflect on the concept of complexity. A case study's complexity could relate to the NRCE framework, where each component includes multiple aspects for the nurse to consider, and where those aspects are unpredictable in nature. For example: the nurse may be unfamiliar with a client's required care and the roles of other health care professionals on the care team; the client may have several described comorbidities or an unstable condition that worsens their overall health and for which they are not compliant; and new monitoring technology may have been introduced to the unit. Think about which changes you suggest will lead to more decision points, increased collaboration, or clearer and more frequent communication with the client, for instance.

### Answers to Review Questions

1. The client's *potential condition* is *diabetic ketoacidosis (DKA)*, which progresses rapidly and requires prompt identification and treatment. The client is exhibiting signs of hyperglycemia (elevated plasma glucose), not hypoglycemia. Clients experiencing hyperosmolar hyperglycemic state (HHS) may exhibit much higher blood glucose levels and no ketones in their urine or blood. Although the client may need reassurance about the staff's comment, physiological status takes priority. The two *actions to take* are *initiation of IV fluid resuscitation* and the *administration of IV potassium*. IV fluid resuscitation with a 0.9% NaCl solution is a priority until blood pressure stabilizes and urine output increases to 30–60 mL/hr. Early potassium replacement is essential because hypokalemia is a significant cause of preventable death during treatment of DKA. The two *parameters to monitor* and *review* are *breath sounds* and the identified *lab values*. Assessment of breath sounds for fluid overload is a priority assessment in the patient with DKA. As the treatment of IV fluid resuscitation and IV potassium are the initial actions, the nurse must monitor the serum levels of serum pH, potassium, and glucose. Abdominal pain and gastrointestinal functioning are important, but they are not priorities for monitoring the identified outcomes (Tyerman & Cobbett, 2023, p. 1295).

2. b
*Rationale:* Although sleep is a physiological concern, the client's most pressing need is to address the partner relationship. There is no indication that the infant's health is an issue, and the client is prioritizing the relationship over the changes at home. In this case, the nurse may address the client's short-term lack of sleep once the primary client need for partner support is explored.

3. c
*Rationale:* A client whose health status is unclear or unpredictable is a priority compared with a client whose condition is stable. A client who has uncontrolled pain and is experiencing undiagnosed confusion requires assessment and monitoring to fully analyze, decide on an action(s), and develop a plan of care. Many complicating conditions do not represent the complete reason for focusing on the second client, and the independence and stability of the second client is not a reason for prioritizing the first client.

## CHAPTER 8

### Notes on Think-Aloud Pair Problem Solve (TAPPS)

Problem A may benefit from the six steps for prioritizing safety during an instance of microaggression. Review the steps and apply them to this situation, which relates to equity, diversity, inclusion, advocacy, and safety as overarching influences on the provision of care. Consider how training and support of nurses in similar circumstances would improve overall client care and staff retention.

In Problem B, knowledge of Sustainable Development Goal 5, "gender equality," would inform correction of the clinic form. A group to examine changes to policy and implement more inclusive practice may be suggested.

### Notes on the Case Study Review

Recall that deliberate practice is focused, repeated activities that are aimed at improving optimal performance, with feedback from a skilled practitioner. Meaningful feedback is received from a skilled nurse. The feedback is reflected on over time by the student as they prepare to continue learning and practising.

## Answers to Review Questions

1. a
*Rationale:* First and foremost, the nurse's obligation is to the client. Find information on the client first, and continue with the thinking process. Use assessment information to inform others (manager and physician) and perform appropriate treatments or actions. Reflect on the entire process for what occurred, and use available educational supports.

2. a, b, c, d, e
*Rationale:* Reflection is a broad skill that applies to all thinking processes and their phases. It enables an examination of bias and supports cultural sensitivity and humility.

3. b
*Rationale:* Most directly, advocacy in interactions with racialized people should occur in practice and in educational settings. Exclusion and acceptance of unconscious bias do not demonstrate antiracist nursing practice. Policy changes in law are indirect actions.

## REFERENCES

Keenan-Lindsay, L., Sams, C. A., & O'Connor, C (2022). *Perry's maternal child nursing care in Canada* (3rd ed.). Elsevier, pp. 434, 479.

Levett-Jones, T., Hoffman, K., Dempsey, J., et al. (2010). The "five rights" of clinical reasoning: An educational model to enhance nursing students' ability to identify and manage clinically "at risk" patients. *Nurse Education Today, 30*(6), 515–520.

Panchuk, J., & Thirsk, L. M. (2021). Conscientious objection to medical assistance in dying in rural/remote nursing. *Nursing Ethics, 28*(5), 766–775. doi:10.1177/0969733020976185.

Tyerman, J., & Cobbett (2023). *Lewis's medical-surgical nursing in Canada: Assessment and management of clinical problems* (5th ed.). Elsevier, pp. 225, 421, 622–624, 1295.

Note: Page numbers followed by "*f*" indicate figures, "*t*" indicate tables, and "*b*" indicate boxes.